GOT HEALING?

GOD'S WAY?

Dwaine Thomas Martin

Got Healing?

Other books by Dwaine Thomas Martin

Whatcha' Got? Series

Got Love?   Got Patience?   Got Hope?   Got Faith?
Got Peace? Got Wisdom?   Got Trust?   Got Him?
Got Healing?   Got Spirit?   Got Grace?   God Dominion?
Got Answers!   Got Seed! Got Surrender? Got Light?

By The Mercies of God   His Will, His Way
How To Find Solutions – Volumes 1 & 2
Shaping the Instrument – Volume 3
Ebb N`Flow   (Study of Spirit, Soul, & Body)
Fitting the Parts   (The Functional Gifts)
In The Eye of The Storm
A Place Called, "REFUGE"
Numbering the Finished Work
Process Proves Grace
Surrender Broken Parts
The Dimension Called "PURPLE"
The Invitation (The Mechanics of Intercession)

<u>BIBLICAL **SERIES:**</u>

Proverbs: $\left\{ \begin{array}{l} \text{Wisdom's Fruit – Volume 1} \\ \text{Wisdom's Grace – Volume 2} \\ \text{Wisdom's Mercy – Volume 3} \end{array} \right.$

Nahum –<u>EQUALITY</u> Courting the Favor of God
James – <u>EFFECTIVENESS</u> Living To Prevail
2 Peter – <u>NATURE</u> God's Word Exalted
Philemon – <u>GRACE</u> – Living To Serve
Hebrews – <u>PATTERN</u> – In His Image
Philippians – <u>RESOLVED</u> – Living By Reigning
Ephesians – <u>PERMITTED</u> – Living In The Spiritual

BIBLICAL <u>SERIES SOON TO COME!</u>

Genesis – <u>BEGINNINGS</u> – Reaching Beyond Purpose
Luke – <u>COMPASSION</u> – Whom Do You Say I AM?

http://www.amazon.com/dwainethomasmartin

Unless otherwise indicated, all scripture quotations are taken from the King James Version of the Bible.

GOT HEALING?

GOD'S WAY

Volume 1 of 2

ISBN-13: 978-1548486891

Published by
SPIRIT-WIND HOUSE
Printed in U.S.A.

Table of Contents

E X P L A N A T I O N   O F
T H I S   W R I T I N G

The language of the Bible has long been a topic of discussion among those desiring to know the truth. The difficulty in accepting most translations, though, is that they primarily all say the same thing. Yet, all translations are at best the conviction of the translators.   In other words, the differences are inserted because of personal convictions, or doctrines taught to them since birth. Most commentaries are the "*parroting*" of other previous generations. I mean no disrespect; but, I am looking and searching for the Eternal God; not the copy of another man's thinking.

When a translation is commissioned for the scrolls of Hebraic/Aramaic writings, the scholars doing the translation imply their own beliefs and convictions by the manner of the word(s)they use to translate the ideas written. If the pattern of mindsets or thought-patterns does not choose to follow the layout of the original text, then error can ensue because of a translator's individual belief.

There are many such translations. The scholars translating the scrolls, for the purpose of providing a Bible that the common person could have, were consistently prideful in their interpretation, not believing the common person could understand the deeper things of God's Word. This is still the skeptical ideas of those schooled and educated today, towards those who are not. The scholars believed that the unlearned, untrained, uneducated, would accept and adopt convictions that may or may not be the original thought of God in the mix. The attempt in every translation is one of religious ideas and convictions taught out of pulpits listening intently to what others have said; while never going to the Source of Who spoke the Word from the start.

The search of this volume is for the reality of knowing the God of the Ages, the Rock of Salvation, and the Ancient of Days. What we read in most translations, most commentaries are the opinions and ideas of those who seek man's approval, instead of God's. The ONLY criterion for TRUTH is whether what is taught, and passed on, produces the LIFE of GOD in the living of the believer.

My search found originality when investigation presented the facts that those who first wrote of biblical happenings and events were not men of education, as much as they were just common folk God choose to become His prophets and scribes. This led us in our search to find the ARAMAIC translation from original scrolls found in the caves of the Dead Sea, giving us an original writing by the work of the everyday person serving the One True God. Therefore, the original PICTOGRAPH of the Semitic early language was discovered to be the original writings of those to whom God spoke in the earliest of man's times. Investigation revealed that the Semitic (origin *of Shem, son of Noah)* tribes were the originators of this language and alphabet. Believing this to be the earliest representation of unspoiled, uncontaminated thoughts of God, the writings following this preface are an introduction and suggestion offered as a result of a 45 year search for the TRUTH expounded in each biblical writing.

While the alphabet of the Hebraic and the Aramaic are the same 22 letters, it follows that both the old and new testament contain a more clear and concise reckoning of God's Word to His Creation than those translations that arrogantly focus efforts on a man-centered writing and teaching. It is this God-focused, God-centered, Christocentric gospel that reveals the TRUTH about God's intentions toward His Creation. And how joyous those intentions are when revealed in the *"original thought"* of original language and writings.

We offer these biblical volumes as a means to come to know the LOVE of the Father to His own. This writer will not engage in anything but the pursuit of truth as it concerns God in the living of every believer. Doctrines, dogmas, liturgies, and the like will not be accepted as though God spoke and wrote them down. Save your breath. Examine your life and living, after you have read the volume that follows, and investigate as to whether the God you believe is the God of the ages who makes His message known through original language. You are the only one who will give an accounting of their living to God. You are the only one responsible for WHO it is you believe; God or man!

May God Bless You in all Your Endeavors for HIM!
Dwaine Thomas Martin
December, 2013

Got Healing?

Where Is the Author Coming From?

Jesus the Messiah spoke Aramaic. Of course, this was two thousand years ago, the language has evolved and today it is like the old English of the King James Version, in that it sounds very different. It is called, "***Ancient Aramaic***". The Ancient Church of the East, that emerged out of Jerusalem at the end of the Apostolic Age, referred to it as "***Leeshana Ateeqah***" or the "*old tongue*." Nobody speaks this language anymore -- not the ancient form of it. Those who claim to speak Aramaic are only speaking modern versions of the language, just as nobody speaks Old English or even Middle English anymore. Nobody speaks Koine Greek, Old Norse, or Old German, and so on. These languages have all evolved. And so today one also finds Hebrew and Aramaic spoken by millions of people in the Middle East, but these are modern versions of the language. The roots of many words are the same and the old form can be learned. This I have done, so I can read the Scriptures and translate them faithfully. I offer the "***Original Thoughts***" as a suggestion of what I consider the true, and original thought of God's speaking. Actually, the Scriptures have preserved the Ancient Aramaic language, and the language has preserved the Scriptures.

The difficulty I see, as an author/mentor/teacher /pastor, is that the clergy/church allows the changing of Scriptures by translations that do not carry the original thoughts of God through to the people. In short, the reason for the languishing of the church's influence throughout the world is the lacking of purpose, depth, and explanation as to the original thought of God through what He spoke to the early believers from the beginning. Our age seems more adept at handing out punishment and judgment than elevating the fact that these things were paid-in-full at Calvary, through the Blood of the Lamb offered, without spot to God!

All religions are great when it comes to celebration, success, and victory; but when it comes to sickness, failure, and death, religions have nothing to offer, except to express sorrow and consolation. When Jesus walked the earth, He fed the thousands with a few fish, and a few loaves of bread, He healed the sick and raised the dead; but His purpose in coming was not merely to demonstrate His ability to feed the masses or prevent them from dying. He had not come to lead His followers in battle against their enemies. He could have done all that from heaven. He did not need to set foot on earth.

Jesus came to the world to teach us how to deal with failure, sickness and death. We all do very well when successful, healthy and alive. When there are failures in life, no solutions, insurmountable problems and opposition, there is no greater example than that set by Jesus, the Christ, as He instructed His disciples to deal with each and every difficulty.

Why Another Bible Language?

Got Healing?

The Scriptures were placed in the order we find them because of the spiritual progression toward revealing Jesus, the Messiah. The Lord, *Himself* writes His teachings over the hearts of men and women. It is not by the greatness of men's visions or their magnificent intellects that the truth is preserved. It is in The Lord's own words that the truth is revealed throughout the ages. It is men's responsibility to point the way to the truth.

Aramaic is the ancient language of the Semitic family group, which includes the Assyrians, Babylonians, Chaldeans, Arameans, Hebrews, and Arabs. In fact, a large part of the Hebrew and Arabic languages is borrowed from Aramaic, including the Alphabet. The Peshitta is the official Bible of the Church of the East. The name Peshitta in Aramaic means "Straight", in other words, the original and pure New Testament. The Peshitta is the only authentic and pure text, which contains the books in the New Testament that were written in Aramaic, the Language of the Messiah and His Disciples.

Why ANOTHER ParaPhrase?

If there is but one person who would understand one verse, or even one word about Jesus, the Christ, and come to know Him as Messiah, Redeemer, Savior, Lord, Master, Teacher, Mentor, Deliverer, or any of the other 192 names He is, besides the eternal only He knows about, then it is worth the effort, the time, the frustration, in dealing with those who say it is but a waste of good paper. To them this writer defers to the Gospel of Jesus Christ. Remember the parable of the *"LOST SHEEP"* LUKE 15

How To Approach This Book

Teach me Holy Spirit, **to see** as Jesus sees, **hear** as Jesus hears, **speak** as Jesus speaks, and **do** as Jesus does.

This is the premise, the foundation of the eternal "NOW". The *"teaching"* is the surrender of our will to His. The *"seeing"* is the vision of Him as He is within us. The *"hearing"* is about the sound of His voice to lead, to guide, and to direct our living. The *"speaking"* is about our agreement, first within our will; second, from the resolve to follow; and third, through the action to walk in His LIGHT. The *"doing"* is about the initiative settled by the choice within, and the follow-through in living it out. This is the eternal *"NOW"* from which we live in Kingdom Living.

THE DEVOUT RECOGNITION OF GOD SHOULD PRECEDE ALL PHILOSOPHIES. The God whom we worship is not a metaphysical idea; a form of thought; a philosophical abstraction; but a living, personal, eternal Being, apart from and prior to all human thought. He is not a creation of the intellect, but the intellect's Creator. We must begin with Him. Is not this one of the child's first thoughts and one which life's long experience but deepens and confirms — that it was God who created all things? Does not the bare statement carry with it its own conviction? What need is there of proof? Who agrees that there is a solid earth on which he stands; a sun shining in midday sky? Who constructs arguments to prove his own existence? And does not God stand at the beginning of all thought and all argument? And is not the denial of Him a sheer and willful absurdity which no attempt at proof can make even plausible?

How To Understand the Format

Understand first, that the Aramaic/Hebraic alphabets are 22 letters, each. Each of the 22 letters retains their own meaning through a root composite of three terms. These terms define the various areas that each letter involves and can be followed when translation or paraphrasing options are involved. Below is an example of how this author proceeds from the original manuscript provided from internet files found at www.biblehub.com.

In the example below: ... ...

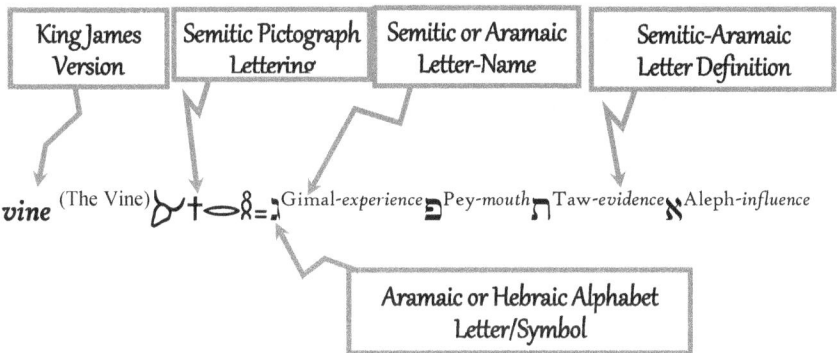

What we have interpreted, or suggest throughout the writings, is not so much a scholar's approach, but a suggested paraphrase of what might actually apply to living today. We understand, some will disdain, or seek to prove us wrong. However, **the ONLY criterion/measure/gauge for TRUTH is what, or <u>WHO</u> does such teaching reveals**? Obviously, the terrorist preaching and teaching of a **"hell-fire and damnation"** theory began in the dark ages, is completely false and man-centered with the idea of controlling the masses. The Bible is NOT man-centered! It is completely, through-and-through GOD–FOCUSED, GOD-CENTERED! We must return to this focus when we teach **"Jesus, the Christ, the Son of the Living God"**. For it is only as our gaze is set upon Him, our hearts fixed upon Him, our walk transcending beyond ourselves, and locked upon Him...that we will completely, and utterly find the fullness of Him that filleth all-in-all!

May God richly bless your endeavors FOR HIM!
Dwaine Thomas Martin
December, 2013

Chapter ONE

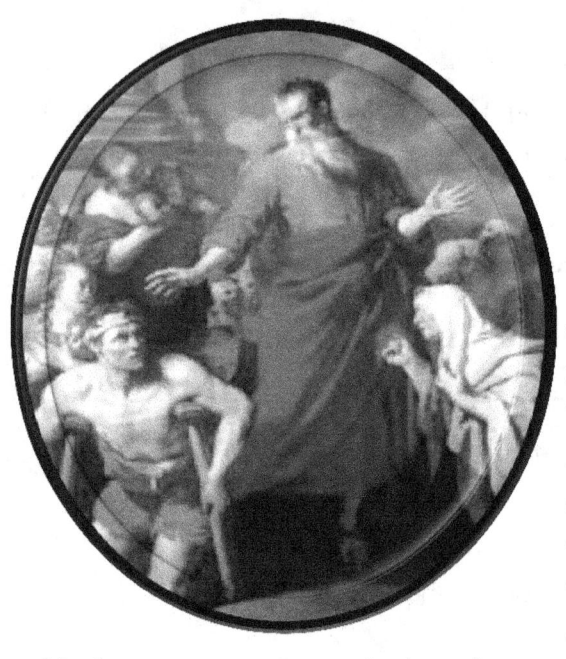

Healing: A Challenge?

Is HEALING a valid promise or just an illusion created by some magician, or minister wanting a *"fast buck"*? Charlatans abound; and magicians like *"Simon [Acts 8:9]"* constantly mesmerize the unwitting soul into believing what their ministry has, is what everyone needs.

*W*ith many organized churches within the world's religious systems, there is touted the theology that *"God helps those who help themselves"*. This has never been a Scriptural Premise. The question that follows such rhetoric is, *"what kind of help; from where does such help come; and/or if we're the helper, what is God's part?"* NONE OF THIS IS SCRIPTURAL, much less God-inspired! Either what Jesus did at Calvary <u>revealed</u> <u>ALL</u> <u>as finished</u>, or not!

*R*ESTORATION of Health is about a GREAT EXCHANGE in one's LIVING! By many creeds and dogmas, the pilgrim in pursuit of God begins an arduous excursion, leading them toward many pitfalls of unsound and unscriptural beliefs. Most dogmas are about one man's control over others. These things are <u>NOT OF GOD</u>! WHY? Because they do not produce a lifestyle that exemplifies THE RESURRECTED LIFE OF CHRIST JESUS through the believer.

<u>2 CORINTHIANS 3:2-3 KJV</u>
*"2 You are our epistle written in the heart,
known and read of all men:
3 Forasmuch as ye are manifestly*

Got Healing?

declared to be the epistle of Christ
ministered by us, written not with ink,
but with the Spirit of the living God;
not in tables of stone,
but in fleshy tables of the heart".

The Church must continue to become the *"written epistle"* of Christ; not the doctrines and traditions of those hirelings who desire to make another corporation, or write another book providing for themselves alone.

No other agency on earth has been able to match the Body of Christ's record of success in caring for the sick and afflicted. How many atheistic hospitals do you know about? How many Buddhist hospices have you discovered? At a time when Western culture desperately needs the church's ministry of healing, it is the charismatic-Pentecostals who proclaim it regularly but it is almost absent or invisible in most churches of every evangelical persuasion.

Too much doctrine tries to establish baseless facts. Yes, if you choose, you CAN make the Bible say whatever suits your purpose. *"But strong meat belongeth to them that are of full age, even those who by __reason of use__ have __their senses exercised__ to discern both good and evil".* HEBREWS 5:14 KJV The clearest method of discerning *good and evil*, is to KNOW THEIR (GOD'S) LIFE; and The *Tree of Life* that is beyond what the *Tree of Death* is about.

To name one of those baseless facts is: *The Action Of "__Contrition__"*; which is never to be involved with thoughts of unworthiness in any way, shape, form, or fashion, about the child of God's Creation, or about their lacking of proper choices made. *"__Contrition__"* is not about an apology, but about a *"change of the mind's direction, in Whom to believe".*

"Who hath believed our report? And to whom is the arm of the LORD __revealed__?" ISAIAH 53:1 KJV

Healing is a subject of intense scrutiny, yes! However, *a complete and honest look from a spiritual foundation,* __trying to make it line up with the physical__, is still an improper method of examination. Since God's Word will interpret itself; why not allow the Scriptures to present, to clarify, and to magnify the One Who is at the focus of the healing He offers?

After all, there is NO HEALING without JESUS!

No Healing, Without His Word

*T*he thought a believer can never dismiss is that ***IT IS GOD'S WILL TO HEAL!*** Scripture proves this TRUTH! Therefore, if healing does not, or is not manifesting through one's use of the Scriptures *"rightly divided"*, then there is something wrong, and it is never God that is in the wrong!

*L*ook with us over three areas concerning this subject of: HEALING, HEALED, and HEALTH. Remember, the Old Covenant <u>conceals</u> the New; and the New Covenant <u>reveals</u> the Old. What is seen as being done in the Old Testament/Covenant, has in fact, since Calvary, been revealed as FINISHED in the New Testament/Covenant, and continues to offer that which IS FINISHED, as the WORK continually and consistently continues to give. Where many a believer falls short of manifesting is that wherein they fail to REALIZE AS BEING ALREADY THEIRS!

The Law of First Mention

A fundamental idea of study begins by seeing a topic or message from its FIRST MENTION.

*L*ooking to find the first time the word itself has use is a more complete way than just reading words first written in 1611, which was the year the King James Version was offered.

*I*t goes without saying that societal ideas presented, through the use of words, has drastically changed in use and definition over the years.

Refusing to study and examine, what was the ***original thought,*** places one's self in a precarious position.

The worst place to be is where God is no longer <u>present</u>.

As He is ETERNAL, so He is ever moving, not for change, but to continually reveal HIS LOVE to His Creation.

<u>OLD TESTAMENT PARADIGMS</u>

<u>*Abraham's Example; God's Concept*</u>

Dominion's Pattern Increases By Revelation Of His Triumph Through The Spoken Word Providing Instruction For Discovering/Exposing His Truth

GENESIS 20:17
KJV+SM

So Abraham[H85] prayed[H6419] [H8691] unto God[H430]: and God[H430] healed[H7495] [H8799] Abimelech[H40], and his wife[H802] and his maidservants[H519]; and they bare[H3205] [H8799] children.

ORIGINAL THOUGHTS

...(20:17) Dominion's pattern increases by revelation of His Triumph, through the Spoken Word, providing instruction for discovering/exposing His Truth. Confirm every true increase of discovery, as Dominion examines each measure revealed; while practicing the Spoken Word as accomplished, by confirming evidence/witness. Mastery of His Pattern postures remembrance, providing sacrifice of the Kingdom as sown. Purpose needs revelation, to confirm the change displayed; because actions provide His Faith.

JOHN 16:24 KJV

Hitherto have you asked nothing in my name:
ask, and you shall receive, that your joy may be full.

Dominion's pattern increases by revelation of His Triumph through the Spoken Word, providing instruction for discovering/exposing His Truth.

The significance of noting any triumph or success is found in acknowledging/realizing the PATTERN through which one's Dominion acquires such success, or triumph. **DOMINION** *is the action of the believer, agreeing with, then allowing the Word of God to present the appearing of Christ to any/every observer.* Dominion is an action of REST, TRUST, and PATIENCE at work in the believer's living, bringing them into an ever deepening and widening experience of FELLOWSHIP, FIRST WITH GOD!

On the Pattern of Healing, Dominion is asserted FIRST. This offers the thought that the believer will need to become dominant by embracing the POWER OF HIS PRESENCE and PERSON. *We must continually* _realize that Christ in us is the HEALING being performed in our living._ If living in Christ is not a continual, consistent, and continuing **PATTERN** embraced, why would we even think that "_a shot amongst the bushes_" would ever even "_hit the trees_"? In other words, if our living His LIFE is a "_hit 'n miss_" operation/attitude/fearful flight, why would we ever think we would realize ANYTHING from God? This is not to speak of a "_non-reality_", never occurring in one's living. This is teaching the EXPERIENCE of REALIZING that through HIS WORD we HAVE HIM; WHO then becomes what was before only a wish, or a hope, or even just a prayer!

It is through the **PATTERN** called, **PRAYER**, the believer finds access, and a waiting ear to hear their agreement. Abraham resorted to what _HE HAD COME TO KNOW_. He could PRAY; God would LISTEN. The outcome is in His control; but Abraham knew God would listen to a petition of concern and care, yet, be devoid of personal appeal. Notice, his prayer did not include a plea for his wife to be returned; just healing for the king in whose land he dwelt. Yet, when all was said and done, his wife was returned to him unharmed.

Notice, his prayer for Lot's family to be released from captivity, was _not a prayer to change God's mind, but to find God's Will in the matter_. Either we use Prayer for what God has intended it to be used for; or we fail in our efforts to influence an outcome that will glorify Him, and Him alone! "_For it is God which worketh in you both to will and to do of His good pleasure_". PHILIPPIANS 2:13 KJV

JAMES 1:5-9 KJV
"_...5 If any of you lack wisdom, let him ask of God, that giveth to all men liberally, and upbraideth not; and it shall be given him. 6 But let him ask in faith, nothing wavering. For he that wavereth is like a wave of the sea driven with the wind and tossed. 7 For let not that man think that he shall receive any thing of the Lord. 8 A double minded man is unstable in all his ways. 9 Let the brother of low degree rejoice in that he is exalted:_"

Any Of You, is a phrase that is not just talking about the multitudes you rub shoulders with every day. You, my friend, are a three-part being;

Got Healing?

YES? Then, what about examining/studying yourself to see if there is a *fault-line* in your belief system. You may be SAYING everything that is right; however, your belief in times of silence may be eschewed/off balance. Since we know there is no lack in the character of your enjoined spirit with His Spirit; it must be that the lack, or *hiccup* is part of your soul, or your body being in control, instead of HIM! Ask for the Spirit's discernment! She will never lead you astray by/through His Word. When we substitute the LITERAL TRANSLATION of men's thoughts, rather than examine the **original thought** before God, this is where TRUTH becomes clouded, and PRESUMPTION, or ACCUSATION, or IGNORANCE begins.

Confirm every true increase of discovery, as Dominion examines each measure revealed; while practicing the Spoken Word as accomplished.

*A*rmed with the Dominion given man at Creation, the believer is able to use what has been made available for use. Dominion is the *art of directing/commanding/ordering a situation, condition, or circumstance; according to what the Word of God says about it. Set your thoughts to agree with what the Lord has said, and change what you speak to match with what He has spoken. "God is not a man, that He should lie; neither the son of man, that He should repent: hath He said, and shall He not do it? or hath He spoken, and shall He not make it good"?* NUMBERS 23:19 KJV

*E*ven though you might be in an examination mode, do not let up on speaking the Word of God's measure from the spiritual-realm. As the spiritual is always above that which is physical, remain on point with the Law of the Spiritual held~to. Speak the Word of God as the Law of the Spirit of Life in Christ Jesus. The Law of sin and death from the physical realm HAS NO POWER, since the Blood of the Lamb was shed, spilled, and offered at Eternity's altar. *That which has no POWER OF GOD to be alive, carries no LIFE to express one's LIVING, which God has promised!*

Mastery of His Pattern postures remembrance, providing sacrifice of the Kingdom as sown; wherein purpose needs revelation, to confirm the change being displayed; because actions provide His Faith.

*T*he positioning of REMEMBRANCE comes at the grasping by the believer of the untold half of God's Majesty in charge, as large and in control.

$\mathcal{F}$or centuries, the Word of God has been USED to control men's minds for purposes that are less than godly. Larger buildings; greater control of choices; expanded power through finances; these are but a few of the areas, men have sought to work from, in order to have the power over other men's lives. *If it walks like a duck, quacks like a duck, looks like a duck, guess what~~IT'S A DUCK!*

$\mathcal{Y}$et, it is always a necessity by REMEMBRANCES made that the WILL OF GOD is always SUPREME, FIRST, because of the Sovereign One Who spoke it, and the believing believer who hears/accepts it and agrees and applies it into the physical by God's own Faith at work in their living.

SEMITIC~ARAMAIC~HEBRAIC THESAURUS
Aramaic before first {
Semitic Root before first =
Lettering for ParaPhrase after second =

...(20:17) So Abraham H85 〜〜〼〥‐ロ〥{ㄥ〥=the strength of the house}=ℵAleph-dominion ability confirm-ꓶ Beyt-[in/by] pattern thought existing-in-principle-ꓶ Resh-practice beginning strength-ꓶ Hey-[the/His] character reveal grace-ꓶ Final-Mem-weight fashions prevail- prayed H6419 ∪∪∘{∪∘=speaking with confidence}=ꓶ Pey-mouth SpokenWord speak-ꓶ Lamed-[to/toward] instruct truth provide-ꓶ Lamed-[to/toward] instruct truth provide-ꓶ fragrance reveal grace-ꓶ Lamed-[to/toward] instruct truth provide- unto H413 ∪∪∘{∪〥=looks toward something/someone}=ꓶ Hey-[the/His] character reveal grace-ꓶ Lamed-[to/toward] instruct truth provide-ꓶ Vav-[and] identity intensity counsel- God: H430 〥{∪〥=strongly}=ℵAleph-dominion ability confirm-ꓶ Lamed-[to/toward] instruct truth provide-ꓶ Vav-[and] identity and God H430 〼〥∪〥{∪〥=strengthening}=ℵAleph-dominion ability confirm-ꓶ Lamed-[to/toward] instruct truth provide-ꓶ intensity counsel-ꓶ Hey-[the/His] character reveal grace- healed H7495 〼〥∪〥{∘〥=to mend/cure/make whole}=ꓶ Resh-practice beginning strength-ꓶ Pey-mouth SpokenWord speak-ꓶ Final-Aleph-ending finish maturity- H853 〼〥∪〥=ℵAleph-dominion ability confirm-ꓶ Taw-evidence prove signify- Abimelech H40 〰∪〜〜‐ロ〥{〰∪〜〜‐ロ〥=my father is king}=ℵAleph-dominion ability confirm-ꓶ Beyt-[in/by] pattern thought existing-in-principle-ꓶ Yud-purpose posture actions-ꓶ Mem-change challenge remembered-ꓶ Lamed-[to/toward] instruct truth provide-ꓶ Final-Kaph-acknowledge offer allow- and his wife H802 〼〜〜⅃〥{〥=in order to get healed}=ℵAleph-dominion ability confirm-ꓶ Nun-seed patience continue-ꓶ Yud-purpose posture actions-ꓶ Shin-pressure exchange disperse-ꓶ Hey-[the/His] character reveal grace- and his maidservants H519 〼〜〜{〜〥=and the point of departure/division}=ℵAleph-dominion ability confirm-ꓶ Mem-[from/out of] temper challenge remembered-ꓶ Hey-[the/His] character reveal grace- and they bare H3205 ㄸ∪〥{ㄸ∪=travails}=ꓶ Yud-purpose posture actions-ꓶ Hey-[the/His] character reveal grace-ꓶ Dalet-[that/which/of] faith establish presence- ~~children.~~

The Semitic Emphasis

The strength of the house speaking with confidence looks toward something/someone strongly and strengthening~~to mend/cure /make whole~~my father is king in order to get healed and the point of departure/division travails.

Humanity has a two-fold nature. They are both a material and a spiritual being.

Both natures have been equally affected by the fall.

His body is exposed to disease; His unrenewed soul is corrupted by sin.

We would therefore expect that any complete scheme of redemption would include both natures, and provide for the restoration of the physical as well as the renovation of the spiritual life.

We are never disappointed with God's part.

The Redeemer appears among men with both hands stretched out to such misery and need.

In the one He holds salvation; in the other, Healing.

He offers Himself to us as a complete Saviour; His indwelling Spirit, being His LIFE of our spirit; His resurrection body, being His LIFE to our mortal flesh.

He begins His ministry by healing all that had need of healing.

He closes it by making on the Cross a full atonement for our sin.

This was "*the faith once delivered unto the saints.*"

What has become of it?

Why is it not still universally taught and realized?

Did it disappear with the Apostolic age?

Was it withdrawn when Peter, Paul, and John were removed?

BY NO MEANS!

It remained in the Church for centuries and only disappeared gradually in the growing worldliness, corruption, formalism and unbelief of the early Christian centuries.

With a reviving faith, with a deepening spiritual life, with a more marked and Scriptural recognition of the Holy Spirit and the Living Christ, and with the nearer approach of the Master Himself, this blessed Gospel of physical redemption is beginning to be restored to its ancient place, and the Church is slowly learning to reclaim what she never should have lost.

Pattern-Thought Adjusts Practice
Piercing With Counsel Strengthened
By The Nature Of His Purpose/Focus
Through Grace

Got Healing?

KJV+SM
The flesh[H1320] also, in which[H3588], even in the skin[H5785] thereof, was a boil[H7822], and is healed[H7495] [H8738],

ORIGINAL THOUGHTS
...(13:18) His Pattern-Thought adjusts every practice piercing with His Counsel strengthened by the nature of His Purpose/Focus through Grace. Pressure determines actions keeping-hold-of one's living; rather practicing/repeating the Spoken Word as His Finished Work.

His Pattern-Thought adjusts every practice piercing with His Counsel strengthened by the nature of His Purpose/Focus through Grace.

*T*he influence of His THOUGHT is higher than that of this physical realm.

The BODY of CHRIST must allow/focus their mind to think upon things that are above, and not on the earth/physical.

"*Set your affection on things above, not on things on the earth*". COLOSSIANS 3:2 KJV

Our living displays, or proves what manner of things we are thinking upon.

Either we make this our habit, or we flail and flounder in our own demise.

When a believer's living becomes instinctive, or predictable, as far as their "*walk of Faith*", then, provides the ABUNDANT LIVING as promised.

JOSHUA 24:15 KJV
And if it seem evil unto you to serve the LORD, choose you this day whom ye will serve; whether the gods which your fathers served that were on the other side of the flood, or the gods of the Amorites, in whose land ye dwell: but as for me and my house, we will serve the LORD.

Pressure determines actions keeping-hold-of one's living; rather, practicing/repeating the Spoken Word as His Finished Work.

*W*hether our actions produce life or death, portrays with GOD it is that we follow after.

The pressures of Life that which is around you, displays by actions what a person believes.

Examining the day's actions determines where, what, and WHOM a

GOT HEALING?   *Page 18*

person follows!

*H*ere is where the *"rubber-meets-the-road"*!

To say what you believe, and yet follow a course that contradicts what you have spoken; is life and death coming out of the same outlet.

"Out of the same mouth proceedeth blessing and cursing. My brethren, these things ought not so to be". JAMES 3:10 KJV

*H*EALING must be a part of our <u>living</u>, not just a subject amongst our thought-processes.

HEALING is but the beginning/revealing of the expression we call, HEALED; which in turn, produces/reveals the HEALTH granted from the beginning of God's edict to His Creation.

Man has a two-fold capacity. He is both a material and a spiritual being.

Both capacities have been equally affected by the fall.

Our body is exposed to disease; our soul is corrupted by sin.

The ONLY decided DIFFERENCE is the proportion by which we choose to live our living IN HIM!

SEMITIC~ARAMAIC~HEBRAIC THESAURUS

Aramaic before first {
Semitic Root before first =
Lettering for ParaPhrase after second =

...(13:18) The flesh H1320 =blood relationship} also, in which H3588 =wherever} even in the skin H5785 =an adversary} thereof was H3588 =wherever} =there exists/endures} H7822 =thoughts} and is healed, H7495 =of inheritance}

The Semitic Emphasis

<u>Blood relationship wherever an adversary~~wherever there exists/endures thoughts of inheritance.</u>

Original thoughts tend to lead the soul back, again, to God.

This verse explains the actions of the believer (SEE LEVITICUS 13:17) when facing a malady in the flesh that appears to oppose the Word of God's Promises.

"And the blood shall be to you for a token upon the houses where ye are: and when I see the blood, <u>I will pass over you, and the plague shall not be upon you</u> to

destroy you, when I smite the land of Egypt." EXODUS 12:13 *KJV*

The earliest promise of healing is in <u>EXODUS XV. 25, 26</u>: *"There He made for them a statute and ordinance, and there he proved them, and said, If thou wilt diligently hearken to the voice of the Lord thy God, and wilt do that which is right in His sight and wilt give ear to His commandments, and keep all His statutes, I will put none of these diseases upon thee, which I have brought upon the Egyptians: for I am the Lord thy God which healeth thee."*

The place of this promise is most marked.

It is at the very outset of their journey, like Christ's healing of disease at the opening of His ministry.

It comes immediately after the passage of the Red Sea.

And we know that this event was distinctly typical of our redemption, and their journey of our pilgrimage.

"These things happened unto them for examples, and are written for our admonition, on whom the ends of the world are come." FIRST CORINTHIANS 10:11 *KJV*

This promise, therefore, becomes ours, as the redeemed people of God.

And God meets us at the very threshold of our pilgrimage with *the covenant of healing,* declaring that <u>as we walk in holy and loving obedience</u>, we shall be kept from sickness, which belongs to the old life of bondage we have left behind us forever.

Sickness <u>belongs</u> to the mess it represents, not to the people of God.

And only as we return spiritually to the mess ^(EGYPT) do we return to its maladies and perils.

Nay, this is not only a promise; it is *"a statute and an ordinance."*

And so the Lord Jesus has left for us *a distinct ordinance of healing* in His name as sacred and binding as any of the other ordinances/decrees of the Gospel.

<u>Consider Intent As His Prevail</u>
<u>Perpetuating Evidence/Witness In Parallel</u>

<u>LEVITICUS 13:37</u>
KJV+SM

But if the scall[H5424] be in his sight[H5869] at a stay[H5975] [H8804] and that at a stay[H5975] **and that there is black**[H7838] there is black[H7838] hair[H8181] grown[H6779] [H8804] up therein; the scall[H5424] is healed[H7495] [H8738] he is clean[H2889]: and the priest[H3548]

---

shall pronounce him clean[H2891] [H8765].

ORIGINAL THOUGHTS

...(13:37) Consider intent as His prevail, perpetuating evidence/witness in parallel, wisely posturing/positioning progress. Perceiving reflection by His Faith enlarges determined counsel, as practiced by apprehending wisely His strength anticipating challenge appropriately, to perpetuate evidence/witness; in parallel of practice/repeating His Spoken Word as His Finished Work. Reveal/Discover the Identity of His Finished Work; and balance His Character, as His counsel becomes the Beginnings consenting to every portion revealed and remaining with the blending of Grace as for strength.

It is a continuing marvel to this writer that after 50+ years of being involved in ministry, people CONTINUE to challenge the Wisdom and Authority of the Living God that CREATED them.

When a believer ASSERTS their WILL over HIS, they find turmoil, upset, anxiety, and stress on the increase, EVERY TIME!

How is it that ANYONE would contest the WISDOM of the Eternal ONE, Who created them?

YET, it is a continuing fact that we choose our WAY, instead of waiting ON HIS!

JOB 38:1-15 KJV

1 Then the LORD answered Job out of the whirlwind, and said, 2 ***Who is this that***
darkeneth counsel by words without knowledge*? 3 Gird up now thy loins like a man;*
for I will demand of thee, and answer thou Me. 4 Where wast thou when I laid the
foundations of the earth? Declare, if thou hast understanding. 5 Who hath laid the
measures thereof, if thou knowest? Or who hath stretched the line upon it? 6
Whereupon are the foundations thereof fastened? Or who laid the corner stone
thereof; 7 When the morning stars sang together, and all the sons of God shouted for
joy? 8 Or who shut up the sea with doors, when it brake forth, as if it had issued out
of the womb? 9 When I made the cloud the garment thereof, and thick darkness a
swaddlingband for it, 10 And brake up for it my decreed place, and set bars and
doors, 11 And said, Hitherto shalt thou come, but no further: and here shall thy proud
waves be stayed? 12 Hast thou commanded the morning since thy days; and caused
the dayspring to know his place; 13 That it might take hold of the ends of the earth,
that the wicked might be shaken out of it? 14 It is turned as clay to the seal; and they
stand as a garment. 15 And from the wicked their light is withholden, and
the high arm shall be broken.

Consider intent as His prevail, perpetuating evidence/witness in parallel, wisely posturing/positioning progress.

Got Healing?

*D*o you take the Word of God as real, or just maybe, or even *"just make believe"* as some?

Or, do you take the Word of God as He has spoken what He has prepared, and is prepared to reveal?

It is not the persuasiveness of men that makes the argument sustained.

It is the heart and mind of your own **BE**-ing that determines WHO you believe about what!

*O*f you see by God's Word that there is the INTENT of His desire to see PREVAIL; then, WHY do sit on your *"blessed assurance"* and remain unchanged?

What is it that makes you contemplate as to whether or not HE is telling you the TRUTH?

Or, is it that we have failed at holding men, as being messengers, accountable for their actions, as well as the message they present?

Or, is it that we have not held ourselves accountable for HOW we believe what He has spoken?

After all, it is not men that have shed their blood for our freedom to live as HE HAS ORDAINED and PREPARED US TO LIVE!

Perceiving reflection by His Faith enlarges determined counsel, as practiced by apprehending wisely His strength to perpetuate evidence/witness; in parallel of practice/repeating His Spoken Word as His Finished Work.

*W*hat is the evidence/witness that we hold to?

Is it the words of our parents, or our pastors, or our friends, our mentors/teachers?

Or, is it the WORD OF THE LIVING GOD having found a place in our heart and mind, and established His PLACE BY THE FOUNDATION HE HAS MADE within us?

*U*ntil the foundation of WHO WE BELIEVE is made up of those WORDS He has spoken, any storm will shipwreck the untested, untried, unproven persuasion/conviction we hold onto!

It is even by the repetitious actions of speaking/declaring His WORD that we find we are persuaded that HE IS THE ONE to WHOM we hold, and none other.

"And he said, LORD God of Israel, there is no God like thee, in heaven above,

or on earth beneath, Who keepest covenant and mercy with Thy servants that walk before Thee with all their heart:" FIRST KINGS 8:23 KJV

<u>Reveal/Discover the Identity of His Finished Work; and balance His Character, as His counsel becomes the Beginnings consenting to every portion revealed and remaining with the blending of Grace as strength</u>.

Discovering WHO HE IS, becomes paramount in the developing of the believer's experience.

He has blessed us with ALL spiritual blessings, yes! EPHESIANS 1:3

However, we have not EXPERIENCED the fullness of what He has prepared for us TO experience.

If you feel you HAVE experienced what He spoke, but it is/was not an experience to your liking; ~~~

QUESTION: was it not to YOUR liking, or were you flexible at seeing God's purpose for bringing these things to pass, the way that He did?

Experience can be a great window to see through, and note different occurrences as happenings He is seeking to reveal His preparedness through our own reactions or responses.

Here becomes the work of Grace in blending toward the balance of His Word at work in us.

Can you learn to say, "I'm NOT mad at you God, for the WAY that YOU have brought; because it is YOUR FAITH that has brought me through"!

Again, HEALING is about HIS WORD WORKING IN US; not just giving us what we want!

Before anyone can have a steadfast faith for the healing of their body, they must **be rid of all uncertainty** concerning God's will in the matter.

Before attempting to exercise faith for healing, one needs to know what the Scriptures plainly teach; **THAT** it is just as much God's will to heal the body as it is to heal the soul.

Until we know what God's will is, there is nothing to base our faith upon.[1]

There are, of course, three lies you have been told, or you will continue to be told.

[1]-You cannot have it!

Got Healing?

2]-You can have it, but not right now.
3]-You can have it now, but it won't last.

Appropriating the Faith of God, when allowed to work within the believer's living, can go no further than WHAT/WHO the believer believes is true. Actually, the TRUTH declares,

1]-You can have it!
2]-You can have it right now.
3]-You can have it, and it will last, forever.

SEMITIC~ARAMAIC~HEBRAIC THESAURUS

Aramaic before first {
Semitic Root before first =
Lettering for ParaPhrase after second =

...(13:37) But if H518 {ﬦﬦ}ﬠ =blunting the faculty of perception} actions- Final-Mem-weight fashions prevail- the scall H3424 =external eruption}= Nun-perpetuate patience persist- Taw-evidence prove signify- Quph-contrast parallel structure- be in his sight H5869 =of mental and spiritual faculties}= Ayin-pierce perceive wisdom-practice beginning strength- at a stay, H5975 =to stand/remain/endure}= Ayin-pierce perceive wisdom- Mem- transform encounter remembrance- Dalet-faith establish presence- and that there is black H7838 =seeking earnestly/looking for diligently}= Shin-pressure exchange disperse- Hhet-specific share beyond- Vav-increase degree assure- Resh- process beginning strength- hair H8181 =to storm/shiver}= Samech-adjust apprehend resource- Ayin-pierce perceive wisdom- Resh-practice beginning strength- grown up H6779 =to sprout/spring up}= Tsad-pursuit journey anticipate- Mem-[from/out of] temper challenge remembered- Hhet-specific appropriate beyond- therein; the scall H5424 =to pull/tear/draw off}= Nun-perpetuate patience persist- Taw-evidence prove signify- Quph-contrast parallel structure- is healed, H7495 =to heal/make healthy}= Resh-practice beginning strength- Pey-mouth SpokenWord speak- Final- Aleph-ending finish maturity- he H1931 =resuming with evidence}= Hey-character reveal grace- Vav-intensify degree counsel- Final-Aleph-perfected finished matured- is clean H2889 =to shine/be bright}= Thet-restraint mixture balance- Hey-character reveal grace- Vav-intensify degree counsel- Resh-practice beginning strength- and the priest H3548 =to mediate}= Kaph-surrender making consent- Vav-intensify degree counsel- Hey-character reveal grace- Final-Nun-keep-hold-of-living foundation progress- shall pronounce him clean H2891 =being firm/extensive in resources}= Thet-restraint mixture balance- Hey-character reveal grace- Resh-practice beginning strength-

The Semitic Emphasis

Blunting the faculty of perception~~external eruption of mental and spiritual faculties~~to stand/remain/endure seeking earnestly/ /looking for diligently to storm/shiver~~to sprout/spring up~~to pull/tear/draw off~~to heal/make healthy resuming with evidence~~to shine/be bright to mediate being firm/extensive in resources.

The story of Job is one of the oldest records of history.

It gives us an unmistakable view of the source from which sickness comes—the accuser/the adversary; and the course which brings healing, taking the place of humble self-judgment at the mercy-seat.

If ever a sick chamber was unveiled it was that of Uz.

However, we see no physician there, no human remedy, but only a looking unto God as his Avenger.

And when Job renounces his self-righteousness and self-vindication,

and takes the place where God is seeking to bring him~~that of self-renunciation and humility~~he is healed.

"Bless the Lord, oh my soul, and forget not all His benefits: who forgiveth all thine iniquities, who healeth all thy diseases." The Psalms of David are a continual record of affliction." *PSALMS 103: 2-3 KJV*

But God is always the deliverer and God alone.

We see no human hand.

As directly does he look to Heaven for the healing as he does for the pardon, and in the same breath, he cries, *"Who forgiveth all thine iniquities, who healeth all thy diseases."*

And it is a complete healing, ALL his diseases, as universal and lasting as the forgiveness of his sins.

And how glorious and entire that was, is evident enough.

"As far as the East is from the West, so far hath He removed our transgressions from us."

But here, as in the case of Job, there is an intimate connection between the sickness and the sin; and both must be healed together.

"And Asa, in the thirty and ninth year of his reign, was diseased in his feet, until his disease was exceeding great: yet in his disease he sought not to the Lord, but to the physicians. And Asa slept with his fathers." *SECOND CHRONICLES 16:12-13 KJV*

Here was a king who had begun his reign by an act of simple implicit trust in God, when human resources utterly failed him; and by that trust, *SECOND CHRONICLES 14:9-12 KJV*, he won one of the most glorious victories of history.

However, success corrupted him, and taught him to value too highly the arm of flesh.

So that in his next great crisis *SECOND CHRONICLES 16:7-8 KJV*, he formed an alliance with Syria, and lost the help of God.

He refuses to take warning from the prophet, and rushes on to the climax of his earthly confidence.

He becomes sick.

Here is a greater foe than the Ethiopians, but again he turns to man.

"He sought not to the Lord, but to the physicians."

And more sad or sarcastic could not well be the vivid picture of the ending of the issue.

"*And Asa slept with his fathers.*"

Making His Counsel To Reveal Progress Out Of Purpose Pursuing As Though Finished

LEVITICUS 14:3
KJV+SM

...(14:3) *And the priest*[H3548] *shall go forth*[H3318] [H8804=S=A simple/causal action M=referring to a time, or the present] *out*[H2351] *of the camp*[H4264]; *and the priest*[H3548] *shall look*[H7200] [H8804=S=A simple/causal action M=referring to a time, or the present] *and, behold, if the plague*[H5061] *of leprosy*[H6883] *be healed*[H7495] [H8738=S=Simple, sometime reflexive completed action M=referring either to a time, or the present] *in the leper*[H6879] [H8803=S=Expresses the "simple" or "causal" action of the root in the active voice; M=represents an action or condition in its passive unbroken continuity; in its passive/inert/in-active/reflexive activity];

ORIGINAL THOUGHTS

...(14:3) *Making His Counsel to reveal progress out of purpose; pursuing as though finished, while revealing/discovering Truth, and renaturing focus to keep-hold-of one's living. Specifying the Intensity of His journey; while reflecting the specific/determined persistence in character/nature/name, making counsel to reveal progress. Practicing/Repeating Dominion of Grace, restates the influence of His Grace, while discovering the single-minded patience of any atmosphere. Gather wisely to anticipate strength of Wisdom signifying practice/repeating of the Spoken Word as His Finished Work. Challenge position with progress, and pursue for the strength of His Wisdom.*

*U*ntil the person seeking healing is *sure* from God's Word that it is God's will to heal *them*, they are trying to reap a harvest where there is no seed planted.

Would it not be impossible for a farmer to have faith for a harvest, before he was *sure* that the seed had been planted?

From the scope, or position of the word/place that "**healing**" represents; is there not a bridge of awareness necessary to grasp or apprehend, or take hold of that which God requires to be understood?

Does not God request that we know WHOM we believe in, before we step into the Day before us?

"*For the which cause I also suffer these things: nevertheless I am not ashamed: for I know Whom I have believed, and am persuaded that He is able to keep that which I have committed unto Him against that day*". 2 TIMOTHY 1:12 KJV

Healing is not about the action, but about the foundation upon which the HEALING rests.

Knowing that the Body is HEALED, already, is the foundation upon which the HEALTH of the Body realizes its HEALING.

HEALTH is the ultimate.

If one's HEALTH is not something accepted as important that which is HEALED becomes weakened by the doubts that attend to one's uncertainty of the foundation of their HEALTH in God's promise.

Making His Counsel to reveal progress out of purpose; pursue as though finished, while revealing/discovering Truth, and renaturing focus to keep-hold-of one's living.

*R*emaining true to the influence toward the effort causes one to examine, "*whether they be in the faith*", or not!

The counsel of His Word determines the stride of each step taken.

The progress attained by such steps reveals the purpose of one's pursuit to begin with.

It is not the sustaining of the steps, but the determined continuing of the journey ahead.

If a believer is void of God's Word, how will they maintain where they attain to without a secure anchor in Whom they chose to believe in the first place?

*M*aintaining the course prescribed and prearranged by the Father is not finished by continually looking at the horizon ahead.

Revealing/Discovering His Truth, changes the atmosphere of the journey; enhancing the moment-by-moment experience of the pursuit at hand.

Each time we adjust our attitudes, to comply with the territory we have walked into; we find the strength of His Breath in the atmosphere of His Presence; and decide to pursue Him from the clearing of our eyes to behold HIM!

Vs.1
He washed my eyes with tears that I might see,
The broken heart I had was good for me;
He tore it all apart and looked inside,
He found it full of fear and foolish pride.

Got Healing?

He swept away the things that made me blind
And then I saw the clouds were silver lined;
And now I understand 'twas best for me
He washed my eyes with tears that I might see.
Vs.2
He washed my eyes with tears that I might see
The glory of Himself revealed to me;
I did not know that He had wounded hands
I saw the blood He spilt upon the sands.
I saw the marks of shame and wept and cried;
He was my substitute for me He died;
And now I'm glad He came so tenderly;
And washed my eyes with tears that I might see.

Specifying the Intensity of His journey; while reflecting the specific/determined persistence in character/nature/name, making counsel to reveal progress.

*F*or anyone battling sickness, there is a need to know that it is God's **will** to heal them; for this is the **seed** to be planted in their mind and heart.

The coming forth of the *seed* becomes the fruit of the harvest, at the time ordained.

For the seed is not *planted* until He[*the Seed*] is known, received and trusted.

No looking back; no questioning His times or seasons; His purposes or reasons; just saying, "*Yes, my Lord*".

It is not the knowing, remembering, or memorizing of the Seed that is necessary.

It is apprehending, grasping, and taking-hold of the IDEA that HE IS THE SEED.

It is a knowing, receiving, and trusting of HIM WHO IS THE SEED; this magnifies Him, and manifests the harvest/product of the SEED as sown, in the living of any believer believing.

Practicing/Repeating Dominion of Grace, restates the influence of His Grace, while discovering the single-minded patience of any atmosphere.

*I*t is never about what is going on around us that "*frazzles*" our brain, or makes us anxious. It is not taking-hold of the Anchor in our senses that is HIM!

Praying for healing with words destroying faith is like saying, "*if it be*

Thy Will, I believe He can heal me"!

That's like a farmer saying, "*I know God can give me a harvest, so I'll just believe the seed is in the ground*".

Such words do not make any connection with the validity necessary to acquire the package with your name on it.

Present your IDENTIFICATION; the matter at hand requires the presence of Your DECISION backed by the WORD OF HIS SPEAKING!

The prayer of faith, which heals the sick, is to FOLLOW [*not precede*] the planting of the Seed.

Gather wisely to anticipate strength of Wisdom signifying practice/repeating of the Spoken Word as His Finished Work.

𝒯he Wisdom of knowing God's Word about *healing*, requires that a person have a firm grasp of the benefits promised, and provided to those who know WHOSE THEY ARE.

Instead of saying, "*Pray for me*", there should first be the acknowledgement, requesting that "*someone teach me which be the first principles, that I may grow thereby*".

We must know what the BENEFITS of Calvary are, before we can accept, approve, and appropriate them by faith.

The first level of Salvation is the developing of attitude toward SIN!

After being sufficiently enlightened, our attitude toward *being sick* becomes the same as one's attitude toward sin.

Our purpose out of desiring to be healed should be as concrete in its existence as is our purpose out of desiring to see the fullness of God abound in our mentalities, and mindsets.

"*In every thing give thanks: for this is the will of God in Christ Jesus concerning you*". *1 Thessalonians 5:18 KJV*

Challenge position with progress, and pursue for the strength of His Wisdom.

𝒲here you may be, according to your belief, must needs have added the Strength of God's Wisdom, in order to attain to where you want to be IN HIM!

Again, while we have all been blessed with ALL SPIRITUAL BLESSINGS; we have yet to experience the rush of ETERNAL

Got Healing?

EXPERIENCE, transcending the pull of the physical to remain where we might be, at the moment.

HEBREWS 10:35-36 KJV

"Cast not away therefore your confidence, which hath great recompense of reward. For ye have need of patience, that, after ye have done the will of God, ye might receive the promise".

MARK 11:23-26 KJV

"For verily I say unto you, That whosoever shall say unto this mountain, Be thou removed, and be thou cast into the sea; and shall not doubt in his heart, but shall believe that those things which he saith shall come to pass; he shall have whatsoever he saith. Therefore I say unto you, What things soever ye desire, when ye pray, believe that ye receive them, and ye shall have them. And when ye stand praying, forgive, if ye have ought against any: that your Father also which is in heaven may forgive you your trespasses. But if ye do not forgive, neither will your Father which is in heaven forgive your trespasses".

SEMITIC~ARAMAIC~HEBRAIC THESAURUS

Aramaic before first {

Semitic Root before first =

Lettering for ParaPhrase after second =

...(14:3) **And the priest** H3548 {=and one burnt with Fire}= Kaph-surrender making consent- Vav-[and] identity intensity counsel- Hey-[the/His] character reveal grace- Final-Nun-keep-hold-of-living foundation progress- **shall go forth** H3318 {=will bring to an end}= Yud-purpose posture actions- Tsad-pursuit journey anticipate- Final-Aleph-perfected finished matured- Hey-[the/His] character reveal grace- Lamed-[to/toward] instruct truth provide- H4480 **out of** {=and remove}= Hey-[the/His] character reveal grace- Yud-purpose posture actions- Final-Nun-keep-hold-of-living foundation progress- H351 **portion** {=to sever}= Hey-[the/His] character reveal grace- Vav-[and] identity intensity counsel- Tsad-pursuit journey anticipate- Hhet-specific appropriate beyond- **the camp;** H4264 {=the encampments}= Mem-[from/out of] temper challenge remembered- Nun-perpetuate patience persist- Hey-[the/His] character reveal grace- **and the priest** H3548 {=and one burnt with Fire}= Kaph-surrender making consent- Vav-[and] identity intensity counsel- Hey-[the/His] character reveal grace- Final-Nun-keep-hold-of-living foundation progress- **shall look** H7200 {=will perceive the face of God}= Resh-practice beginning strength- Aleph-dominion ability confirm- Hey-[the/His] character reveal grace- and, **behold,** H2009 {=looking at what is here}= Hey-[the/His] character reveal grace- Yud-purpose posture actions- Nun-perpetuate patience persist- Hey-[the/His] character reveal grace- Ayin-pierce perceive wisdom- **of leprosy** H6883 {=infection of skin/cloth/a building}= Tsad-pursuit journey anticipate- Resh-practice beginning strength- Ayin-pierce perceive wisdom- Taw-evidence prove signify- **if the plague** H5061 {=touching}= Gamel-walk gather carry- **be healed** H7495 {=repairing}= Resh-practice beginning strength- Pey-mouth SpokenWord speak- Final-Aleph-ending finish maturity- H4480 **in** {=in kind}= Mem-renature challenge remembered- Yud-purpose posture actions- Final-Nun-keep-hold-of-living foundation progress- **the leper** H6879 {=of infection}= Tsad-pursuit journey anticipate- Resh-practice beginning strength- Ayin-pierce perceive wisdom-

The Semitic Emphasis

And one burnt with Fire will bring to an end and remove portion to sever the encampments and one burnt with Fire will perceive the face of God looking at what is here touching infection of skin/cloth/a building repairing in kind of infection.

ISAIAH 53:4~5 KJV *"Surely He hath borne our griefs, and carried our sorrows and with His stripes we are healed."*

This the great Evangelical vision, the Gospel in the Old Testament, the very mirror of the coming Redeemer.

And here in the front of it, prefaced by a great AMEN-the only *"surely"* in the chapter is the promise of healing; the very strongest possible statement of complete redemption from pain and sickness by his life and death, and the very words which the Evangelist afterwards quotes, under the inspired guidance of the Holy Ghost-MATTHEW 8:17 KJV, as the explanation of His universal works of healing.

The translation in our English version does very imperfect justice to the force of the original.

The translation in MATTHEW 8:17 is much better: *"Himself took our infirmities, and bare our sicknesses."*

The literal translation would be," surely He hath borne away our sicknesses and carried away our pains."

Any person who will refer to such a familiar commentary as that of Albert Barnes on Isaiah, or any other Hebrew authority, will see that the two words here used denote respectively sickness and pain, and that the words for "bear" and "carry," denote not mere sympathy, but an actual substitution and the removal utterly of the thing borne.

Therefore, in the same full sense as He has borne our sins, Jesus Christ has SURELY BORNE AWAY and CARRIED OFF our sicknesses; yes, and even our PAINS, so that abiding in Him, we may be fully delivered from both sickness and pain.

Thus *"by His stripes we are healed."*

Blessed and glorious Gospel!

Blessed and glorious Burden Bearer.

Agree/ Accept/ Apply ~~ Repeat As Needed...

LEVITICUS 14:48
KJV+SM

And if the priest[H3548] shall come in [H935] [H8799=S=A simple/causal action, or process, or condition of the root, M=which is incomplete] [H935] [H8800=S=A combination of a word plus a verb, M=expressing an action or a state of being], and look[H7200] [H8804=S=A simple/causal action M=referring to a time, or the present] upon it, and, behold, the plague[H5061] hath not spread[H6581] [H8804=S=A simple/causal action M=referring to a time, or the present] in the house[H1004], after[H310] the house[H1004] was plaistered[H2902] [H8736=S=Simple, sometimes reflexive M=uncompleted action, process, or condition]: then the

---

Got Healing?

priest^{H3548} shall pronounce the house^{H1004} clean^{H2891} [H8765=S= Simple expressing intensive/intentional, repeated/extended action; M=completed referring to a time, or the present] because the plague^{H5061} is healed^{H7495} [H8738= S=Simple, sometime reflexive completed action M=referring either to a time, or the present]

ORIGINAL THOUGHTS

...(14:48) Consider the intent of His prevail, while consenting to every portion revealed and remaining. For as the pattern-thought, existing-in-principle intensifies every portion of His Finished Work; strengthen the Dominion of His Grace. Develop the focus of His witness discovered, while perpetuating your walk wisely, providing the counsel of His Finished Work. The Spoken Work exchanges with Grace, existing-in- principle/precept working to signify, and confirm the appropriate beginnings. Confirming evidence/witness, reinforces the appropriate beginnings that fortify evidence//witness; as existing-in-principle/precept, while working to signify the blending of intensity determined. Consent/Agree with every portion revealed, while remaining in balance of disclosing the practice//strength of deepening evidence/witness, as existing-in-principle/precept. Work to signify surrender/agreement with purpose, while perpetuating your walk wisely. Practice/Repeat the Spoken Word as His Finished Work.

HEBREWS 6:11-12 KJV

And we desire that every one of you do shew the same diligence to the full assurance of hope unto the end: That ye be not slothful, but followers of Him, who through faith and patience inherit the promises.

<u>Consider the intent of His prevail, while consenting to every portion revealed and remaining</u>.

*H*idden purposes always reveal undisclosed benefits and rewards waiting.

His intent is always revealed through understanding the higher thoughts of His design and ultimate purpose.

The believer's agreement remains the *"lynch-pin"* of discovery.

The opening of Heaven, since Calvary, provides any believer, willing and obedient, to become able to be a minister/servant of the New Covenant sealed, and activated by the offering of His Blood on the Eternal Altar of Heaven.

<u>For as the pattern-thought, existing-in-principle, intensifies every portion of</u>

His Finished Work; strengthen the Dominion of His Grace.

*F*inding those thoughts that reciprocate/respond to the strengthening of His gracious Dominion given, provides the believer with an untold arsenal of abilities and strategies for overcoming, as well as maintaining what has been received and embraced already.

That which exist-in principle follows the same of constructing the line to an Anchor that keeps the soul safe even in the midst of the storm's raging.

Develop the focus of His witness discovered, while perpetuating your walk wisely, providing the counsel of His Finished Work.

*O*bserving His moving amongst His people, defines the need for focus; but, also provides the insight giving wise counsel to every step that lies ahead of the believer's journey.

What He exhibits and exudes becomes the map that leads to the fullness of Who He is, and what He has finished.

There can never be a misguided approach, when observing His actions provides a clearer understanding of His example.

The Spoken Work exchanges with Grace, existing-in-principle/ /precept working to signify, and confirm the appropriate beginnings.

*A*fter Jonah had prayed for mercy, he did not cast away his confidence, because there was, as yet, no visible proof that his prayer was answered.

He held fast his confidence, and added to it, in advance, the sacrifice of thanksgiving.

"But I will sacrifice unto thee with the voice of thanksgiving; I will pay that that I have vowed. Salvation is of the LORD". JONAH 2:9 KJV

God's promises work their wonders, while we observe and respond by/through *eternal* realities, [*such as His faithfulness, His refuge of peace/safety, etc.*]; refusing to be affected by *temporal* things to the contrary.

"With long life will I satisfy him, and shew him My salvation". PSALMS 91:16 KJV

PROVERBS 4:20-22 KJV
My son, attend to My words; incline thine ear unto My sayings.
Let them not depart from thine eyes; keep them in the midst of
thine heart. For they are life unto those that find them, and

Got Healing?

health to all their flesh.

Confirming evidence/witness, reinforces the appropriate beginnings that fortify evidence/witness; as existing-in-principle/precept, while working to signify the blending of intensity determined.

The Word of God cannot be healing, and then, health to the soul or the body, before it is heard, received, and ATTENDED TO.

It is one thing to agree that we have HEARD, and RECEIVED His Word; and yet, another to ATTEND TO what we heard and received!

If it is your need to receive the HEALING, and HEALTH promised; then make your living to ATTEND to finding the words of LIFE that promise such results.

Consent/Agree with every portion revealed, while remaining in balance of disclosing the practice/strength of deepening evidence/witness, as existing-in-principle/precept.

ENOUGH with the "_fast-food_" promises of charlatans seeking only to take offerings, and sell their books and tapes; while little or no results follow their journeys.

There is a divine method to receiving the blessings which God has provided.

Many continue to fail at receiving healing, and health, because they have taken the time necessary to follow His methods/His strategies; finding that what they seek for is always PRESENT IN HIM!

Work to signify surrender/agreement with purpose, while perpetuating your walk wisely.

On Proverbs 4:20-22; He tells how to "ATTEND TO" His Words.

"_Let them NOT depart from your eyes; keep them in the midst of your heart/thoughts_".

So, instead of having your focus kept on your symptoms; becoming pre-occupied with them, instead of HIM; look to HIS WORDS continually, consistently, and closely.

Practice/Repeat the Spoken Word as His Finished Work.

Abraham grew strong in FAITH by continually accessing the Word of God from the memories of what was said in their meetings together.

Got Healing?

Each time you pick up your Bible; each time you bask in His Presence; each time the negative seeks to control your thinking; _think_ _on_ _things_ _above_.

"_Finally, brethren, whatsoever things are true, whatsoever things are honest, whatsoever things are just, whatsoever things are pure, whatsoever things are lovely, whatsoever things are of good report; if there be any virtue, and if there be any praise, think on these things. Those things, which ye have both learned, and received, and heard, and seen in me, do: and the God of peace shall be with you_".
PHILIPPIANS 4:8-9 KJV

SEMITIC~ARAMAIC~HEBRAIC THESAURUS
Aramaic before first {
Semitic Root before first =
Lettering for ParaPhrase after second =

...(14:48) And if H518 〰〰 =conditional whenever}= Aleph-dominion ability confirm- Yud-purpose posture actions- Final-Mem-weight fashions prevail- the priest H3548 =to mediate}= Kaph-surrender making consent- Vav-intensify degree counsel- Hey-character reveal grace- Final-Nun-keep-hold-of-living foundation progress- shall come in, H935 =to enter/to attain to}= Beyt-pattern thought existing-in-principle- Vav-intensify degree counsel- Final-Aleph-perfected finished matured- H935 =to enter/to attain to}= Beyt-pattern thought existing-in-principle- Vav-intensify degree counsel- Final-Aleph-perfected finished matured- and look H7200 =inspect/perceive/consider}= Resh-practice beginning strength- Aleph-dominion ability confirm- Hey-character reveal grace- upon it, and, behold, H2009 =though}= Hey-character reveal grace- Yud-purpose posture actions- Taw-evidence prove signify- Hey-character reveal grace- the plague H5061 =to touch/reach/strike}= Nun-perpetuate patience persist- Gamel-walk gather carry- Ayin-pierce perceive wisdom- hath not H3808 =without/nothing}= Lamed-instruct truth provide- Vav-intensify degree counsel- Final-Aleph-perfected finished matured- spread H6581 =to spread}= Pey-mouth SpokenWord speak- Shin-pressure exchange disperse- Hey-character reveal grace- in the house H1004 =to build/establish/cause to continue}= Beyt-pattern thought existing-in-principle- Yud-purpose posture actions- Taw-evidence prove signify- after H310 =afterwards/behind}= Aleph-dominion ability confirm- Hhet-specific appropriate beyond- Resh-practice beginning strength- H853 =plowing the furrow to sow}= Aleph-dominion ability confirm- Taw-evidence prove signify- the house H1004 =to build/establish/cause to continue}= Beyt-pattern thought existing-in-principle- Yud-purpose posture actions- Taw-evidence prove signify- was plaistered: H2902 =to spread over/cover over}= Thet-restraint mixture balance- Vav-intensify degree counsel- Hhet-specific appropriate beyond- Hey-character reveal grace- then the priest H3548 =to mediate}= Kaph-surrender making consent- Vav-intensify degree counsel- Hey-character reveal grace- Final-Nun-keep-hold-of-living foundation progress- shall pronounce the house clean, H2891 =turn aside}= Thet-restraint mixture balance- Hey-character reveal grace- H853 =plowing the furrow to sow}= Aleph-dominion ability confirm- Taw-evidence prove signify- H1004 =to build/establish/cause to continue}= Beyt-pattern thought existing-in-principle- Yud-purpose posture actions- Taw-evidence prove signify- because H3588 =since/but rather}= Kaph-surrender making consent- Yud-purpose posture actions- the plague H5061 =to touch/reach/strike}= Nun-perpetuate patience persist- Gamel-walk gather carry- Ayin-pierce perceive wisdom- is healed, H7495 =to make healthful}= Resh-practice beginning strength- Pey-mouth SpokenWord speak- Final-Aleph-ending finish maturity

The Semitic Emphasis

Conditional _whenever_ to mediate to enter/to attain to~~to enter/to attain to inspect/perceive/consider *though to touch/reach/strike without/nothing to spread to build/establish/cause to continue afterwards/behind plowing the furrow to sow to build/establish/ /cause to continue to mediate turn aside appearing to agree to build/establish/cause to continue to touch/reach/strike to make healthful.*

"*Surely He hath borne our griefs, and carried our sorrows~~and with His stripes we are healed.*" ISAIAH 53:4~5 KJV

This is the great Evangelical vision, the Gospel in the Old Testament, the very mirror of the coming Redeemer.

And here in the front of it, prefaced by a great AMEN~~the only "*surely*" in the chapter is the promise of healing.

The very strongest possible statement of complete redemption from pain and sickness by his life and death, and the very words which the Evangelist afterwards quotes, under the inspired guidance of the Holy Ghost~~ MATTHEW 8:17 KJV, as the explanation of His universal works of healing.

The translation in our English version does very imperfect justice to the force of the original.

The translation in **MATTHEW 8: 17 KJV**, is much better: "*Himself took our infirmities, and bare our sicknesses.*"

The literal translation would be," *surely He hath borne away our sicknesses and carried away our pains.*"

Any person who will refer to such a familiar commentary as that of Albert Barnes on Isaiah, or any other Hebrew authority, will see that the two words here used denote respectively sickness and pain, and that the words for "*bear*" and "*carry,*" denote not mere sympathy, but an actual substitution and the removal utterly of the thing borne.

Therefore, in the same full sense as He has borne our sins, Jesus Christ has SURELY BORNE AWAY and CARRIED OFF our sicknesses; yes, and even our PAINS, so that abiding in Him, we may be fully delivered from both sickness and pain.

Thus "*by His stripes we **are** healed.*"

Oh, Blessed and glorious is this Gospel of God and Jesus Christ, the Son of the Most High!

Blessed and glorious is this Burden Bearer~~Jesus, the Beautiful Rose of Sharon, and Fairest of Ten~Thousand to my soul!

Thus the ancient prophet beholds in vision the Redeemer coming first as a Great Physician, and then hanging on the Cross as the Great

Sacrifice.

And thus the Evangelists have also described Him; for three years the Great Healer, and then for six hours of shame and agony, the Dying Lamb.

Focus On Revelation
While Intensifying His Character Continually

DEUTERONOMY 28:7
KJV+SM

The LORD[H3068] shall cause[H5414] [H8799=S=A simple/causal action, or process, or condition of the root, M=which is incomplete] thine enemies[H341] [H8802=S=Expresses the "simple" or "causal" action of the root in the active voice; M=through an action or condition in its unbroken continuity] that rise up[H6965] [H8801=] against thee to be smitten[H5062] [H8737=S=Simple, sometime reflexive uncompleted action, process, or condition ;in its unbroken continuity; M=and may be used of present, past, or future time] before thy face[H6440]: they shall come out[H3318] [H8799=S=A simple/causal action, or process, or condition of the root, M=which is incomplete] against thee one[H259] way[H1870], and flee[H5127] [H8799=S=A simple/causal action, or process, or condition of the root, M=which is incomplete] before[H6440] thee seven[H7651] ways[H1870].

ORIGINAL THOUGHTS

...(28:7) Focus on revelation, while intensifying His Character continually, agreeing with His Nature, pressing beyond actions and proceed with renaturing the journey. Align every portion by keeping-hold-of your living; by perceiving His identity within the Spoken Work provided; and gather strength by pattern of thoughts that determine your practice. Apprehend His Counsel with the Dominion of Faith; through practice of adjusting the provision through the counsel of His Finished Work. Practice/Repeat the Spoken Word as His Finished Work.

$\mathcal{I}$t must be understood that God is not a God of revenge.

His vengeance is about His **BE**-ing, as one of *"longsuffering, not willing that any should perish, but that all should come to repentance"*. [2PETER 3:9]

If a believer is incorrect, and incomplete allowing *"blessing and cursing"* [JAMES 3:10] to come *"out of the same mouth"*; then, it must be acknowledged that neither can God do what He forbids His Creation to do.

If we speak one thing when we around another, and then something opposite when we talk to ourselves, or others; we speak as though being a *"double-minded"* person.

"But let him ask in faith, nothing wavering. For he that wavereth is like a wave of the sea driven with the wind and tossed. For let not that man think that he

---

shall receive any thing of the Lord. A double minded man is unstable in all his ways", JAMES 1:6-8 KJV

Focus on revelation, while intensifying His Character continually; agreeing with His Nature, pressing beyond actions and proceed with renaturing the journey.

Attentively looking after the Word strengthens one's resolve to see the matter through to its triumph.

"*This is my comfort in my affliction: for Thy Word hath quickened me*". PSALMS 119:50 KJV

"*For this cause also thank we God without ceasing, because, when ye received the word of God which ye heard of us, ye received it not as the word of men, but as it is in truth, the word of God, which effectually worketh also in you that believe*". 1 THESSALONIANS 2:13 KJV

When we receive and obey the Word of God, we can say with the Apostle Paul, "*Whereunto I also labour, striving according to his working, which worketh in me mightily*". COLOSSIANS 1:29 KJV

Align every portion by keeping-hold-of your living; by perceiving His identity within the Spoken Work provided; and gather strength by pattern of thoughts that determine your practice.

The previous passage of <u>PROVERBS 4:20-22</u>; provides us the method/plan/strategy for obtaining the results of every portion of His Word's promises.

        1]-*There is need for an* ATTENTIVE HEARING...
        2]-*There must be the gaze of a* STEADFAST LOOK...
        3]-*There must be cultivated an* EMBRACING HEART...

Again, when your gaze remains upon the symptoms and your thinking processes are more occupied with this, than with His Will, through His Word; you are creating the wrong type of soil/ground/atmosphere for the SEED to grow from/out of.

It is this using of one kind of SEED, and yet sowing it in a diverse type of soil/ground/atmosphere, while expecting a fruitful harvest.

Your harvest will be fruitful; but, such fruit will not bring any healing to you, and certainly not bring any glory to God, Himself!

Apprehend His Counsel with the Dominion of Faith; through practice of adjusting the provision through the counsel of His Finished Work.

*O*nce the Word of your petition is sown into the soil of your heart and mind; there is the next provision required that provides the *"evidence of things"* UNSEEN.

Knowing we are IN CHRIST, provides us the perfected evidence of His Faith at work in us.

"Whereby are given unto us exceeding great and precious promises: that by these ye might be partakers of the divine nature, having escaped the corruption that is in the world through lust". SECOND PETER 1:4 KJV

Seeing only what God has said, about our healing, defends and determines, by the evidence He provides, the very healing that we seek; because in HIM we already have what we seek for.

Practice/Repeat the Spoken Word as His Finished Work.

*T*his practice of repeating His Spoken Word, and accepting this evidence presented as being His Finished Work; makes it easier to believe than to doubt.

An old saying is, *"Feed your faith, and you will starve your doubts"*!

While your doubts will change with every wind that blows; HIS FAITH AT WORK IN YOU will never change the evidence He has provided and sown into your being.

SEMITIC~ARAMAIC~HEBRAIC THESAURUS
Aramaic before first {
Semitic Root before first =
Lettering for ParaPhrase after second =

Got Healing?

confirm ⊐Hhet= specific appropriate beyond ⊓Dalet= [that/which/of] faith establish presence H1870 ⊔⅄⊓⌐{⊔⅄⊓⌐=to way, overtake/apprehend}= ⊓Dalet= [that/which/of] faith establish presence ⊏Resh= practice beginning strength-⅃Kaph= surrender obtain desire and flee H512≀⅄⅄{≀⅄=avoid/keep something hidden}=⌐ ⊐Nun= perpetuate patience persist ⅄Vav= [and] identity intensity counsel ⊐Samech= adjust apprehend resource H6440⊓⊐⅄ before ⅄⊐⅄{≀⊐=in the presence of}=⊐ ⊐Pey= mouth SpokenWord speak ⅃Nun= perpetuate patience persist ⊏Hey= [the/His] character reveal foresee thee seven H7651 ⊙⊔⊔{⊙⊔⊔=complete}=⅄. Shin= pressure exchange disperse ⅃Beyt= [in/by] pattern thought existing-in-source ⅄Ayin= experience perceive wisdom ways H1870 ⊔⅄⊓⌐{⊔⅄⊓⌐=overtaking/apprehend-ing}=⌐ ⊓Dalet= [that/which/of] faith establish presence ⊏Resh= practice beginning strength-⅃Kaph= surrender obtain desire

The Semitic Emphasis

The Self-Existent One opportunity/evidence plowing the furrows to sow in direction of/possession of/accuser even to establish/solve a problem hurt/plague appearance turn into/to exclude concerning someone/a certain to overtake/apprehend avoid/keep something hidden in the presence of overtaking/apprehending.

"He healed all that were sick, that it might be fulfilled which was spoken by Esaias the prophet saying, Himself took our infirmities and bare our sicknesses." MATTHEW 8:17 KJV

This is quoted as the reason why He healed all that were sick.

It was not that He might give his enemies a vindication of His Divinity, but that He might fulfill the character presented of Him in ancient prophecy.

Had he not done so, He would not have been true to His own character, and if He did not still do so, He would not be--"*Jesus Christ, the same yesterday, to-day, and forever.*"

These healings were not occasional, but continual; not exceptional, but universal.

He never turned anyone away.

"*He healed all that were sick.*"

"*As many as touched Him, were made perfectly whole.*"

He is still the same.

Now, this was the work of His life.

We have been too ready to sum up all the Redeemer's work in the one act at the close; and in our zeal for the value of His blood, we have forgotten the preciousness of His earthly life.

But God would not have us forget that He spent more than three years in deeds of power and love before He went up to that Cross to die.

And we need that Living Christ quite as much as Christ Crucified.

The Levitical types included the meat offering quite as much as the sin offering; and suffering human hearts need to feed upon the Great Loving

Heart of Galilee and Bethany, as much as on the Lamb of Calvary.

It would take entirely too long to examine in detail the countless records of His healing power and grace, or tell how He cured the leper, the lame, the blind, the palsied, the impotent, the fever stricken, *"all that had need of healing."*

How He linked sickness so often with sin, and forgave before He spake the restoring word.

How He required their own personal touch of appropriating faith, and bade them take the healing by rising up and carrying their bed.

How His healing went far beyond His own immediate presence, and reached and saved the centurion's servant and the nobleman's son.

How sharply He reproved the least question of His willingness to help, and threw the responsibility of man's suffering on his own unbelief.

These and many more such lessons crowd every page of the Master's life, and still reveal to us the secret of claiming His healing power.

And what right anyone can claim to explain away these miracles, as mere types of spiritual healing and blessing, and not as specimens of what He still is ready to do for all who trust Him~~is as inexplicable as the Mythical Theory, as well as the Mystery of the Gospel of Jesus, the Christ!

Such was Jesus of Nazareth.

But was this blessed power to die with Him?

Focus Revelation By Identifying His Character Through Perpetuating Agreement With His Nature

DEUTERONOMY 28:35
KJV+SM

The LORD[H3068] shall smite[H5221] [H8686= S=Simple, causative, sometime reflexive action; M=as an action, process, or condition incomplete] thee in the knees[H1290], and in the legs[H7785], with a sore[H7451] botch[H7822] that cannot[H3201] [H8799=S= A simple/causal action, or process, or condition of the root, M=which is incomplete] be healed[H7495] [H8736=S=Simple, sometimes reflexive M=uncompleted action, process, or condition], from the sole[H3709] of thy foot[H7272] unto the top of thy head[H6936]

ORIGINAL THOUGHTS
...(28:35) Focus revelation by identifying His Character; through perpetuating agreement with His Nature, to perceive His Truth, as existing-

in-principle, and strengthening covenant. Perceive His Truth by pressing the intensity of parallels that are strong in circumstances, while pressuring you beyond actions that proceed to fortify the exchange by practice. Focus your agreement on His Truth, providing the counsel of His Finished Work. Practice/Repeat the Spoken Word as His Finished Work; then, renature your focus to keep-hold-of your living; by yielding-up the Spoken Word. The Beginning Walk teaches and discerns His Faith's parallels, presenting the very structure identified in belief.

Focus revelation by identifying His Character; through perpetuating agreement with His Nature, to perceive His Truth, as existing-in-principle, and strengthening covenant.

The revelations, and inspirations, given by God to His people, only serve to drive the hunger and thirst for more of Him.

Identifying what His Character contains; what He is about; what traits are those that are His alone; this pursuit is not after more knowledge, but desirous of more of HIM!

Knowing He is a merciful God provides every believer with the opportunity of choosing to stand firm as to Who they believe His Person to remain.

QUESTION: *If God is ABSOLUTE TRUTH; how then can Truth bear the LIE, when presented in contrast AGAINST HIS OWN CHARACTER?*

*"And said, If thou wilt diligently hearken to the voice of the LORD thy God, and wilt do that which is right in his sight, and wilt give ear to his commandments, and keep all his statutes, I will put none of these diseases upon thee, which I have brought upon the Egyptians: for I am the LORD that **healeth** thee".* EXODUS 15:26 KJV

How do you seek to balance this verse, against the idea that God makes you sick? Is this argument not bitter vs. sweet; right vs. wrong; life vs. death?

Does such argument not make those who resist patrons of theories that contain no LIFE OF GOD at all?

NO!

Let us read of the Word; examine the **"original thought"** of the Scriptures from the very first of manuscripts; not of Greek, Latin, or even Hebrew; but, of Semitic and Aramaic!

These tell us that our God, Jehovah-Jireh/Rapha/Shalom/Shammah//McKaddesh/Tsidkenu/Adoniah/El-

Elyon/Nissi/Rohi/Shaddai/Elohim, and any other Covenant Name of the Lord God Most High; He is THE GOD THAT DELIVERS US!

Perceive His Truth by pressing the intensity of parallels that are strong in circumstances, while pressuring you beyond actions that proceed to fortify the exchange by practice.

*P*arallels are those concepts and paradigms that exist irrespective of others, and yet run the same course, along-side of one another, showing the diversity and completely differing, though moving toward the same MARK!

Focus your agreement on His Truth, providing the counsel of His Finished Work.

*A*ttention must be given COMPLETELY to His WORD; as these are the only facts in evidence, transcending every experience man may use to deflate, and devaluate the Healing Power of God, Himself.

There is no healing, that lasts, apart from His Word!

Practice/Repeat the Spoken Word as His Finished Work; then, renature your focus to keep-hold-of your living; by yielding-up the Spoken Word.

*T*he sacrifice of PRAISE is about offering up God's Word to Him in a fully-yielded vessel of Praise and Thanksgiving.

This is never about thanking Him for any sickness, or tragedy, or circumstance, for that matter.

This is about exalting Him above every instance that tries the FAITH OF GOD at work in men's souls.

Except a believer hold-fast to the confession/profession of, and by, the Faith deposited by the Father within their own vessel, they have no other hope without hoping in HIM FIRST!

The Beginning Walk, teaches and discerns His Faith's parallels, presenting the very structure identified in belief.

*T*he building of His IDENTITFY within our living provides the fulfilling of the Promise made to be with us.

Confession is an affirmation of a Bible truth we have embraced.

This is simply believing with our hearts, and repeating with our mouths/speech the declaration of God Himself, as to WHOSE we are IN

CHRIST!

SEMITIC~ARAMAIC~HEBRAIC THESAURUS
Aramaic before first {
Semitic Root before first =
Lettering for ParaPhrase after second =

...(28:35) The LORD H3068 יהוה {אתא=the Self~Existing One} = Yud=purpose possess actions- Hey=-[the/His]
character reveal foresee- Vav=-[and] identity intensity counsel- Hey=-[the/His] character reveal foresee- **shall smite** H5221 נכה {ש=with thee**
seed in the palm} = Nun-seed patience continue- Kaph-surrender obtains consent- Hey-quality reveal grace-
in H5921 על {◉=experiencing the staff/knowledge/experience} = Ayin-pierce perceive wisdom- Lamed-instruct truth
provide- **the knees,** H1290 ברך {◉=filling with a gift} = Beyt-pattern thought existing-in-principle- Resh-practice beginning
strength- Kaph-surrender making consent- **and in** H5921 על {◉=concerning} = Ayin-pierce perceive wisdom- Lamed-instruct truth
provide- **the legs,** H7785 שוק {◉=repeating a cycle} = Shin-pressure exchange disperse- Vav-intensify degree counsel- Quph-
contrast parallel structure- **with a sore** H7451 רע {אא=piling together} = Resh-practice beginning strength- Gimal-circumstances
understanding encounter- **botch** H7822 שחין {◉=sharp walls} = Shin-pressure exchange disperse- Hhet-specific appropriate beyond-
Yud-purpose posture actions- Final-Nun-keep-hold-of-living foundation progress- **that** H834 אשר {◉=press the
beginning} = Aleph-dominion ability confirm- Shin-pressure exchange disperse- Resh-practice beginning strength-
cannot H3201 יכל {◉=bending/subduing the will} = Yud-purpose posture actions- Kaph-surrender making consent- Lamed-
instruct truth provide- H3808 לא {◉=to be without anything such as no~thing} = Lamed-instruct truth provide- Vav-
intensify degree counsel- Final-Aleph-perfected finished matured- **be healed,** H7495 רפא {◉=taking medicine through the
mouth} = Resh-practice beginning strength- Pey-mouth SpokenWord speak- Final-Aleph-ending finish maturity- **from the
sole** H4480 מן {◉=indicating the origin of directional movement} = Mem-renature challenge remembered- Yud-purpose
posture actions- Final-Nun-keep-hold-of-living foundation progress- H3709 כף {◉=in measure} = Kaph-surrender making consent- Pey-
mouth Spoken Word speak- **of thy foot** H7272 רגל {◉=of following} = Resh-practice beginning strength- Gamel-walk gather carry-
Lamed-instruct truth provide- **unto** H5704 עד {◉=up to the time that} = Ayin-pierce perceive wisdom- Dalet-faith establish
presence- **the top of thy head,** H6936 קדקד {◉=inclining oneself out of honor & reverence} = Quph-contrast
parallel structure- Dalet-faith establish presence- Quph-contrast parallel structure- Vav-intensify degree counsel- Dalet-faith establish presence-

The Semitic Emphasis

The Self~Existing One with seed in the palm/hand~~knowing from experience filling with a gift concerning repeating a cycle piling together~~sharp walls press the beginning~~bending/subduing the will to be without anything such as no~thing taking medicine through the mouth~~indicating the origin of directional movement in measure of following seeing the door inclining oneself out of honor & reverence.

Scripture is replete/repetitive with stories of God's Healing Power.

The unfortunate system of our day, however, entails that these stories cannot be believed as though being evidence to us today that the same God then, is the same God today!

It would take entirely too long to examine in detail the countless records of His healing power and grace, or tell how He cured the leper, the lame, the blind, the palsied, the impotent, the fever stricken, *"all that had need of healing"*.

Of how He linked sickness so often with sin, and forgave before He spake the restoring word; how He required their own personal touch of appropriating faith, and bade them take the healing by rising up and carrying their bed; how His healing went far beyond His own immediate presence, and reached and saved the centurion's servant and the nobleman's son; and _how sharply He reproved the least question of His willingness to help, and threw the responsibility of man's suffering on his own unbelief_.

These and many more such lessons crowd every page of the Master's life, and still reveal to us the secret of claiming His healing power.

And what right anyone can claim to explain away these miracles, as mere types of spiritual healing and blessing, and not as specimens of what He still is ready to do for all who trust Him-is as inexplicable as the Mythical Theory.

"Verily, verily, I say unto you, He that believeth on Me, the works that I do shall he do also; and greater works shall he do, because I go to my Father." JOHN 14:12 KJV

Here is another "VERILY," nay a "VERILY, VERILY."

Then it must be something emphatic, and something man was sure to doubt.

Now, it is no use to tell us that this meant that the Church after Pentecost was to have greater spiritual power, and do greater spiritual works by the Holy Ghost than Jesus Himself did, __inasmuch as the conversion of the soul is a greater work than the healing of the body__; because Jesus says, "_The works that I do, shall he do also_," as well as the "_greater works than these:_" that is, he is to do the same works Christ did, and greater also.

So we know they did the same works that He did.

Even during His life He sent out the twelve Apostles, and then He sent out the seventy as forerunners of the whole host of the Christian Eldership (for the seventy were just the first Elders of the Christian Age, corresponding to the seventy Elders of Moses), with full power to heal.

And when He was about to leave the world, He left on record both these Commissions in the most unmistakable of terms.

We write again: _Healing IS for today as much as it was for yesterday._

The reason for its not being seen today, as in yesterday, is not due to the lacking of His Promises; but the lacking of belief to step out on those promises by His Body, the Church of which all of Creation is part.

His Dominion Restores By His Truth
And Considers His Intent As
The Prevail/Triumph Of Pressing His Truth

1 SAMUEL 6:3
KJV+SM

And they said[H559] [H8799] If ye send away[H7971] [H8764] the ark [H727] of the God[H430] of Israel[H3478] send[H7971] [H8762] it not empty[H7387]; but in any wise[H7725] [H8687] return[H7725] [H8686] him a trespass offering[H817]: then ye shall be healed [H7495] [H8735] and it shall be known[H3045] [H8738] to you why his hand [H3027] is not removed[H5493] [H8799] from you.

ORIGINAL THOUGHTS

...(6:3) His Dominion restores by His Truth, and considers His Intent as the prevail/triumph of pressing His Truth, to appropriate the settling of His Evidence/Witness. Dominion strengthens His Counsel, as proven; while deepening His Truth, as identifying His character. Focusing exchange with strength, and conforming to Truth pressing Truth to appropriate confirming evidence/witness promised by His Finished Work. Beginnings posture/position contrasts, through prevail/triumph; consenting to purpose pressing exchange of identifying counsel, while existing-in-principle/precept. Conform every exchange with/through His prevail, by deepening the methods of practicing the Spoken Word as His Finished Work. Focus His Faith by perceiving/discerning reflections of His Grace; arranging/locating His Presence by providing the counsel of His Finished Work. Apprehend every portion of strength renaturing focus to keep-hold-of your living.

Dominion restores by Truth, and considers His intent as the prevail/triumph of pressing His Truth, to appropriate the settling of His Evidence/Witness.

The strength of Dominion, given by God, matches every stride, every pull, every ebb~n`~flow, when Truth comes to validate WHO HE IS, in the believer!

Notice, that the confession, which is saying the same thing God says, is by FAITH!

That is, believing and confessing comes BEFORE experiencing the results.

As with Salvation, confession comes after believing, but before receiving the manifestation. It does work in reverse!

FAITH is always about acting on GOD'S WORD!

Dominion strengthens His Counsel, as proven; while deepening His Truth, as identifying His character.

$\mathcal{A}$ COMMAND/Dominion of His Word is the counsel proving the deepening of one's belief; while identifying the character/integrity of God's WORK in the heart and living of the believer!

Focusing exchange with strength, and conforming to Truth pressing Truth to appropriate confirming evidence/witness promised by His Finished Work.

"*Beat your plowshares into swords, and your pruning-hooks into spears: let the weak say, I am strong*". *JOEL 3:10 KJV*

Whenever the "*confession*" is used, many instinctively think upon confessing sin, weakness, and failure.

However, that is only the negative side of God's operation in a person's confession.

When the positive side of a believer's confession is made, there is a way opened up, so that the soul of man is embraced by the Will of God, through the speaking/confessing of His Word in FAITH.

Beginnings posture/position contrasts, through prevail/triumph; consenting to purpose pressing exchange of identifying counsel, while existing-in-principle/precept.

$\mathcal{T}$he successive BEGINNINGS that a believer starts/commences, defines/displays the successive FORMS of the working of SALVATION'S MANIFESTATION.

1st~ in the form of the new birth, it is even in the form of every blessing promised us in the Word of God.

The BELIEVER is call upon by God, to ACT on every part/portion of the SALVATION GIVEN THEM BY GOD that he is aware of because of hearing, reading, and believing the teachings of HIS WORD!

2nd~ we are to believe with heart, and continue confessing with our mouth by the extent that the Word of God continues forming such petitions, and outlining such prayers, so as to consistently form the DESIRE through the platform of HIS WORD SPOKEN IN BELIEF.

Conform every exchange with/through His prevail, by deepening the methods of practicing the Spoken Word as His Finished Work.

Got Healing?

*A*ll that Jesus did in His substitutionary work is the private property of the believer for whom Jesus did what He did.

So, throughout the believer's living for God, God wants the believer to believe with their heart, and then continuously SPEAK with their mouth, all that He says we are IN CHRIST!

Conforming our speech patterns and words to His Promises provided, causing the formation of not only a defense against NOT receiving; but, it is the basis for the acts of Faith which puts God to work fulfilling His Word in us, to us.

Focus His Faith by perceiving/discerning reflections of His Grace; arranging/locating His Presence by providing the counsel of His Finished Work.

*T*he reflections of Grace are about what we see in HIM, as US.

When we see HIM in us, we are to reflect the image that we see.

This IMAGE of GOD IN the believer, is the responsible reflecting of HIS WORD, coming alive in the mind, with imaginations that glorify GOD, every time!

Make the following verse, yours!

"*And YE ARE COMPLETE IN HIM, which is the head of all principality and power.*" COLOSSIANS 2:10 KJV

Make your confession as this: "*I AM COMPLETE IN HIM*"!

Apprehend every portion of strength renaturing focus to keep-hold-of your living.

*T*aking hold of His WORD, with the grasp of FAITH at work in your imaginations, creates the flow of His Presence, moving within your own, to present the fullness of His *BE*-ing through the greatness of what you say in FAITH, through His WORD!

SEMITIC~ARAMAIC~HEBRAIC THESAURUS
Aramaic before first {
Semitic Root before first =
Lettering for ParaPhrase after second =

...(6:3) *And they said,* H559 〔carefully wrapped〕= Aleph-dominion ability confirm- Mem-renature challenge
remembered- Lamed-instruct truth provide- *If* H518 〔conditionally when〕= Aleph-dominion ability confirm- Final-Mem-weight fashions prevail- disperse- Lamed-instruct truth provide- Hhet-specific appropriate beyond- *ye send away* H7971 〔to let loose/dismiss/release〕= Shin-pressure exchange dominion ability confirm- Taw-evidence prove signify- *the ark* H727 〔plowing the furrow to sow〕= Aleph-dominion ability confirm- Resh-practice beginning strength- Vav-intensify degree counsel- Taw-evidence prove signify- *of the God* H430 〔behaving like〕

God}=⟨ Aleph-dominion ability confirm-⟨ Lamed-instruct truth provide-⟨ Vav-intensify degree counsel-⟨ Hey-character reveal grace-⟨ of Israel, H3478 ⟨ Yud-purpose posture actions-⟨ Shin-pressure exchange disperse-⟨ Resh-practice, beginning strength-⟨ Aleph-dominion ability confirm-⟨ Lamed-instruct truth provide-⟨ =God prevails}=⟨ send H7971 ⟨ =to let loose/dismiss/release}=⟨ Shin-pressure exchange disperse-⟨ Lamed-instruct truth provide-⟨ Hhet-specific appropriate beyond-⟨ it H853, ⟨ =plowing the furrow to sow}=⟨ Aleph-dominion ability confirm-⟨ Taw-evidence prove signify not H408 ⟨ =without/nothing}=⟨ Lamed-instruct truth provide-⟨ Final-Aleph-perfected finished matured-⟨ empty; H7387 ⟨ =to pour out/down}=⟨ Resh-practice beginning strength-⟨ Yud-purpose posture actions-⟨ Quph- contrast parallel structure-⟨ Final-Mem-weight fashions prevail-⟨ but H3588 ⟨ =certainly}=⟨ Kaph-surrender making consent-⟨ Yud- in any wise return. H7725 ⟨ =to turn back}=⟨ Shin-pressure exchange disperse-⟨ Vav-intensify purpose posture actions-⟨ degree counsel-⟨ Beyt-pattern thought existing-in-principle-⟨ H7725 ⟨ =to turn back}=⟨ Shin-pressure exchange disperse-⟨ Vav- intensify degree counsel-⟨ Beyt-pattern thought existing-in-principle-⟨ him a trespass offering: H817 ⟨ =compensation}=⟨ Aleph-dominion ability confirm-⟨ Shin-pressure exchange disperse-⟨ Final-Mem- weight fashions prevail-⟨ then H227 ⟨ =at that time}=⟨ Aleph-dominion ability confirm-⟨ Zayin-skill alter method-⟨ ye shall be healed, H7495 ⟨ =soundness}=⟨ Resh-practice beginning strength-⟨ Pey-mouth SpokenWord speak-⟨ Final-Aleph-ending finish maturity-⟨ and it shall be known H3045 ⟨ =perceive/distinguish/by experience}=⟨ Yud-purpose posture actions-⟨ Dalet-faith establish presence-⟨ Ayin-pierce perceive wisdom-⟨ to you why ⟨ =of what grace-⟨ challenge remembered-⟨ Hey-character reveal his kind/whatsoever}=⟨ Mem-renature to you why ⟨ =of what hand H3027 ⟨ =strength/power}=⟨ Lamed-instruct truth provide-⟨ Vav-intensify degree counsel-⟨ Final-Aleph-perfected finished matured-⟨ is not removed H5493 ⟨ =turn aside/remove}=⟨ Samech-adjust apprehend resource-⟨ Vav-intensify degree counsel-⟨ Resh-practice beginning strength-⟨ from H4480 ⟨ =portion}=⟨ Mem-renature challenge remembered-⟨ Yud-purpose posture actions-⟨ Final-Nun- keep-hold-of-living-foundation progress-⟨ you.

The Semitic Emphasis

<u>Carefully wrapped</u> <u>conditionally</u> <u>when</u> to <u>let loose/dismiss/release</u> <u>plowing</u> the <u>furrow</u> to <u>sow</u> <u>behaving like God</u>~~<u>God prevails</u> to <u>let</u> <u>loose/dismiss/release</u> <u>plowing</u> the <u>furrow</u> to <u>sow</u> <u>without/nothing</u> to <u>pour out/down</u> <u>certainly</u> to <u>turn back</u>~~<u>to turn back</u> <u>compensation</u> <u>at that time</u> <u>soundness</u> <u>perceives/distinguishes/by experience</u> <u>of what</u> <u>kind/whatsoever</u> <u>strength/power</u> <u>nothing/without</u> <u>turning aside/removing portion.</u>

"*Verily, verily, I say unto you, He that believeth on Me, the works that I do shall he do also; and greater works shall he do, because I go to my Father.*" JOHN 14:12 KJV

Here is another "VERILY," nay a "VERILY, VERILY." Then it must be something emphatic, and something man was sure to doubt.

Now, it is no use to tell us that this meant that the Church after Pentecost was to have greater spiritual power, and do greater spiritual works by the Holy Ghost than Jesus Himself did, inasmuch as the conversion of the soul is a greater work than the healing of the body.

Because Jesus says, "*The works that I do, shall he do also,*" as well as the "*greater works than these:*" that is, he is to do the same works Christ did, and greater also.

And so we know they did the same works that he did.

Even during His life, He sent out the twelve Apostles, and then He sent out the seventy as forerunners of the whole host of the Christian Eldership (for the seventy were just the first Elders of the Christian Age, corresponding to the seventy Elders of Moses), with full power to heal.

And when He was about to leave the world, He left on record both these Commissions in their most unmistakable terms.

Focus Your Pursuit As Though Finished; Discovering/Exposing Truth

2 KINGS 2:21
KJV+SM

...*(2:21) And he went forth*[H3318] *[H8799= S=A simple/causal action, or process, or condition of the root, M=which is incomplete] unto the spring*[H4161] *of the waters*[H4325] *and cast*[H7993] *[H8686=S=Simple, causative, sometime reflexive action; M=as an action, process, or condition incomplete] the salt*[H4417] *in there, and said*[H559] *[H8799= S=A simple/causal action, or process, or condition of the root, M=which is incomplete] Thus saith*[H559] *[H8804=S=A simple/causal action M=referring to a time, or the present] the LORD*[H3068] *I have healed*[H7495] *[H8765=S= Simple expressing intensive/intentional, repeated/extended action; M=completed referring to a time, or the present] these waters*[H4325]*: there shall not be from thence any more death*[H4194] *or barren*[H7921] *[H8764=S= An intensive or intentional action, representing an action or condition in its unbroken continuity, M=and may be used of present, past or future time] land ..*

ORIGINAL THOUGHTS
...*(2:21) Focus your pursuit as though finished; discovering/exposing Truth, and rendering the intensity of your journey as perfected/matured; remembering by Grace the enhancing of Truth consented to. Restore His provision of surrender, and enlarge your prevail/triumph; as Dominion restores Truth; while arranging discoveries that focus revelation upon Authority representing the Truth. Intensify His character by practice/repetition of the Spoken Word as His Finished Work. Enhance, then, by prevail, replenishing by discoveries that provide the counsel of His Finished Work. Renature the focus of prevail/triumph, and replace by overcoming through discerning counsel established; remembering identity of evidence/witness, replacing by surrender with Truth.*

His love is unconditional, but His blessings are conditional. God loves me because of who I am, but He blesses me because of what I do.

Focus your pursuit as though finished; discovering/exposing Truth, and rendering the intensity of your journey as perfected/matured; remembering by Grace the enhancing of Truth consented to.

"Being IN HIM" means we see through His eyes; hear through His ears; speak through His lips; and walk by His feet.

Everything for the believer is seen as finished through Jesus, the

Christ!

"*Thou art snared with the words of thy mouth, thou art taken with the words of thy mouth*". PROVERBS 6:2 KJV

"*Death and life are in the power of the tongue: and they that love it shall eat the fruit thereof*". PROVERBS 18:21 KJV

When doubt rears its ugly head, it is because the believer believes something else directly contrary to His Word, and Plan.

Continually speaking doubt compromises faith, and increases the strength of one's doubt.

Speaking doubt, instead of faith, imprisons the believer by their own words spoken with no accountability, or responsibility.

Restore His provision of surrender, and enlarge your prevail/triumph; as Dominion restores Truth; while arranging discoveries that focus revelation upon Authority representing the Truth.

𝒟is-ease gains the upper hand, when a believer confesses/declares the testimony of their physical senses improperly.

Where a feeling, or an appearing of something may seem important and significant in this physical realm; REMEMBER: the spiritual realm dictates and creates the physical dimension.

"*If any man speak, let him speak as the oracles of God; if any man minister, let him do it as of the ability which God giveth: that God in all things may be glorified through Jesus Christ, to whom be praise and dominion for ever and ever. Amen*". FIRST PETER 4:11 KJV

Intensify His character by practice/repetition of the Spoken Word as His Finished Work.

"*𝓛et no corrupt communication proceed out of your mouth, but that which is good to the use of edifying, that it may minister grace unto the hearers*". EPHESIANS 4:29 KJV

The thoughts of God ONLY exude the person, presence, and power of God Himself! "*(For we walk by faith, not by sight).*" 2 CORINTHIANS 5:7 KJV

The manner, or course of living that best exalts Him, and enhances His Person and Presence in our living is thinking, speaking, and acting through, by, and on the Word of the Living God.

Got Healing?

"For as he thinketh in his heart, so is he: Eat and drink, saith he to thee; but his heart is not with thee". PROVERBS 23:7 KJV

<u>Enhance, then, by prevail, replenishing by discoveries that provide the counsel of His Finished Work.</u>

The spiritual and physical transformations that the Spirit of God transforms and shapes the believer's living, comes by the continual input of His Word.

*"I beseech you therefore, brethren, by the mercies of God, that ye present your bodies a living sacrifice, holy, acceptable unto God, which is your reasonable service. And be not conformed to this world: but be ye transformed by the renewing of your mind, that ye may prove what is that **good**, and **acceptable**, and **perfect**, will of God".* ROMANS 12:1-2 KJV

Notice in these verses, there is implication made that there is more than one level of renewal in the believer's living, unto God.

The *good, and acceptable, and perfect will of God.*

Give attention to this fact: *believers have the choice of which level at which they may serve productively.*

Your healing depends upon your level of commitment, in seeing the hand and presence of God in action within your living.

This is NOT an inference as to one's performance, productivity, or any such kind.

This is the inclusion of understanding that presents the NEED and FACT of living a more complete expression of God's **<u>BE</u>**-ing through their own.

<u>Renature the focus of prevail/triumph, and replace by overcoming through discerning counsel established; remembering identity of evidence/witness, replacing by surrender with Truth.</u>

"(For the weapons of our warfare are not carnal, but mighty through God to the pulling down of strong holds); Casting down imaginations, and every high thing that exalteth itself against the knowledge of God, and <u>bringing into captivity every thought to the obedience of Christ</u>; And having in a readiness to revenge all disobedience, when your obedience is fulfilled. Do ye look on things after the outward appearance? If any man trust to himself that he is Christ's, let him of himself think this again, that, as he is Christ's, even so are we Christ's". [2]

Got Healing?

Whereas plans usually are aimed at reducing the risk of the unknown, spontaneity embraces the risk and excitement of seizing the moment.

In a world where everything seems to have its place and time, it can be a surprising joy to do something~~unexpected.

It might start with something small, but continue to look for those opportunities.

It is easy to fall into the habit of only doing what you are familiar with and convincing yourself that you are simply not good with certain activities. But just as our physical muscles do not develop if we do not use them, so too, neurological development ceases if we do not exercise our brains.

The brain changes itself, shows that learning something new, something challenging, activates neurological activity.

When we learn something new, there are neurons that fire together and wire together.

SEMITIC~ARAMAIC~HEBRAIC THESAURUS
Aramaic before first {
Semitic Root before first =
Lettering for ParaPhrase after second =

...(2:21) And he went forth^{H3318} {Ɔ⌒=to go out/exit/proceed to} = Yud-purpose posture actions- Tsad-pursuit journey anticipate- Final-Aleph-perfected finished matured- unto^{H413} {=concerning/on account of} = Hey-fragrance reveal grace- Lamed-instruct truth provide- the spring^{H4161} {Ɔ⌒=of leading out/of delivering} = Mem-renature challenge remembered- Vav-intensify degree counsel- Tsad-pursuit journey anticipate- Final-Aleph-perfected finished matured- of the waters^{H4325} {⌒=of danger/refreshment} = Mem-renature challenge remembered- Hey-character reveal grace- and cast^{H7993} {=to throw out} = Shin-pressure exchange disperse- Lamed-instruct truth the salt^{H4417} {=maintenance} in there^{H8033} {=} = Shin-pressure exchange disperse- Final-Mem-weight fashions prevail- and said^{H559} {=carefully wrapped} = Aleph-dominion ability confirm- Mem-renature challenge remembered- Thus^{H3541} {=on this manner} = Kaph-surrender making consent- Hey-character reveal grace- saith^{H559} {⌒=carefully wrapped} = Aleph-dominion ability confirm- Mem-renature challenge remembered- Lamed-instruct truth provide- the LORD^{H3068} {=the Self-Existent One} = Yud-purpose posture actions- Hey-character reveal grace- Vav-intensify degree counsel- Hey-character reveal grace- I have healed^{H7495} {⌒=mended/repaired thoroughly} = Resh-practice beginning strength- Pey-mouth SpokenWord speak- Final-Aleph-ending finish maturity- these^{H428} {=removed far away} = Shin-pressure exchange disperse- Final-Mem-weight fashions prevail- waters^{H4325} {⌒=something unknown} = Mem-renature challenge remembered- Hey-character reveal grace- not^{H3808} {=nothing/without} = Lamed-instruct truth provide- Vav-intensify degree counsel- Final-Aleph-perfected finished matured- be^{H1961} {=enduring/existing} = Hey-quality reveal grace- Yud-purpose posture actions- Hey-quality reveal grace- from thence^{H4480} {⌒=the blood continues} = Mem-renature challenge provide- Kaph-surrender making consent- there shall more^{H5750} {=} = Ayin-pierce perceive wisdom- Vav-intensify degree counsel- Dalet-faith establish presence- any death^{H4194} {⌒=chaos marks} = Mem-renature challenge remembered- Vav-intensify degree counsel- Taw-evidence prove signify- or barren^{H7921} {=sorrow from a lack of evidence} = Shin-pressure exchange disperse- Kaph-surrender making consent-**Ⅼ**Lamed-*instruct truth provide-*land.

The Semitic Emphasis

To go out/exit/proceed to concerning/on account of of leading out/of delivering of danger/refreshment to throw out maintenance carefully wrapped on this manner carefully wrapped the Self-Existent One mended/repaired thoroughly removed far away something unknown nothing/without enduring/existing the blood continues chaos marks sorrow from a lack of evidence.

This is a season in which both joy and loneliness can be amplified.

Many will reconnect with families and friends to eat and laugh and relax.

For others loneliness will be intensified.

The very fact that so many families come together and celebrate magnifies their own disconnected lives.

When we don't experience the love of other human beings, the love of God seems equally distant.

But this is exactly what made the life and message of Jesus so significant.

In the midst of people going about their daily lives~~with the same desires and concerns we have today~~while religious thinkers were speculating about a holy god, Jesus confronted us with a new reality.

Those who knew Jesus struggled for years to find better words to describe what they witnessed.

Somehow they glimpsed God in this human.

Somehow, in this person of Jesus, God was no longer a distant or separate being, but a tangible and present reality in His Person, Presence, and Power.

Humility.

We must put our "*self*" and our own voice aside.

We have to get away from the clutter of everything bombarding us and only seek God.

Prayer.

Reading God's Word and praying are two of the very best ways for us to clearly hear His voice.

It is amazing how getting on our knees opens our ears to hear.

Practice.

Hearing God's voice is not a one-time event.

It is ongoing and it takes practice.

Do you think Moses, out in the middle of the desert, had not heard God's voice before he encountered the burning bush?

Do you think that the encounter with the Ethiopian eunuch was was a one-time event with Phillip?

They were men who were humble and in prayer actively seeking God's voice and practicing their hearing skills.

Focus Revelation As Though Intensifying His Character By Pressures Renaturing Perceptions

2 CHRONICLES 30:20

KJV+TVM

And the LORD[H3068] hearkened[H8085] [H8799] to Hezekiah[H3169], and healed[H7495] [H8799] the people[H5971].

ORIGINAL THOUGHTS

...(30:20) Focus revelation as though intensifying His Character by pressures renaturing perceptions. His Character provides purpose, by appropriately altering the parallels of actions; as revealing every portion, practicing the Spoken Word as His Finished Work. Confirming evidence/witness perceives prevail/triumph.

<u>Focus revelation as though intensifying His Character by pressures renaturing perceptions.</u>

𝒯he stronger, and greater one's declarations become, the more that Heaven's Host acts on the believer's behalf.

Believers must become His Word/His Promise; confessing/ declaring every promise with their lips; they confess that Eternity, our former position, frees us from everything external, or outside of the Will of God, while doing everything in their living according to *"thus saith the Lord"*!

Believers confess that their deliverance, and exchange is complete; as they live according to the laws of another dimension; that is, God's own Heaven.

<u>His Character provides purpose, by appropriately altering the parallels of actions; as revealing every portion, practicing the Spoken Word as His Finished</u>

Work.

Man is the only being in God's Creation given the ability to acclimate, activate, and appropriate from two dimensions; Physical and Spiritual; knowing that the Spiritual created, and continues to create the Physical.

The spiritual revelation of the word, "*Remission*", applies the wiping away of anything connected with death, decay, and inactivity.

"*Therefore if any man be in Christ, he is a new creature: old things are passed away; behold, all things are become new*". 2 CORINTHIANS 5:17 KJV

Believers must regard the necessity of confessing/declaring the redemption made available by the offering of His Blood on their behalf.

"*And almost all things are by the law purged with blood; and without shedding of blood is no remission*". HEBREWS 9:22 KJV

Confirming evidence/witness perceives prevail/triumph.

Continually making one's stand upon the Word of God is a foundation that weathers any storm.

"*Let the words of my mouth, and the meditation of my heart, be acceptable in thy sight, O LORD, my strength, and my redeemer*". PSALMS 19:14 KJV

PSALMS 103:2-6 KJV

2 *Bless the LORD, O my soul, and forget not all His benefits:* 3 *Who forgiveth all thine iniquities; Who healeth all thy diseases;* 4 *Who redeemeth thy life from destruction; Who crowneth thee with lovingkindness and tender mercies;* 5 *Who satisfieth thy mouth with good things; so that thy youth is renewed like the eagle's.* 6 *The LORD executeth righteousness and judgment for all that are oppressed.*

SEMITIC ARAMAIC HEBRAIC THESAURUS

...(30:20) *And the LORD* H3068 {=the Self-Existent One} reveal grace- Vav-intensify degree counsel- Hey-character reveal grace- Yud-purpose posture actions- Hey-character *hearkened* H8085 {=hearing to respond} = Shin-pressure exchange disperse- Mem-renature-challenge remembered- Ayin-pierce perceive wisdom- *to* H413 {=looking toward something/someone} = Hey-character reveal grace- Lamed-instruct truth provide- *Hezekiah* H3169 {=Jehovah makes strong} = Yud-purpose posture actions- Hhet-specific appropriate beyond- Zayin-skill alter method- Quph-contrast parallel structure- Yud-purpose posture actions- Hey-character reveal grace- Vav-intensify degree counsel- *and healed* H7495 {=open thoughts} = Resh-practice beginning strength- Pey-mouth Spoken Word speak- Final- Aleph-ending finish maturity- H853 {=plow~pointing furrows for sowing} = Aleph-dominion ability confirm- Taw-evidence prove signify- *the people.* H5971 {=working through imaginations} = Ayin-pierce perceive wisdom- Final- Mem-weight fashions prevail

The Semitic Emphasis

The Self~Existent One hearing to respond looking toward Jehovah makes strong open thoughts plow~pointing furrows for sowing working through imaginations.

Hearing God and responding, is a question that many today are asking.

The problem of such questions arises when we think we are needed, in order for God to accomplish what He has designed and purposed.

If your remedies involve seeking a mentor other than God; or searching for something that will convince you that it is God speaking to you~~you have already stepped in the wrong direction, by taking measures into your own hands!

Never make the mistake that anything or anyone in this physical dimension has an open corner on the market of knowing God's will for you.

God's will is individual, and it will only be revealed through an intimate, close relationship with HIM ALONE.

Learn not to allow outside influences, voices, or other sundry tools that lead you AWAY from God, instead of establishing a better relationship with Him.

Hearing the Holy Spirit takes humility, prayer and practice.

It is a spiritual *art~form* that God calls all His children to perfect over the course of our lives.

OBEYING the Spirit's voice is admittedly more difficult than HEARING, but becoming a mature follower of Jesus requires us to do both.

The Focus On Revelation Intensifies His Character

PSALMS 30:2
KJV+SM

O LORD^{H3068} my God^{H430} I cried^{H7768} [H8765=S=Simple expressing intensive/intentional, repeated/extended action; M=completed referring to a time, or the present] unto thee, and thou hast healed^{H7495} [H8799=S=A simple/causal action, or process, or condition of the root, M=which is incomplete] me.

ORIGINAL THOUGHTS
...(30:2) The Focus on Revelation intensifies His Character.
Deepen His Truth; by identifying His disposition, and exchanging every portion of your perception, while discovering/exposing His Truth, by the practiced repetition of the Spoken Word as His Finished Work.

Got Healing?

The Focus on Revelation intensifies His Character, as deepening the Truth; by identifying His disposition, and exchanging every portion of your perception, while discovering/exposing His Truth, by the practiced repetition of the Spoken Word as His Finished Work.

The spiritual law of Confession is that what comes out of your mouth, in turn, rules your living through what is spoken.

Some believers confess with their lips, while all the while they deny Him in their heart.

"If we suffer, we shall also reign with him: if we deny him, he also will deny us:...". 2 TIMOTHY 2:12 KJV

A believer's confession embraces and envelopes more than just saying, *"I believe I am healed"*!

It is more than *"just trying to hold on"*!

*"Seeing then that we have a great high priest, that is passed into the heavens, Jesus the Son of God, let us **hold fast** our profession".* HEBREWS 4:14 KJV

"My flesh and my heart faileth: but God is the strength of my heart, and my portion forever". PSALMS 73:26 KJV

"Surely he hath borne our griefs ^{weaknesses} *, and carried our sorrows* ^{diseases} *: yet we did esteem Him stricken, smitten of God, and afflicted".* ISAIAH 53:4 KJV

Notice, it was NOT God who looked upon Him, Jesus as stricken, smitten, or afflicted! Just humanity!

1 PETER 2:21-24 KJV

21 For even hereunto were ye called: because Christ also suffered for us, leaving us an example, that ye should follow his steps: 22 Who did no sin, neither was guile found in his mouth: 23 Who, when he was reviled, reviled not again; when he suffered, he threatened not; but committed himself to him that judgeth righteously: 24 Who his own self bare our sins in his own body on the tree, that we, being dead to sins, should live unto righteousness: by whose stripes ye were healed.

When we read His scriptures, we find the Person that He is; not just WHAT He is about.

FOR EVEN HEREUNTO WERE YE CALLED:

The calling/vocation/beckoning of God toward the believer is for the purpose of divulging and proving the fullness of what is offered through Christ's living sacrifice.

The example of Christ's living and ministry serves as the Pattern-Work of God's Will, through every effort made by every believer willing to follow HIM!

BECAUSE CHRIST ALSO SUFFERED FOR US, LEAVING US AN EXAMPLE, THAT YE SHOULD FOLLOW HIS STEPS:

If He leaves us an EXAMPLE, what is the purpose of such an example?

His example is the pattern for every believer to follow, when faced with dilemmas, decisions, or any other decisive actions.

What He suffered/allowed, we must then exemplify.

To follow His steps, we must stay the course of what living for Him requires, and yes, even demands.

WHO DID NO SIN, NEITHER WAS GUILE FOUND IN HIS MOUTH:

A selfish-independent-nature cannot have its place in the confines our heart; so our attitude must exude the Love of His Person present within our heart and mind and thoughts.

Guile is likened to *duplicity*; which is *disguising one's true intentions by deceptive words or actions.*

Whatever is not heard from one's speech, cannot be assumed as being a part of one's living, or belief.

WHO, WHEN HE WAS REVILED, REVILED NOT AGAIN; WHEN HE SUFFERED, HE THREATENED NOT; BUT COMMITTED HIMSELF TO HIM THAT JUDGETH RIGHTEOUSLY:

Notice, He, Jesus, was not the type of person who give what He got! He only returned each insult, each barb, each comeback, with a giving of Himself unto His Father's opinion.

Though He knew He could call ten-thousands of angels; yet, He died alone for you and me!

His living was a commission of righteous perfection. He did not die AS GOD; He died as the perfect man, without sin!

WHO HIS OWN SELF BARE OUR SINS IN HIS OWN BODY ON THE TREE, THAT WE, BEING DEAD TO SINS, SHOULD LIVE UNTO RIGHTEOUSNESS: BY WHOSE STRIPES YE WERE HEALED.

He became the scapegoat, offered upon the altar of two dimensions; in the physical, He was offered at an altar called, Calvary.

Got Healing?

In the spiritual, He was offered at the altar of Prayer, before Heaven, and the Throne of His Father, the Creator of the Universe.

He died not that we should be reminded of our failures; but, that we might have His Robe of Righteousness, accepted as sons and daughters, as His own dear family.

SEMITIC~ARAMAIC~HEBRAIC THESAURUS
Aramaic before first {
Semitic Root before first =
Lettering for ParaPhrase after second =

...(30:2) O LORD H3068 יְהוָה {צוּה}=the Self-Existent One} = Yud-purpose posture actions- Hey-character reveal grace- Vav-intensify degree counsel- Hey-character reveal grace-

my God, H430 אֱלֹהַי {עֲזֻ}=the strength of authority} = Aleph-dominion ability confirm- Lamed-instruct truth provide- Vav-intensify degree counsel- Hey-character reveal grace- Ayin-pierce perceive

I cried H7768 שִׁוַּעְתִּי {שׁ}=carefully observing} = שׁ Shin-pressure exchange disperse- Vav-intensify degree counsel-

wisdom- unto H413 אֵלֶי {שׁ}=looking toward something} = ה Hey-fragrance reveal grace- Lamed-instruct truth provide-

thee, and thou hast healed H7495 רְפָא {ר}=of something man opened} = ר Resh-practice beginning strength- פ Pey-mouth Spoken Word

speak- Final-Aleph-ending finish maturity- me.

The Semitic Emphasis

The Self~Existent One~~the strength of authority carefully observing~~looking toward something~~of something man opened.

It never fails.

Watch some people in their lives, for when nothing transpires as they think it would/should, they become downcast and crestfallen in their attitudes.

Too many Christians endeavor to overcome, by their own ingenuities, and when they fail, want to blame God for not giving them what they THOUGHT was His Will.

The flaw in most of our journeys reveals the lack in our relationship with the Lord God.

Until we learn to accept His thoughts as ours, we will not ascend to the heights of the Destiny He planned for each of us.

It is *The Self~Existent One* in Whom we have our life's essence.

It is *The Self~Existent One* in Whom we have our life's being/existence.

It is *The Self~Existent One* in Whom we have our life's wholeness, and yet we choose to suffer as though we are like the animals of the field, which having nothing make themselves content with nothing.

Beloved, none of the aforementioned ideals contain any of the virtues that make up the Character of the Lord Jesus Christ!

Beloved, never lose sight of ETERNITY; which is what Jesus came to re~member our memories with!

Our thoughts need to be *as a sanctified imagination, yet balanced by God's Truth!*

Talking about heaven or hell is one thing; but laboring to go to either one without realizing what each are TRULY about is futile!

Heaven and Hell are concepts of humanity's imagination against waiting in expectation for the appearance of Christ through the nations and lives that live on this planet!

Looking beyond to anticipate something we have never seen, nor can we prove to be a real tangible place is foolish, ignorant, and uncalled for; when there is a mountain of evidence that depicts both through truth in a more real way!

Read *REVELATION 20:11-15*, and discover by examining the REAL TRUTH about both Heaven and Hell, then decide in this dimension WHOM YOU WILL CHOOSE TO FOLLOW!

Read *PSALMS 139:8,* and uncover the facts about God's Presence being everywhere our living exists!

Then read the substance contained in *SECOND CORINTHIANS 5:6 & 8*, realizing that there is no place where God is not.

Even though we make our own HELL, we never realize that God is there WITH US IN OUR OWN DARKNESS.

If He is there WITH US, why else would He be there except in His desire to deliver us from what we have created for ourselves?

Jesus returned to Heaven, to be with Father, AND to prepare us as a PLACE wherein He, and the Father, and the Spirit might abide and reside throughout eternity.

CHECK IT OUT!

Disperse The Truth Specifically To Establish Pattern-Thought Out Of Beginnings

PSALMS 107:20
KJV+SM

He sent [H7971] [H8799=S= A simple/causal action, or process, or condition of the root, M=which is incomplete] his word [H1697] and healed [H7495] [H8799=S=A simple/causal action, or process, or condition of the root, M=which is incomplete] them, and delivered [H4422] [H8762=S= An intensive or intentional, a repeated or extended action, process, or condition M=which is incomplete] *them from their destructions*[H7825]

ORIGINAL THOUGHTS
...(107:20) Disperse the Truth specifically to establish pattern-thought out of Beginnings. Practice/Repeat the Spoken Word as His Finished Work; and restore by His Truth balanced; while renaturing focus to keep-hold-of one's living, Exchange appropriately actions as evidence/witness.

Disperse the Truth specifically to establish pattern-thought out of Beginnings.

Spreading the Truth throughout one's living, pertains to speaking the Word of God, as though into every portion of one's living.

Three main areas there are that cover every other situation or condition within anyone's living.

[1]Health; [2]Wealth; & [3]Family...these three are the main divisions under which there lies every other interruption, temptation, or decision to change, transform, or transcend a person's will and personal thought-patterns.

If we learn to apply HIS TRUTH into the midst of every portion of beginnings that occur in each of these three areas, then a wall of defense; and yet, greater than defense, an outline of strategy will amass an offence that will parallel every portion of a believer's living, to become the strong refuge of His protection.

"But it is good for me to draw near to God: I have *put my trust in the Lord GOD*, that I may declare all thy works". PSALM 73:28

"Trust in the LORD with all thine heart; and lean not unto thine own understanding". PROVERBS 3:5

"Bind them continually upon thine heart, and tie them about thy neck. When thou goest, it shall lead thee; when thou sleepest, it shall keep thee; and when thou awakest, it shall talk with thee. For the commandment is a lamp; and the law is light; and reproofs of instruction are the way of life." PROVERBS 6:21-23

Practice/Repeat the Spoken Word as His Finished Work; and restore by His Truth balanced; while renaturing focus to keep-hold-of one's living.

The consciousness of righteousness is knowing the fact of His righteousness as your own righteousness.

This must become the Breastplate covering and protecting of your commitment, and allegiance unto the Lord God.

Without righteousness protecting the considerations, meditations, and imaginations of your heart, your Will may be bent toward another.

Exchange appropriately, actions as evidence/witness.

At the times and moments of God's nudging, or empowering; stand up to prove the Word of the Lord as superior to any other man~made obstacle, or hindrance.

Have you ever just wanted to ask God: "*What is the living You want me to live*"?

It is a good question—maybe one of the most important questions we could ever bring to God.

He created us, after all.

He knows why, after all.

He knows what is best for each of us, after all.

If we could learn from Him the living He wants us to live—*the details, the pace, the places* where we are to invest ourselves and the places where we are not to invest ourselves, we would be in His will; and there, we would find our living IN HIM!

1

Lord, You are more precious than silver;
Lord, You are more costly than gold;
Lord, You are more beautiful than diamonds;
And nothing I desire compares with You.

2

Lord, Your life is divine, eternal.
Lord, Your life regenerated me.
Lord, Your life is growing within me,
Until I am fully conformed to Thee.

3

Lord, Your love is wide as the ocean.
Lord, Your love is deep as the sea.
Lord, Your love encompasses the nations,
And that is all I want to live in me.

SEMITIC~ARAMAIC~HEBRAIC THESAURUS

Aramaic before first {

Semitic Root before first =

Lettering for ParaPhrase after second =

...(107:20) He sent H7971 שלח{=to stretch out/let go of}=ש Shin-pressure exchange disperse- ל Lamed-instruct truth provide- ח Het-specific appropriate beyond- his word, H1697 דבר{=order/substance}=ד Dalet-faith establish presence- ב Beyt-pattern thought existing-in-principle- ר Resh-practice beginning strength- and healed H7495 רפא{=as cured/repaired}=ר Resh-practice beginning strength- פ Pey-mouth SpokenWord speak- א Final-Aleph-ending finish maturity- them, and delivered H4422 מלט{=saved/preserved/prepared}=מ Mem-renature challenge remembered- ל Lamed-instruct truth provide- ט Thet-restraint mixture balance- them from their destructions. H4480 מין{= from}=מ Mem-renature challenge remembered- י Yud-purpose posture actions- ן Final-Nun-keep-hold-of-living foundation progress- H7825 שחית{=pit of despair}=ש Shin-pressure exchange disperse-┌Hhet-specific appropriate beyond-╷Yud-purpose posture actions-╻Taw-evidence prove signify-

The Semitic Emphasis

To stretch out/let go of order/substance as cured/repaired~~ saved/preserved/prepared from the pit of despair.

The call of God in any portion of our living should be addressed in worship, humility, and surrender to His Will beyond our own.

With His Gethsemane Prayer, Jesus gave us the example of how we should become, or be, in the midst or beginning or ending of any event in our living for/of HIM!

When Jesus said, "*nevertheless, not my Will but Thine be done*", He committed everything He was and had to the Will of the Father~~above and beyond His own choices otherwise.

We ask you, reader, "*what would Jesus do*"?

The response that should come is, "*whatever be Your Will, O God, show me the way wherein You have made me to walk*"!

Any Healing, Every Healing is about our worship of Him, our humility before Him, and our surrender to Him~~HIM ALONE!

Truth Existing-On-Principle/Precept Through Skillful Discoveries Wisely Overcomes Every Pressure Of Change

ISAIAH 6:10
KJV+SM

Make the heart [H3820] of this people [H5971] fat [H8080] [H8685= S=Simple, causative, sometimes reflexive action; M=as an order, or a command] and make their ears [H241] heavy [H3513] [H8685=S=Simple, causative, sometimes reflexive action; M=as an order, or a command], and shut [H8173] [H8685=S= Simple, causative, sometimes reflexive action; M=as an order, or a command] their eyes [H5869]: lest they see [H7200] [H8799=S= A simple/causal action, or process, or condition of the root, M=which is incomplete] with their eyes [H5869], and hear [H8085] [H8799=S= A simple/causal action, or process, or condition of the root, M=which is incomplete] with their ears [H241], and understand [H995] [H8799=S= A simple/causal action, or process, or condition of the root, M=which is incomplete] with their heart [H3824], and convert [H7725] [H8802=S=Expresses the "simple" or "causal" action of the root in the active voice; M= through an action or condition in its unbroken continuity], and be healed [H7495] [H8804=S=A simple/causal action M=referring to a time, or the present].

ORIGINAL THOUGHTS

...(6:10) Truth existing-in-principle/precept, through skillful discoveries; wisely overcomes every pressure of change, in progress as confirming His identity of method. Holding onto one's consent toward His Pattern/Outline of Belief/Faith, replaces with wise perception/discerning, and the learned

Got Healing?

posturing/positioning of progress through the Spoken Word keeping-hold-of one's living. Strengthening abilities resolved wisely, postures/positions progress to enhance every challenge with Wisdom. Confirming His identity of method, as holding to the outline of His purpose is the enduring/persisting through the provision of pattern-thoughts existing-in-principle/precept, and exchanging the intensity of mindsets, while practicing the Spoken Word as His Finished Work.

Truth, as existing-in-principle/precept, through skillful discoveries; wisely overcomes every pressure of change, in progress as confirming His identity of method.

So long as humanity resides/remains in the earthen/fleshly vessel, there will be circumstances that APPEAR as being greater than what the PROMISES of God provide.

Yet, a healthy study of the Scriptures proves beyond any shadow of doubt that the ETERNAL will always OUTWEIGH the PHYSICAL.

The best offense focuses then upon a person's/soul's CHOICE!

"And if it seem evil unto you to serve the LORD, choose you this day whom ye will serve; whether the gods which your fathers served that were on the other side of the flood, or the gods of the Amorites, in whose land ye dwell: but as for me and my house, we will serve the LORD". JOSHUA 24:15 KJV

Truth always lies in the ETERNAL, never being found real in only the PHYSICAL.

The IDENTITY of the Eternal God always provides clear choice, when the searcher searches from within the FOUNDATIONS of one's own experience.

Of course, it must be mentioned, when a soul only follows what they have been taught from succeeding generational themes and interpretations, there is never found that which provides, must less presents, the ETERNAL WISDOM OF GOD, HIMSELF!

The VOICE of understanding will always present a knowledge that is a *"freeing influence"* awaiting one's plausible, believable, and acceptable CHOICE; while, the VOICE of argument will always fashion its own unsubstantiated IGNORANCE.

A believer has only to look, and identify that which has no LIFE of GOD in its presentation, much less its precepts.

Yet, there will ALWAYS be found in the pages/volume of the BOOK written of HIM that there is LIFE, and THAT LIFE MORE

ABUNDANTLY GIVEN.

Which do you choose, seeker, LIFE or DEATH? The CHOICE is yours!

Holding onto one's consent toward His Pattern/Outline of Belief/Faith, replaces with wise perception/discerning, and the learned posturing/positioning of progress through the Spoken Word keeping-hold-of one's living.

One has only to hold, unequivocally, to the Anchor of their soul, from within the precepts of God's Eternal Majesty; finding the foundation in the ROCK that is higher than all.

There, upon the ROCK, their house/dwelling/refuge will stand firm through the ages.

MATTHEW 7:24-29 KJV

²⁴ Therefore whosoever heareth these sayings of Mine, and doeth them, I will liken him unto a wise man, which built his house upon a rock: ²⁵ And the rain descended, and the floods came, and the winds blew, and beat upon that house; and it fell not: for it was founded upon a rock. ²⁶ And every one that heareth these sayings of Mine, and doeth them not, shall be likened unto a foolish man, which built his house upon the sand: ²⁷ And the rain descended, and the floods came, and the winds blew, and beat upon that house; and it fell: and great was the fall of it. ²⁸ And it came to pass, when Jesus had ended these sayings, the people were astonished at His doctrine: ²⁹ For He taught them as one having authority, and not as the scribes.

Strengthening abilities resolved wisely, postures/positions progress to enhance every challenge with Wisdom.

Out of the Wisdom of God's Words, there is always found the settled, tranquil understanding that as He has spoken, thus will it always be about His RIGHTEOUSNESS as being ours!

Wisdom makes no apologies for complaining, or lethargy, or inattentiveness on the part of another's ill-conceived CHOICES.

Wisdom provides the PRECEPT.

Wisdom explains the PRINCIPLE, and the outcome of one's PARTICIPATION will always yield the PROFITABLE.

Confirming His identity of method, as holding to the outline of His purpose is the enduring/persisting through the provision of pattern-thoughts existing-in-principle/precept, and exchanging the intensity of mindsets, while practicing the

Spoken Word as His Finished Work.

His WISDOM always confirms/affirms HIS IDENTITY in the mix/blend of any circumstance that is examined in the LIGHT of WHO HE IS!

His Word HOLDS to the PATTERN of His IDENTITY; always IDENTIFYING the PERSON of His PRESENCE, even within the midst of every anxiety, or turmoil, or upset.

The focus of every one of HIS PURPOSES, provides indomitable proof/evidence that HIS SPOKEN WORD, with reference to the need of any one person, or many thereof; always provides motive/reason for triumph when CHOICE is made to follow HIS REPORT, and not another's.

The INTENSITY of one's mindset follows the outline of HIS PURPOSE when allowed, agreed with, and applied.

No person has the RIGHT to assert that God does not honor His WORD; when, they in fact, do not HOLD TO HIS WORD without wavering!

JAMES 1:4-8 KJV

⁴ But let patience have her perfect work, that ye may be perfect and entire, wanting nothing. ⁵ If any of you lack wisdom, let him ask of God, that giveth to all men liberally, and upbraideth not; and it shall be given him. ⁶ But let him ask in faith, nothing wavering. For he that wavereth is like a wave of the sea driven with the wind and tossed. ⁷ For let not that man think that he shall receive any thing of the Lord. ⁸ A double minded man is unstable in all his ways.

The perfect work of Patience is for the believer to become mature/perfect, and of a finished form/entire.

What God desires for His Creation, He outlines in the PATTERN or government of His WORD!

However, the precept of perfection hinges upon a person's CHOICE to remain stable, or become/remain undecided and unstable.

CHOOSING Him and His Word ALWAYS creates a stability unparalleled in any portion of mere human existence.

God is BIGGER THAN ANY MOUNTAIN/PROBLEM that I can, or cannot see!

HEALING, then, is a WORD from God defining HIS WILL for any believer who remain willing and obedient.

Got Healing?

Follow Christ's example!

"Though he were a Son, yet learned he obedience by the things which He suffered". HEBREWS 5:8 KJV

"This book of the law shall not depart out of thy mouth; but thou shalt meditate therein day and night, that thou mayest observe to do according to all that is written therein: for then thou shalt make thy way prosperous, and then thou shalt have good success". JOSHUA 1:8 KJV

SEMITIC~ARAMAIC~HEBRAIC THESAURUS

Aramaic before first {

Semitic Root before first =

Lettering for ParaPhrase after second =

...(6:10) *Make the heart* H3820 לב{שמל =understanding/mindful}= Lamed-instruct truth provide- Beyt-pattern thought existing-in-principle- *of this* H2088 זה{ =at the place where}= Zayin-skill alter method- Hey-character reveal grace- *people* H5971 *of this* עם{ =imaginations}= Ayin-pierce perceive wisdom- Final-Mem-weight fashions prevail- *fat* H8082 שמן{ =in *direction of/in possession of}*= Shin-pressure exchange disperse- Mem-renature challenge remembered- Final-Nun-keep-hold-of-living foundation progress- *and make their ears* H241 אזן{ =with a handle}= Aleph-dominion ability confirm- Vav-intensify degree counsel- Zayin-skill alter method- Final-Nun-keep-hold-of-living foundation progress- *heavy,* H3513 *presence-* כבד{ שמל =difficult}= Kaph-surrender making consent- Beyt-pattern thought existing-in-principle- Dalet-faith establish- *and shut* H8173 שעע{ =of *holding tight}*= Shin-pressure exchange disperse- Ayin-pierce perceive wisdom- Ayin-pierce perceive wisdom- *their eyes;* H5869 עין{ =with regard to appearance/spring/fountain}= Ayin-pierce perceive wisdom- Yud-purpose posture *eyes;* actions- Final-Nun-keep-hold-of-living foundation progress- *lest* H6435 פן{ =the one without}= Pey-mouth SpokenWord speak- Final-Nun-keep-hold-of-living foundation progress- *they see* H7200 ראה{ =the ability to see/perceive/have a *vision}*= Resh-practice beginning strength- Aleph-dominion ability confirm- Hey-character reveal grace- *with their eyes,* H5869 עין{ =with regard to appearance/spring/fountain}= Ayin-pierce perceive wisdom- Yud-purpose posture *eyes,* actions- Final-Nun-keep-hold-of-living foundation progress- *and hear* H8085 שמע{ =to hear and respond}= Shin-pressure exchange disperse- Mem-renature challenge remembered- Ayin-pierce perceive wisdom- *with their ears,* H241 אזן{ =with a *handle}*= Aleph-dominion ability confirm- Vav-intensify degree counsel- Zayin-skill alter method- Final-Nun-keep-hold-of-living foundation progress- *and understand* H995 בין{ =continuing the house/dwelling/abiding}= Beyt-pattern thought existing-in-principle- Yud-purpose posture actions- Final-Nun-keep-hold-of-living foundation progress- *with their heart* H3824 לבב{ שמל =understanding/mindful}= Lamed-instruct truth provide- Beyt-pattern thought existing-in-principle- Beyt-pattern thought existing-in-principle- *and convert* H7725 שוב{ שמל =pressing to the dwelling}= Shin-pressure exchange disperse- Vav-intensify degree counsel- Beyt-pattern thought existing-in-principle- *and be healed* H7495 רפא{ =as *cured/repaired}*= Resh-practice beginning strength- Pey-mouth SpokenWord speak- Final-Aleph-ending finish maturity-

The Semitic Emphasis

<u>Having understanding/being mindful at the place where imaginations~~in direction of/in possession of with a handle difficult of holding tight~~with regard to appearance the one without the ability to see/perceive/have a vision~~with regard to appearance to hear and respond with a handle continuing the abiding~~having understanding/being mindful while pressing to the dwelling as cured/repaired/healed.</u>

Where there are difficulties in one's living, there are imaginations conceiving such difficulties as being hard to deal with, or hard to overcome.

Note then that the understanding, or being mindful of such~~is an indicator of an area lacking in one or more of the needed/necessary elements of character toward the Living God.

In other words, when things are difficult in our living, it usually involves things that we cannot control.

Being healed, or gaining a healing is what many are after; and yet, these are not attained because of our performance, but because of a way that our body accepts and responds toward.

Medical science aids healing through physical means by administering medicine into the physical body. God's Divine Healing is Spiritual.

It is administered through the human spirit. *FIRST CORINTHIANS 2:9-12 KJV*

PSALM 107:20, tells us that God sent His Word and healed THEM.

Notice that it didn't say that God sent his Word to heal but He sent His Word and HEALED.

God considers it done.

God is no respecter of persons, but He does respect FAITH in His Word.

Reveal/Discover The Identity Of His Finished Work And Appropriate His Truth

ISAIAH 53:5
KJV+SM

But He was wounded[H2490] [H8775=S=Represents an action or condition in its unbroken continuity, and corresponds to the English verb, "to be" with the present participle. M=It may be used of present, past or future time] for our transgressions[H6588], He was bruised[H1792] [H8794=S=Passively expressing a causative action being intensive or intentional, as repeated or extended; action or condition in its unbroken continuity, M=and may be used of present, past or future time] for our iniquities [H5771]: the chastisement [H4148] of our peace[H7965] was upon Him; and with His stripes[H2250] we are healed[H7495] [H8738=S=Simple, sometime reflexive completed action M=referring either to a time, or the present] .

ORIGINAL THOUGHTS

...(53:5) Reveal/Discover the Identity of His Finished Work; and appropriate His Truth, as provided; while renaturing your Focus to keep-hold-of your living. Establish your consent/agreement with His Finished Work, and re-nature/restore motive/reason to keep-hold-of your living, even when encountering the intensity of His Counsel remaining. Remember His Identity as apprehended from each beginning; perceiving His Truth beyond His Pattern/ Outline, as existing-in-principle/precept of His Counsel. Strengthen Grace, by practice/repetition of His Spoken Word as being His

Got Healing?

Finished Work. Change the attitude of progressing to understand identifying His Counsel through the Grace of His Truth. Out of Identity adjusts the practice of exchanging provision by His Counsel to Prevail/Triumph. The Wisdom of His Truth applies by the Pattern~of~His~Thought increasing strength in the Unseen life-force through the Spoken Word of His Finished Work.

ISAIAH 53: 4, cannot refer to disease of the soul, and neither of the words translated "*sickness*" or "*pain*" have any reference to spiritual matters, but to bodily sickness alone.

This is proven by MATTHEW 8: 16~17: "~~~and He cast out the spirits with His WORD, and healed all that were sick"~~that it might be fulfilled which was spoken by Esaias/Isaiah, the prophet", saying, "Himself took our infirmities, and bare our sicknesses".

This is an inspired commentary on this fourth verse of ISAIAH 53.

It plainly declares that the prophet refers to bodily ailments.

Therefore, the word *sickness*, **choli**, must be read literally in Isaiah.

The same Holy Spirit, Who inspired this verse, quotes it again in MATTHEW as the explanation of the universal application by Christ of His power to heal the body.

To take any other view is equal to accusing the Holy Spirit of making a mistake in quoting **Her** own prediction.

Reveal/Discover the Identity of His Finished Work; and appropriate His Truth, as provided; while renaturing your Focus to keep-hold-of your living.

*R*eveal what you discover, and see WHO HE IS remains being about WHO HE IS!

God does not change in WHO HE IS; whether amid each storm, or the prevail of peaceful living; He remains the SAME.

"*Jesus Christ the same yesterday, and today, and forever*". HEBREWS 13:8 KJV

Yesterday, today, forever, Jesus is the same.
All may change, but Jesus never! Glory to His Name!
Glory to His Name! Glory to His Name!
All may change, but Jesus never! Glory to His Name!
[1]
O how sweet the glorious message simple faith may claim
Yesterday, today, forever Jesus is the same.
Still He loves to save the sinful, heal the sick and lame
Cheer the mourner, still the tempest, glory to His Name.
[2]

Got Healing?

He, who was the Friend of sinners, seeks the lost one now
Sinner come, and at His footstool penitently bow
He Who said "I'll not condemn thee, go and sin no more,"
Speaks to thee that word of pardon as in days of yore.
[3]
Oft on earth He healed the sufferer by His mighty hand
Still our sicknesses and sorrows go at His command
He who gave His healing virtue to a woman's touch
To the faith that claims His fullness still will give as much.

Establish your consent/agreement with His Finished Work; and renature/restore motive/reason to keep-hold-of your living; even when encountering the intensity of His counsel remaining.

Without a divine revealing, no one can rightfully share to a person the specific reason why their prayer(s) remain delayed, or even unanswered.

A delay in receiving one's healing, in one point, may appear as though being "*good news*".

However, the believer's lives are always in the hand and power of the Almighty.

"*Where He leads me, I will follow; What He feeds me, I will swallow*".

Remember His identity as apprehended from each beginning; perceiving His Truth beyond His Pattern/Outline, as existing-in-principle/precept of counsel.

No believer ought ever to RUSH-IN to a circumstance, without FIRST having met with Lord about it.

Not only should a believer INVITE His Person into the storm rising on the horizon; but, He should be ALLOWED/ PERMITTED to step into the *controls* at any time, without there being a hesitation on the part of the believer.

It is, at these times, there is a need to KNOW the Father's VOICE, to HEAR His SOUND above all others, even the din of the noise abounding around them.

"*Preach the word; be instant in season, out of season; reprove, rebuke, exhort with all longsuffering and doctrine*". 2 TIMOTHY 4:2 KJV

This verse is not speaking of just when you are in front of people, but He speaks with regard to either just living His WORD, or caught in a moment when you are asked to explain.

INSTANT IN SEASON and OUT OF SEASON takes on the purpose of ETERNAL THINGS, when the flesh is obstinately holding on to what has already been dealt with.

Often, our living is about only us; and we become caught in a vortex; a swirling mountain of wind, or adversity, that seems to keep sucking us into its despair.

This is the "*instance*" of the Word becoming used to offset the pull, and instead, take advantage of the *heat of the moment* to spread our wings and make the *heat of the moment* becomes the lifting up into the Presence of God's Grace and Mercies.

"*Wherefore lift up the hands which hang down, and the feeble knees; And make straight paths for your feet, lest that which is lame be turned out of the way; but let it rather be healed. Follow peace with all men, and holiness, without which no man shall see the Lord: Looking diligently lest any man fail of the grace of God; lest any root of bitterness springing up trouble you, and thereby many be defiled;...*". HEBREWS 12:12-15 KJV

Strengthen Grace, by practice/repetition of the Spoken Word as His Finished Work.

Except the believer continually, repetitiously regain what is offered, and Whom it is offered through, failure becomes an option many fall into.

The unfortunateness of living IN this world, finds the believer fighting, and waging a war, that in the spiritual realm, has already been finished.

The *good-fight of Faith* is neither about bringing the *old man Adam into subjection*; nor is it about *overcoming the enemy by prayer*! The Good-Fight of FAITH is just that.

This refers to the believer allowing, trusting, resting IN HIM to fight every battle that is not ours to fight; which is all of them.

Every struggle, every controversy, every antagonistic thought that comes our way is a matter settled IN HIM, the Christ, the LORD OF OUR LIVING!

It is by the repetitious usage of HIS WORD that creates HIS FAVOR on our BEHALF!

If we continue *circling the problem*, we fail at allowing HIM the opportunity to prove HIMSELF to the world around us.

BELIEVERS ARISE; realize that IN HIM we overcome; IN HIM we rise above the situation, to REST IN HIM, thereby ALLOWING HIM to BE WHO HE IS IN US!

Got Healing?

Change the attitude of progressing to understand, while identifying His Counsel through the Grace of His Truth.

How does the old hymn go?

"Trust and obey, for there's no other way to be happy in Jesus, but to trust and obey".

Our attitude can be the greatest of allies, or it can be the most challenging of oppositions.

Except we remain convinced of His Word, and believe beyond any shadow of doubt that God's Word is real, and is as PROMISED, we stand the chance of FAILING with regards to whatever the instance we are endeavoring to stand in Faith regarding.

Out of Identity adjusts the practice of exchanging provision by His Counsel to Prevail/Triumph.

If you've been taught that God doesn't speak to you, then you're probably not going to be listening for His voice.

This all comes down to what kind of relationship you think God offers.

You should ALWAYS question and investigate what others say, especially pastors, ministers, or television evangelists.

Often, they operate out of their memories, which can or cannot be up to date with what God is doing in the NOW!

This takes time and opportunity provided to the Spirit to familiarize you with *Her Voice*.

If you want to make music, you have to learn how to play an instrument. In the beginning, it doesn't sound too good—all the squawks and squeaks and bad timing.

But, you really are on your way to making music.

It just sounds like you're strangling a pig.

If you stick with it, something beautiful begins to emerge. Or how about snowboarding—learning to do that is really awkward at first.

You fall down a lot.

You feel like an idiot.

But, if you hang in there, you come to enjoy it. You get better. It starts to feel natural.

That's when it becomes fun.

This holds true for anything in life, including our walk with God.

It takes time and practice. It's awkward at first, and sometimes we feel stupid.

But if we hang in there, we do begin to get it, and as it becomes more and more natural, our lives are filled with His PRESENCE and all the joy and beauty and pleasure that come with it.

The Wisdom of His Truth applies by the Pattern~of~His~Thought increasing strength in the Unseen life-force through the Spoken Word of His Finished Work.

An intimate, conversational walk with God is available. It is normal, even.

Or, at least, is meant to be normal.

This writer is well aware that a majority of people do not enjoy that~~yet.

However, it is certainly what God desires and what He offers.

Our assumption must be based on the nature of God and the nature of man~made in His Image.

We are communicators.

Our assumption is also based on the nature of relationship, and it requires communication.

It is based on the long record of God speaking to His People of various ranks in all sorts of situations.

And finally, it is based on the teachings of Jesus, who tells us that we hear _His Voice_!

Dr. Young, in his version of the Bible:
3 He is despised, and left of men, A man of pains [Heb., makob], and acquainted with sickness [choli], And as one hiding the face from us, He is despised and we esteemed Him not. 4 Surely our sicknesses [choli] He hath borne, and our pains [makob] He hath carried them, And we— we have esteemed Him plagued, smitten of God and afflicted. 5 And He is pierced for our transgressions, Bruised for our iniquities, the chastisement of our peace is on Him, And by His bruise there is healing to us. 6 All of us like sheep have wandered, each to his own way we have turned, And Jehovah hath caused to meet on him The punishment of us all. 10 And Jehovah hath delighted to bruise him; He hath made him sick [choli]; If his soul doth make an offering for guilt, He seeth seed— He prolongeth days.

Got Healing?

12 With transgressors He was numbered, And He the sin of many hath borne, and for transgressors He intercedeth.

Dr. Isaac Leeser, translator of the Hebrew English Bible, renders these verses as follows:

3 He was despised and shunned of men: a man of pains and acquainted with disease. 4 but only our diseases did He bear Himself, and our pains He carried. 5 and through His bruises was healing granted to us. 10 but the Lord was pleased to crush Him through disease.

SEMITIC~ARAMAIC~HEBRAIC THESAURUS
Aramaic before first {
Semitic Root before first =
Lettering for ParaPhrase after second =

...(53:5) But He H1931 אוה {ↄↄ=looking toward something/someone} = ה Hey-character reveal grace- ו Vav-intensify degree counsel- א Final-Aleph-perfected finished matured- was wounded H2490 ללח {ᒻᒻ=common/defiled} = ח Hhet-specific appropriate beyond- ל Lamed-instruct truth provide- ל Lamed-instruct truth provide- מ Mem-renature challenge remembered- י Yud-purpose posture for our transgressions, H4480 ןמ {ᒻᒻ=indicating the origin of directional movement} = מ actions- ן Final-Nun-keep-hold-of-living foundation progress- H6588 עשפ {ↄↄↄ=causing incorrect actions} = פ Pey-mouth SpokenWord speak- ש Shin-pressure exchange disperse- ע Ayin-pierce perceive wisdom- He was bruised H1792 אכד {ↄↄ= pushing back and forth to crush} = ד Dalet-faith establish presence- כ Kaph-surrender making consent- א Final-Aleph-perfected finished matured- for our iniquities: H4480 ןמ {ᒻᒻ=indicating the origin of directional movement} = מ Mem-renature challenge remembered- י Yud-purpose posture actions- ן Final-Nun-keep-hold-of-living foundation progress- H5771 ןויע {ↄↄ=resulting in twisted actions} = ג Gimal= circumstances understanding encounter ו Vav= [and] identity intensity counsel ו Vav= [and] identity intensity counsel ן Final-Nun= evident grace/truth remain the chastisement H4148 רסומ {ↄↄ= rebellious/stubborn} = מ Mem= [from/out of] image encounter remembered ו Vav= [and] identity intensity counsel ס Samech= adjust apprehend resource ר Resh= practice beginning strength- of our peace H7965 םולש {ᒻᒻ=made whole or complete by adding or subtracting} = ש Shin= pressure exchange disperse ל Lamed= [to/toward] instruct truth provide ו Vav= [and] identity intensity counsel ם Final-Mem= weight fashioning prevail was upon H5921 לע {ↄ=in measurement} = ע Ayin= experience perceive wisdom ל Lamed= [to/toward] instruct truth provide him; and with his stripes H2250 הרובח {ↄↄↄ=to join one thing to another} = ח Hhet= specific appropriate beyond ב Beyt= [in/by] pattern thought existing-in-source ו Vav= [and] identity intensity counsel ר Resh= practice beginning strength- ה Hey= [the/His] character reveal foresee we are healed. H7495 אפר {ↄↄ=as cured/repaired/healed} = ר Resh= practice beginning strength- פ Pey= mouth SpokenWord speak א Final Aleph= perfected finished mature

The Semitic Emphasis

Looking toward something/someone common/defiled indicating the origin of directional movement causing incorrect actions pushing back and forth to crush~~indicating the origin of directional movement resulting in twisted actions rebellious/stubborn~~made whole or complete by adding or subtracting in measure~~to join one thing to another as cured/repaired/healed.

Notice at the end of the Emphasis, the writer alludes to the *measure of adding or subtracting* those things that cause the infirmities to abound.

Everything Jesus did for needy humanity during His earthly ministry was a direct revelation of the perfect will of God for the human race.

Perhaps no one could be more conservative than the scholars of the

Episcopalian church.

Yet, the commission appointed to study the subject of spiritual healing for the body, after three years of study and research in both the Bible and in history, reported back to the church.

Their findings were as follows: *The healing of Jesus was done as a revelation of God's will for humanity.*

Because they discovered that His will is fully revealed, they reported further:

No longer can the church pray for the sick with that faith-destroying phrase, If it be your will.

The message taught in the Gospels is one of complete healing for spirit and body, for all who will come to Him.

Many today say, "*I believe in healing, but I do not believe it is for everyone.*"

If it is not for everyone, then how could we ever pray the prayer of faith?

Among all those who sought healing from Christ during His earthly ministry, there is only one who prayed for healing with the words, If it be your will.

This was an outcast leper, in **MARK 1:40**, who did not know what Christ's will was in healing.

The first thing Christ did was to correct this uncertainty by assuring him, "*I will*".

It is no longer, if it be your will~~it is God's will.

The leper said: If you will, you can.

Jesus answered, "*I Will*".

Let that settle it forever with you: God will heal the sick.

If He wills to heal one, then He wills to heal all.

He is not willing that any should perish.

Practice The Spoken Word As His Finished Work
Confirming By Evidence/Witness
The Pressuring Of His Pattern-Thought As Practiced

JEREMIAH 6:14 & 8:11

KJV+SM [*reference made to identical verses*]
They have healed[H7495] [H8762] *also the hurt*[H7667] *of the daughter*[H1323] [H8676] *of my*

Got Healing?

$people^{H5971}$ $slightly^{H7043\,[H8738]}$, $saying^{H559\,[H8800]}$ $Peace^{H7965}$, $peace^{H7965}$; when there is no $peace^{H7965}$.

ORIGINAL THOUGHTS

...(6:14 & 8:11) Practice the Spoken Word as His Finished Work; confirming by evidence/witness by the pressuring of His Pattern-Thought as practiced. Perceive Truth, contrasting/com-paring His Truth to His Provision. Dominion restores by Truth ex-changing for promise His counsel that prevails; exchanging for promise His Counsel that prevails; for His Ability to act in keeping-hold-of your living, exchanging for promise, His counsel that prevails.

Practice/Repeat the Spoken Word as His Finished Work; confirming by evidence/witness, the pressuring of His Pattern-Thought as practiced.

As the pattern of HIS thoughts engender, or provide the evidence and witness of His SPOKEN WORD, out of the believer's mouth; the evidence/witness provided is realized.

Instead of WAITING for the manifestation of what has already been given you; lift your hands, your voice, your eyes TOWARD HIM, and embrace the TRUTH that the FACT of your healing is completely provided through HIS FINISHED WORK!

Perceive Truth, contrasting/comparing His Truth to His Provision.

The FACT of His TRUTH is the comparison of the PROVISION that has ALREADY BEEN PROVIDED through HIS PROMISES.

In the PROMISE is PROVIDED the PROVISION!

It is never the REPORT of the world THAT WE ACCEPT; it is ALWAYS the REPORT OF THE LORD that we TURN TO; finding the provision provided through His promise completed within/because of His FINISHED WORK!

Dominion restores by Truth exchanging for promise, His counsel that prevails; exchanging for promise, His counsel that prevails; His Ability to act in keeping-hold-of your living, then, exchange for promise, His counsel that prevails.

Three times the word for PEACE presents the idea of FAITH.

Exchange His PROMISE through the COUNSEL of His WORD!

Here is completed this portion of His FINISHED WORK.

When a believer hears, processes, embraces, and applies HIS WORD to the matter, there is formed the foundation of HIS WORD through PROMISE PROVIDING THE PROVISION for your, and my HEALING!

Got Healing?

SEMITIC~ARAMAIC~HEBRAIC THESAURUS

Aramaic before first {
Semitic Root before first =
Lettering for ParaPhrase after second =

...(6:14 & 8:11) *They have healed* H7495 א פ {ר פ =as cured/repaired} = Resh-practice beginning strength- Pey-mouth
SpokenWord speak- Final-Aleph-ending finish maturity- *also* H853 את {ע =the plow~pointing of furrows for*
sowing} = א Aleph-dominion ability confirm- Taw-evidence prove signify- *the hurt* H7667 שבר {שנ ר ש =bursting open} = ש Shin-
pressure exchange disperse- Beyt-pattern thought existing-in-principle- Resh-practice beginning strength- of the
daughter H1323 בנת {ב =the continuing of the house} = ב Beyt[within/in/inside]-pattern thought
inhabit- Nun-seed patience continue- Taw-evidence prove sign- of my people H5971 עמ {מ ע =gathering
together} = ע Ayin-pierce perceive wisdom- Final-Mem-trial fashions prevail- *slightly,* H5921 על {ע =experiencing the*
knowing} = ע Ayin-pierce perceive wisdom- Lamed-instruct truth provide- H7043 קלל {ע ל =gathering authority} = ק Quph-
contrast parallel structure- Lamed-instruct truth provide- Lamed-instruct truth provide- *saying,* H559 אמל {מ =carefully
wrapped} = א Aleph-dominion ability confirm- Mem-renature challenge remembered- Lamed-instruct truth provide-
Peace, H7965 שלומ {מ ל ש =making whole/complete by adding/subtracting} = ש Shin-pressure peace
H7965 שלומ {מ ל ש =making whole/complete by adding/subtracting} = ש Shin-pressure exchange disperse- Lamed-
instruct truth provide- Vav-intensify degree counsel- Final-Mem-weight fashions prevail- *when there is no* H369 אינ {ר ל =Have
you not?} = א Aleph-dominion ability confirm- Yud-purpose posture actions- Final-Nun-keep-hold-of-living foundation progress- *peace.* H7965
שלומ {מ ל ש =making whole/complete by adding/subtracting} = ש Shin-pressure exchange disperse- Lamed-instruct
truth provide- Vav-intensify degree counsel- Final-Mem-weight fashions prevail-exchange disperse- Lamed-instruct truth provide- Vav-
intensify degree counsel- Final-Mem-weight fashions prevail-

The Semitic Emphasis

As cured/repaired the plow~pointing of furrows for sowing bursting open gathering together the
continuing of the house experiencing the knowing gathering authority carefully wrapped making
whole/complete by adding/subtracting~~Have you not? made whole/complete by adding/subtracting

What we add is Jesus + nothing, and that together equals everything!

Where we often fail is when we try to add, or subtract something in/out of the mix that is NOT HIM!

Healing is not always the miraculous episode we may have been taught.

Healing is not always what includes the medicines that man has been given by the Wisdom of God to provide.

Healing is, however, always God's influence, effort, and effect appropriating what His DOMINION given provides.

On the supposition that sickness is a divine discipline and chastening; it is still more evident that its removal must come, not through mechanical appliances, but through spiritual causes.

From whatever side we look at disease, it becomes more and more evident that its remedy must be found alone in God and the Gospel of His Redemption.

His own life was a complete summary of Christianity; and from His words and works we may surely gather the great intent of His Redemption.

And what was the testimony of His life to physical healing?

He went about their cities healing all manner of sickness and disease among the people.

He healed all that had need of healing, that it might be fulfilled which was spoken by Esaias the Prophet, "*Himself took our infirmities, and bare our sicknesses.*"

Now, when we remember that this was not an occasional incident, but a chief part of His ministry; that He began His work with it, that He continued it to the close of His life; that He did it on all possible occasions and in every variety of cases, that He did it heartily, willingly, and without leaving any doubt or question of His will; that He distinctly said to the doubting leper, "*I will,*" and was only grieved when men hesitated to fully trust Him.

We realize that in all this He was but unfolding the real purpose of His great redemption, and revealing His own unchanging character and love, and that He has distinctly assured us that He is still "*the same yesterday, today, and forever*"~~surely we have a great principle to rest our faith upon, as secure as the Rock of Ages.

Modify/Challenge Revelation
Inspiring Purpose By His Character/Integrity

JEREMIAH 15:18
KJV+SM

Why is my pain[H3511] perpetual[H5331], and my wound[H4347] incurable[H605]
[H8803=S=Expresses the "simple" or "causal" action of the root in the active voice; M=represents an action or condition in its passive unbroken continuity; in its passive/inert/inactive/reflexive activity]
[H8765=S=Simple expressing intensive/intentional, repeated/extended action; M=completed referring to a time, or the present] which refuseth[H3985] to be healed[H7495] [H8736=S=Simple, sometimes reflexive M=uncompleted action, process, or condition]?
wilt thou be altogether unto me as a liar[H391], and as waters[H4325] that fail[H539]
[H8738=S=Simple, sometime reflexive completed action M=referring either to a time, or the present]?

ORIGINAL THOUGHTS
...(15:18) Modify/Challenge Revelation, inspiring Purpose by His Character/Integrity. Make Dominion to exist-in-principle/precept, by perpetuating/continuing anticipation specifically remembering persistently the surrender to Grace. His abilities perpetuate exchange modifying dominion to keep-hold-of living, by practicing/repeating the Spoken Word as His Finished Work. Inspire Purpose by His Character/Integrity; Inspire

Got Healing?

Purpose by His Character/Integrity. Reflect single-mindedness, agreeing methodically with His Pattern of Thought. Realign with His nature, providing the counsel of His Finished Work; and confirming progress made.

Modify/Challenge Revelation, inspiring Purpose by His Character/Integrity.

Revelation does not change; but what is revealed, often appears as though being changed; when it is only an expression more complete that appears, the more a person experiences the fullness of Christ, in the Father.

We have the FULLNESS of Christ within our being; yet, we have not experienced the FULLNESS of WHO HE IS in our living.

Like the groceries, or gasoline, or new clothing you may purchase; though bought and paid for, you have yet to experience the fullness of what is made available, in your everyday living!

Make Dominion to exist-in-principle/precept, by perpetuating/continuing anticipation, specifically remembering persistently the surrender to Grace.

Grace is a foundational building block, yes!

However, it is as well, an integral, working part of one's growth and consistent well-being.

As Grace balances one's beginnings; it also blends other elements into the experience, portraying the image of God in a believer's living.

While the precept of Grace may provide foundation, continually; the principle of Grace is applied to every step, every turn, and every choice we make in our journey with the Lord God.

His abilities perpetuate exchange modifying dominion to keep-hold-of living, by practicing/repeating the Spoken Word as His Finished Work.

The abilities of God; whether Grace, Mercy, Love, etc.; replace what is us, in favor of what is HIM; never can we forget that HE FIRST LOVED US.

Lest we become as the church of Ephesus, in REVELATION 2:1-7, in particular verse 4; having departed from the realization that HE FIRST LOVED US; not vice-versa.

The humbling effect of God's LOVE, when accepted from an ever-increasing awareness of His LOVING US FIRST; keeps the pride of life at bay, and in control of His guidance, and directions.

Inspire Purpose by His Character/Integrity; Inspire Purpose by His

---

Character/Integrity.

KNOWING HIM is fuel to the Fire of His **BE**-ing within our own.

The inspiration of His Purpose envelopes, and develops a certain focus, and single-mindedness, and motive/reason, considering actions and choices to come.

When the Spirit prompts us to call someone, or go by and visit someone, or just pray for them; this is a working of the Holy Spirit to provide a different member of the Body, other than yourself, with what they have need of, at the time.

"From whom the whole body fitly joined together and compacted by that which every joint supplieth, according to the effectual working in the measure of every part, maketh increase of the body unto the edifying of itself in love". EPHESIANS 4:16 KJV

Reflect single-mindedness, agreeing methodically with His Pattern of Thought.

What most believers wrestle with is the authority figures in their living that they believe are trying, or seeking to control their living.

Yet, _no one person can MAKE you do something, as an adult, that you do not choose to do!_ RIGHT? RIGHT!

However, we reflect these same attitudes, sometimes more than we want to admit; instead of holding to those viewpoints that would rather offer SUGGESTIONS, instead of projecting a _"know-it-all"_ approach. _Your attitudes and actions, sometimes, speak so loudly that others in need cannot hear what you are trying to say!_

Realign with His nature, providing the counsel of His Finished Work; and confirming progress made.

Choose at any juncture, TO CHANGE!

It does not matter whether it is NOW, or later; just do it!

Become the person God has destined YOU TO BE! The gospel is the power of God to everyone that believes.

When believed and acted upon, any promise of God is transformed into the power of God.

Every promise of God contains the power of God necessary to produce what it promises, when it is believed and acted upon.

God's promises are life to those that find them, and health to all their flesh.

Got Healing?

"And ye shall serve the LORD your God, and He shall bless thy bread, and thy water; and I will take sickness away from the midst of thee. There shall nothing cast their young, nor be barren, in thy land: the number of thy days I will fulfil".
EXODUS 23:25-26 KJV

SEMITIC~ARAMAIC~HEBRAIC THESAURUS
Aramaic before first {
Semitic Root before first =
Lettering for ParaPhrase after second =

...(15:18) Why H4100 {unknown chaos}= Mem-modify challenge remembered- Hey-character reveal grace- Hey-character reveal grace- Yud-purpose posture actions- Hey-character reveal grace- is H1961 {happens}= Kaph-surrender making consent- Aleph-dominion ability confirm- Bey- my pain H3511 {covering the house/dwelling}= pattern thought existing-in-principle- perpetual H5331 {continually}= Nun-perpetuate patience persist- Tsad-pursuit journey anticipate- Hhet-specific appropriate beyond- and my wound H4347 {seed in hand}= Mem-modify challenge remembered- Nun-perpetuate patience persist- Kaph-surrender making consent- Hey-character reveal grace- incurable, H605 {whosoever}= Aleph-dominion ability confirm- Nun-perpetuate patience persist- Shin-pressure exchange disperse- which refuseth H3985 {the blood continues}= Mem-modify challenge remembered- Aleph-dominion ability confirm- Final-Nun-keep-hold-of-living foundation progress- to be healed? H7495 {causing to heal}= Resh-practice beginning strength- Pey-mouth SpokenWord speak- Final-Aleph-ending finish maturity- wilt thou be altogether H1961 {becoming}= Hey-character reveal grace- Yud-purpose posture actions- Hey-character reveal grace- H1961 Hey-character reveal grace- Yud-purpose posture actions- Hey-character reveal grace- unto me as H3644 {the vain words likes of which}= Mem-modify challenge remembered- Yud-purpose posture actions- a liar, H391 {spoken to deceive/cause failure/disappoint}= Kaph-surrender making consent- Zayin-skill alter method- Beyt-pattern thought existing-in-principle- and as waters H4325 {unknown chaos}= Mem-modify challenge remembered- Hey-character reveal grace- reveal grace- that fail? H3808 {without}= Lamed-instruct truth provide- Vav-intensify degree counsel- Final-Aleph- perfected finished matured- H539 {the blood continuing}= Aleph-dominion ability confirm- Final-Nun-keep-hold-of-living foundation progress-

The Semitic Emphasis

Unknown chaos happens covering the house/dwelling continually~~ seeding in hand whosoever~~the blood continues causing to heal becoming the likes of which vain words spoken to deceive/cause failure/disappoint~~unknown chaos without the blood continuing.

The first principle of healing is an understanding of belief anchored in His Word.

If Jesus healed all that came to Him, when He walked this earth; why would He not heal those of us who come to Him now for healing?
MATTHEW 12:15; ACTS 10:34 KJV

Redemption is synonymous with Calvary.

Therefore, we are redeemed from the entire curse, body, soul and spirit, solely through Christ's Atonement.

Since disease is a part of the curse, how could God justly remove this part of the curse by healing the sick without first redeeming us from it?

Again, since *"Christ redeemed us from the curse of the law,"* how can God justify us and at the same time require us to remain under the law's curse?

The apostle Paul says, *"Ye are not under the law, but under grace."* ROMANS 6: 14 KJV

In short, why should anyone remain under the law's curse who is not under the law?

Practice/Repeat the Spoken Word as His Finished Work

JEREMIAH 17:14
KJV+TVM

Heal[H7495] [H8798= S=*Expressing a causative action; M=by a command/directive/mandate*] me, O LORD[H3068] *and I shall be healed*[H7495] [H8735=S=*Simple, sometimes reflexive action, either a verbal noun with verb; M=expressing a verbal idea; or expressing a finite form of the verb*]; save[H3467] [H8685] me, and I shall be saved[H3467] [H8735=S=Simple, sometimes reflexive action, either a verbal noun with verb; M=expressing a verbal idea; or expressing a finite form of the verb]: for thou art my praise[H8416].

ORIGINAL THOUGHTS

...(17:14) Practice/Repeat the Spoken Word as His Finished Work; focus on revelation, when intensifying character; practice/repeat the Spoken Word as His Finished Work. Position/Locate/Identify so as to enlarge/enhance His Wisdom; exhibiting the enlarging/enhancing wisely. Consent with actions affirming meaningful attitudes/viewpoints signifying to uphold every purpose of Truth revealed.

Practice/Repeat the _Spoken_ _Word_ as _His_ _Finished_ _Work; focus_ on _revelation, when_ _intensifying_ _character; practice/repeat_ the _Spoken_ _Word_ as _His_ _Finished_ _Work_.

*R*ecognizing/Realizing that the Spoken Word, from the mouth of a believing believer, is destined by God to be the most resourceful tool in a believer's arsenal.

By the Spoken Word, as spoken in Faith out of the mouth of a believing believer; mountains are moved, the sick are healed, the deaf hear, the blind see, the lame walk; and those who seek the LIGHT find HIM!

Position/Locate/Identify so _as_ to _enlarge/enhance_ _His_ _Wisdom; exhibiting_ the _enlarging/enhancing_ _wisely_.

Wisdom's purpose is to impart the essence of His **BE**-ing in the believer. Arrogance/Pride tends to cause one to become self-important; when, in fact, God Himself is the only important personage in all of history; now, then, and whenever!

Consent with actions affirming meaningful attitudes/viewpoints signifying to uphold every purpose of Truth revealed.

King Solomon declared himself to be the natural man who knew it all, had it all, and did it all.

He epitomized life as being *"under the sun"*, but knew nothing of true worship.

Essentially empty on the inside, Solomon focused his building on the external realm, but lacked any internal soundness.

Until you are fully convinced that God wants you to be well, there will always be a doubt in your mind as to whether or not you will be healed.

As long as there is that doubt in your mind, perfect faith cannot exist; and until faith is exercised, without doubt or wavering, you may never be healed.

SEMITIC~ARAMAIC~HEBRAIC THESAURUS

Aramaic before first {

Semitic Root before first =

Lettering for ParaPhrase after second =

(17:14) Heal^H7495 אָפֵּ{רַ=causing to heal}= Resh-practice beginning strength- Pey-mouth SpokenWord speak- Final-Aleph-ending finish maturity- me, O LORD, ^H3068 יְהֹוָה{הַוֹהֹ=the Self~Existent One}= Yud-purpose posture actions- Hey-character reveal grace- Vav-intensify degree counsel- Hey-character reveal grace- and I shall be healed;^H7495 אָפֵּ{רַ=causing to heal}= Resh-practice beginning strength- Pey-mouth SpokenWord speak- Final-Aleph-ending finish maturity- save^H3467 יַשַׁ{שַׁ=persevering to observe}= Ayin-pierce perceive wisdom- me, and I shall be saved:^H3467 יַשַׁ{שַׁ=reducing to inactivity}= Yud-purpose posture actions- Shin-pressure exchange disperse- Ayin-pierce perceive wisdom- for^H3588 כִּ{שַׁ=because}= Kaph-surrender making consent- Yud-purpose posture actions- thou^H859 אַתָּ{עַ=signifying His dominion/authority}=א Aleph-dominion ability confirm- Taw-evidence prove signify- Hey-character reveal grace- art my praise.^H8416 תְּהִלָּ{תַ=looking toward someone/something}=ת Lamed-instruct truth provide- Hey-character reveal grace- Taw-evidence prove signify- Hey-character reveal grace- Yud-purpose posture actions-

The Semitic Emphasis

causing to heal the Self~Existent One~~causing to heal persevering to observe reducing to inactivity because signifying His dominion/authority looking toward someone/something.

"Whom God hath set forth to be a propitiation through faith in His blood, to declare His righteousness for the remission of sins that are past, through the forbearance of God." ROMANS 3:25 KJV

"And He is the propitiation for our sins: and not for ours only, but also for the sins of the whole world." FIRST JOHN 2:2 KJV

Herein is love, not that we loved God, but that He loved us, and sent His Son to be the propitiation for our sins." FIRST JOHN 4:10 KJV

In other words, were it not for the Atonement, God would be unjust in justifying the lost.

Likewise He would be unjust in healing the sick without first redeeming them from the sickness.

The fact that God ever healed anyone is the best proof that healing was provided by the Atonement.

If healing was not provided for all in redemption, how did all in the multitude obtain from Christ the healing that God did not provide?

"He healed them all."

By The Indwelling Of Foundation/Support His Dominion Establishes His Prevail On Exchange Of Existence Practiced And Conforming To Every Proof

EZEKIEL 30:21

KJV+TVM

Son ^{H1121} of man ^{H120}, I have broken $^{H7665\,[H8804]}$ the arm ^{H2220} of Pharaoh ^{H6547} king ^{H4428} of Egypt ^{H4714}; and, lo, it shall not be bound up $^{H2280\,[H8795]}$ to be healed ^{H7499} $^{H5414\,[H8800]}$, to put $^{H7760\,[H8800]}$ a roller ^{H2848} to bind $^{H2280\,[H8800]}$ it, to make it strong $^{H2388\,[H8800]}$ to hold $^{H8610\,[H8800]}$ the sword ^{H2719}.

ORIGINAL THOUGHTS

...(30:21) By the Indwelling of Foundation/Support, His Dominion establishes His Prevail, in exchange of existence practiced and conforming to every proof. Each skill of His Strength directs the Wisdom of His Spoken Word beginning experiences that identify the revelation of His Imaginations, providing each desired encounter in pursuit of beginnings with purpose and prevail. Through every unseen purpose, there perpetuates/continues the revelations of Truth by His Counsels out of His Finished Work appropriating every persistent exchange of Peace proving the Grace of His Truths. The practice of His Spoken Word identifies the perfections of His Efforts, and reveals, through every adjusting, the intensities that fashion specific actions in evidence of His Counsel provided.

In Scripture, a broken arm = no protection or preparation.

<u>Knowing God's will concerning sickness provides the ground on which perfect faith can act</u>.

Got Healing?

Once people are fully convinced that God wants to heal them and that it is not God's will for them to be sick, they almost always receive healing when prayed for, if not before.

By the Indwelling of Foundation/Support, His Dominion establishes His Prevail, in exchange of existence practiced and conforming to every proof.

God announced Himself to be the healer of His people with these words: "*I am the Lord who heals you*".

He spoke those words to about three million people. Every one of them believed God's words were true.

The result: Every one of them who needed healing was made perfectly whole.

We are told: "*He (God) brought them forth and there was not one feeble person among their tribe*". PSALMS 105:37

Can you imagine three million people all well and strong?

Not one feeble, not one weak, and not one sick?

The major choice before us at every beginning involves one fact: *Do we believe God, and take Him at His Word, OR NOT?*

*If that was true in Israel, under the law, it is much **more true** for you and I, who under His GRACE, have been redeemed by the blood of God's Lamb and are living by His Faith, Mercy, and Truth.*

Each skill of His Strength directs the Wisdom of His Spoken Word beginning experiences that identify the revelation of His Imaginations, providing each desired encounter in pursuit of beginnings with purpose and prevail.

It is God's will for every individual to be well and strong~~*when His conditions are met and His word is believed.*

If there is a justified "*maybe*" in your case, then we are compelled to apply a "*maybe*" in every case, because God is no respecter of persons.

If God will heal anyone, He will heal you.

The tragedy is that these sicknesses and diseases affect the bodies of thousands of Christians, while preachers and teachers, influenced by theological traditions, often stand by with little more than words of sympathy and pity, assuring the sufferer that it must be God's will; that it will work out for the best; that God is teaching the patient some lesson in humility; that possibly it is God's chastisement; or that by it, the sick person is being drawn closer to Him who often works His will in our lives through sickness.

Christians need never be sick, any more than they need to be sinful.

It is always God's desire to heal you.

Through every unseen purpose, there perpetuates/continues the revelations of Truth by His Counsels out of His Finished Work appropriating every persistent exchange of Peace proving the Grace of His Truths.

The only reason those three million Israelites became well and strong was that they believed what God said: "*I am the Lord who heals you*".

That was said to them, and they believed it.

The only reason disease takes such a toll among Christians today is that many do not believe what God has spoken.

They know that God said, "*I am the Lord who heals you*".

Somehow they have failed to believe that He meant what He said, which is basically what the accuser said to Adam and Eve: "*God did not mean what he said*".

Influenced by tradition, people have changed God's "*I am*" to "*I was*".

The practice of His Spoken Word identifies the perfections of His Efforts, and reveals, through every adjusting, the intensities that fashion specific actions in evidence of His Counsel provided.

If, under the old covenant, three million of God's people could be well at one time, then how much more may God's people be well today who are living under the new covenant of mercy, grace, and truth, established on better promises, with a better priesthood, through a more excellent ministry.

SEMITIC~ARAMAIC~HEBRAIC THESAURUS

Aramaic before first {

Semitic Root before first =

Lettering for ParaPhrase after second =

...(30:21) Son^H1121 בֻ{לְ=the continuing of the house/dwelling}=בּ Beyt-pattern-thought indwelling existence- Final-Nun= foundation grace/truth remain- of man^H120 םדֻ{אֻ=the moving back and forth of the blood}=אֻ Aleph-dominion ability confirm- Dalet-faith establish presence- Final-Mem-weight fashions prevail- I have

broken^H7665 שבר{=breaking through}=שׁ Shin= pressure exchange disperse Beyt= [in/by] pattern-thought indwelling existence- Resh= practice beginning strength- ^H853 תאֻ{אֻ=plow~pointing furrows for sowing}=אֻ Aleph-dominion ability confirm- Taw-evidence prove signify- the arm^H2220 עורז{אֻ=the strength}=וֻ Zayin= skill after method Resh= practice beginning strength- Vav= [and] identity intensity counsel Ayin= experience perceive wisdom of Pharaoh^H6547 הערפ{=great house/dwelling~place}=פּ Pey= mouth SpokenWord speak Resh= practice beginning strength- Ayin= experience perceive wisdom Vav= [and] identity intensity counsel Hey= [the/His] character reveal foresee king^H4428 ךלמ{=reigning over}=מ Mem=

Got Healing?

[from/out of] image encounter remembered ⌐Lamed= [to/toward] instruct truth provide ⌐Kaph= surrender obtain desire of

Egypt; H4714 מִמִּצְרָיִם{ΛΥ☉ᴍ=limited mess}=מ Mem= [from/out of] image encounter remembered ⌐Tsad= pursuit journey anticipate ⌐Resh= practice beginning strength-ᴗYud= purpose possess actions ⌐Final-Mem= weight fashioning prevail and,

lo, H2009 הִנֵּה{ΥΧ=the one here!/look!}=ה Hey= [the/His] character reveal foresee ᴗYud= purpose possess actions ⌐Nun= perpetuate patience persist ⌐Hey= [the/His] character reveal foresee it shall not H3808 לֹא{☉Ʋ=without}=ל Lamed-instruct truth provide-ᴗVav-intensify degree counsel-⌐Final-Aleph-perfected finished matured be bound up H2280 חֲבֹשׁ{ᴗᴡᴥ=to wrap firmly/to rule over}=ח Hhet= specific appropriate beyond ᴗNun= perpetuate patience persist ᴡShin= pressure exchange disperse to be

healed, H5414 נָתַתָּ{†=removing}=נ Nun= perpetuate patience persist ⌐Taw= evidence prove signify ᴗFinal-Nun= foundation grace/truth remain H7499 רְפֻאָה{☉ᴖ=through headship with an open mouth}=ר Resh= practice beginning strength-ᴗPey= mouth SpokenWord speak ᴗVav= [and] identity intensity counsel ᴗFinal Aleph= perfected finished mature ⌐Hey= [the/His] character reveal foresee to

put H7760 שִׂים{ᴍᴥ=pressing through chaos unknown/thorny}=ס Samech= adjust apprehend resource ᴗVav= [and] identity intensity counsel ⌐Final-Mem= weight fashioning prevail a roller H2848 חִתּוּל{Ʋᴛ=to entwine/enwrap/to be involved}=ח Hhet= specific appropriate beyond ᴗYud= purpose possess actions ⌐Taw= evidence prove signify ᴗVav= [and] identity intensity counsel ⌐Lamed= [to/toward] instruct truth provide to bind H2280 חֲבֹשׁ{ᴗᴡᴥ=to wrap firmly/to rule over}=ח Hhet-specific appropriate beyond-ᴗBeyt-pattern thought existing-in-principle-ᴡShin-pressure exchange disperse-it, to make it

strong H2388 חֲזַק{☉ᴛ=grabbing hold of strongly to restrain/support}=ח Hhet-specific appropriate beyond-ᴗZayin- skill alter method-ᴗQuph-contrast parallel structure- to hold H8610 תָּפַשׂ{ᴥᴛ=taking hold by force, if necessary}=ת Taw-evidence prove signify-ᴗPey-mouth SpokenWord speak-ᴗSamech-adjust apprehend resource- the

sword. H2719 חֶרֶב{ᴍᴛ=to reduce to inactivity}=ח Hhet-specific appropriate beyond-ᴗResh-practice beginning strength-ᴗBeyt-pattern thought existing-in-principle-

The Semitic Emphasis

The continuing of the house/dwelling~~the moving back and forth of the blood breaking through plow~pointing furrows for sowing~~the strength of a great house/dwelling~place reigning over limited mess~~by the one here!/look!~~without to wrap firmly/to rule over removing through headship with an open mouth pressing through chaos unknown/thorny to entwine/enwrap/to be involved to wrap firmly/to rule over grabbing hold of strongly to restrain/support taking hold by force~if necessary to reduce to inactivity.

If the body were not included in redemption, how can there be a resurrection?

How can "corruption put on *incorruption*" or "*mortal* put on immortality"?

If we have not been redeemed from sickness, would we not be subject to disease in heaven, if it were possible to be resurrected irrespective of redemption?

Someone has well remarked, "*Man's future destiny being both spiritual and bodily, his redemption must be both spiritual and bodily.*"

Why should not the "last Adam" take away all that the "first Adam" brought upon us?

Consider then, a few parallels:

The Inward Man   **The Outer Man**

Got Healing?

Adam, by his fall, brought Selfish~Independent~Nature into our souls and minds...

Selfish~Independent~Nature is therefore, the work of a selfish will or choice...

Jesus was "*manifested*" to reduce to inactivity the works of dis~ease, in the soul/mind by providing REST IN HIM!

He was made "sin for us" SECOND CORINTHIANS 5: 21 KJV when He "bare our sins, in His own body" FIRST PETER 2: 24 KJV

"*For ye are bought with a price: therefore glorify God glorify God in your~~~spirit*" FIRST CORIN~ THIANS 6: 20 KJV

The spirit is bought with a price.

Adam, by his fall, brought a dis~ease into our bodies...

Dis~ease is therefore the offspring or product of selfish thoughts...

Jesus was "*manifested*" to reduce to inactivity the works of dis~ease, in the body by providing REST IN HIM!

He was "*made a curse FOR us*" GALATIANS 3:13 when He "*bare our sicknesses*" MATTHEW 8:17

"*For ye are bought with a price: therefore in your body*" FIRST CORINTHIANS 6: 20 KJV

The body is bought with a price.

If these things be true, and they are; it is because the Bible says so.

If the Bible says such things are so, then we must be just as sure of receiving healing in our being and in our body, as in comparison to when we knelt at an altar and were made sure of His Salvation on our behalf!

These views are not new, and certainly they are not isolated to only a few in the Body of Christ!

The atoning death of Jesus Christ secured for us not only physical healing, but the resurrection, perfecting and glorifying of our bodies as well.

The Gospel of Christ declares as available, salvation for the body as well as for the soul.

Just as one gets the first-fruits of their spiritual salvation in the life that now is, so we get the first-fruits of our physical salvation in the life that now is.

Individual believers, whether Elders or not, have the privilege and the duty to "*pray one for another*" in case of sickness/anxieties, with the expectation that God will hear and heal.

Enabling His Evidence To Confirm Signifies His Truth Through Every Degree Of His Finished Work

EZEKIEL 34:4
KJV+SM

(H853) The diseased[H2470] have ye not[H3808] strengthened,[H2388] neither[H3808] have ye healed[H7495] that which was sick,[H2470] neither[H3808] have ye bound up[H2280] that which was broken,[H7665] neither[H3808] have ye brought again[H7725] that which was driven away,[H5080] neither[H3808] have ye sought[H1245] that which was lost;[H6] but with force[H2394] and with cruelty[H6531] have ye ruled[H7287] them.

ORIGINAL THOUGHTS

...(34:4) Enabling His Evidence to confirm signifies His Truth through every degree of His Finished Work. The unseen skillfulness of each parallel is in the Truth of His Counsel finished from each beginning of His Spoken Word perfected. With specifics acquired, reveal the Truth of His Counsel effecting the determining of His Pattern~of~Thought exchanging each pressure fo the essence of His Strength. Learning each decree of His Finished Work exchanges the increase of His Pattern~Thought within His Faith to determine the Truths of every portion of His Finished Work. In the pattern of each parallel, enlarge the abilities of abiding in His Strength, and share the methods of building every quality of His Grace. His Spoken Word practices allowing the beginnings of His Faith in disclosure.

Enabling His Evidence to confirm signifies His Truth through every degree of His Finished Work.

Healing is a parallel of His Finished Work.

While His Finished Work is the epitome of all that HE IS, Healing define the aspect of His Creation living in the full freedom of His Fullness.

Anything that hinders such a wondrous condition cannot be from HIM Who gives us the very best of ALL THAT HE IS!

"Who hath believed our report? and to whom is the arm of the LORD revealed?" ISAIAH 53:1 KJV

"That the saying of Esaias the prophet might be fulfilled, which he spake, Lord, who hath believed our report? and to whom hath the arm of the Lord been revealed?" JOHN 12:38 KJV

"But they have not all obeyed the gospel. For Esaias saith, Lord, who hath *believed our report?"* ROMANS 10:16 KJV

Believing the WORD OF GOD is the same as believing the Report of The Lord!

How is it that we cannot, or we refuse to see such simplicities?

The unseen skillfulness of each parallel is in the Truth of His Counsel finished from each beginning of His Spoken Word perfected.

The perfecting of His Spoken Word is when the Spirit utters His Person and Presence, through the Power of His Spoken Word to our heart and mind!

When the Spirit discloses the hidden secrets that ages have passed over, missing the primary design of God's Eternal Plan, this makes cause for those who hear Her Voice, to shout from the housetops the joy of His Decree.

Isaiah begins the redemption chapter with the question, *"Who hath believed our report? and to whom is the arm of the Lord revealed?"* ISAIAH 53: 1 KJV

And the report follows that He bore our sins and sicknesses.

The answer to the question is, only those who have **heard the report** could believe it, because *"faith cometh by hearing."*

Since Jesus died to save and to heal, it is surely worth reporting.

With specifics acquired, reveal the Truth of His Counsel effecting the determining of His Pattern~of~Thought exchanging each pressure fo the essence of His Strength.

The greatest barrier to the faith of many seeking bodily healing in our day *is the uncertainty in their minds* as to it being the will of God to heal all.

Nearly everyone knows that God does heal some, but there is much in modern theology that keeps people from knowing what the Bible clearly teaches~~that *healing is provided for all.*

It is impossible to boldly claim, by faith, a blessing that we are not sure God offers.

The power of God can be claimed only where the will of God is known.

Learning each decree of His Finished Work exchanges the increase of His Pattern~Thought within His Faith to determine the Truths of every portion of His Finished Work.

It would be next to impossible to get a sinner to "believe unto righteousness" before you had fully convinced him that it was God's will to save him.

Faith begins where the will of God is known.

If it is God's will to heal only some of those who need healing, then none have any basis for faith unless they have a special revelation that they are among the favored ones.

Faith must rest on the will of God alone, not on our desires or wishes.

Appropriating faith does not believe that God can, **BUT THAT GOD WILL!**

Because of not knowing it to be a redemptive privilege for all, most of those in our day, when seeking healing, _add to their petition the phrase_, "If it be Thy will."

In the pattern of each parallel, enlarge the abilities of abiding in His Strength, and share the methods of building every quality of His Grace.

Among all those who sought healing from Christ during His earthly ministry, we read of only one who had this kind of theology.

This was the leper, who said, "_Lord, if Thou wilt, Thou canst make me clean._"

The first thing Christ did was to correct his theology by saying, "_I will, be thou clean._"

Christ's "_I will_" cancelled his "_if._"

This added to his faith that Christ could heal him, the fact that He would.

If when a believer prays for another, and the healing does not immediately appear, do not be shy when casting down words of imagination.

If Jesus said, I BELIEVE IT; His Word cannot lie! NUMBERS 23:19 KJV

His Spoken Word practices allowing the beginnings of His Faith in disclosure.

The word testament, legally speaking, means a person's will.

The Bible contains God's last will and testament, in which He bequeaths to us all the blessings of redemption.

Since it is His "_last will and testament,_" anything later is a forgery.

A man never writes a new will after he is dead.

If healing is in God's will for us, then to say that the age of miracles is past is virtually saying what is the opposite of the truth, that a will is no good after the death of the testator.

Jesus is not only the testator, who died; He was resurrected and is also the Mediator of the will. He is our lawyer, so to speak.

He will not cheat us out of the will, as some earthly lawyers do.

He is our Representative at the right hand of God.

SEMITIC~ARAMAIC~HEBRAIC THESAURUS

Aramaic before first {
Semitic Root before first =
Lettering for ParaPhrase after second =

...(34:4) [H853] אֶת־ {צֲלע} =plow~pointing furrows for sowing} Aleph-dominion ability confirm- Taw-evidence prove signify- **The diseased** [H2470] { חֶ=the profane/common} = Aleph-authority ability confirm- Taw-evidence prove sign- **have ye not** [H3808] {ולא =without} = Lamed-instruct truth provide- Vav-intensify degree counsel- Final-Aleph-perfected finished matured- **strengthened,** [H2388] { חזק =strongly grabbing hold to restrain/support} = Hhet-specific share beyond- Zayin-skill alter instrument- Quph-contrast parallel structure- **neither** [H3808] {ולא =without} = Lamed-instruct truth provide- Vav- intensify degree counsel- Final-Aleph-perfected finished matured- **have ye healed** [H7495] {רפא =causing to heal} = Resh- practice beginning strength- Pey-mouth SpokenWord speak- Final-Aleph-ending finish maturity- *that which was* **sick** [H2470] {חֶ=the profane/common} = Hhet-specific share beyond- Lamed[to/toward]-instruct acquire provide- Hey[behold/the]-quality reveal grace- **neither** [H3808] {ולא =without} = Lamed-instruct truth provide- Vav-intensify degree counsel- Final-Aleph-perfected finished matured- **have ye bound up** [H2280] {חבשתם =wrapping firmly/govern- ing/restraining} = Hhet-specific share beyond- Beyt[within/in/inside]-pattern thought inhabit- Shin-pressure exchange disperse- *that which was broken,* [H7665] {שבר =braking through} = Shin-pressure exchange disperse- Beyt[within/in/inside]-pattern thought inhabit- Resh-process beginning strength- **neither** [H3808] {ולא =without} = Lamed-instruct truth provide- Vav-intensify degree counsel- Final-Aleph-perfected finished matured- **have ye brought again** [H7725] {שוב =pressing the dwelling~place} = Shin-pressure exchange disperse- Vav-[and/in addition]increase degree assure- Beyt[within/in/inside]-pattern thought inhabit- *that which was driven away* [H5080] {חדח =compelling/withdrawing} = Beyt[within/in/inside]-pattern thought inhabit- Dalet-faith establish presence- Hhet-specific share beyond- **neither** [H3808] {ולא =without} = Lamed-instruct truth provide- Vav-intensify degree counsel- Final-Aleph-perfected finished matured- **have ye sought** [H1245] {בקש =searching for something/someone} = Beyt[within/in/inside]-pattern thought inhabit- Quph-contrast parallel structure- Shin-pressure exchange disperse- *that which was lost,* [H6] {אבד =the door/opening to the dwelling~place/house} = Aleph-authority ability confirm- Beyt[within/in/inside]-pattern thought inhabit- Resh-process beginning strength- **but with force** [H2394] {חזקה =strongly grabbing holding to restrain/support} = Hhet-specific share beyond- Zayin-skill alter instrument- Quph-contrast parallel structure- Hey[behold/the]-quality reveal grace- **and with cruelty** [H6531] {פרך =breaking apart} = Pey-mouth SpokenWord speak- Resh-process beginning strength- Final-Kaph acknowledge offer allow- **have ye ruled** [H7287] {רדה =headship through the opening} = Resh-process beginning strength- Dalet-faith establish presence- Hey[behold/the]-quality reveal grace- **them.**

The Semitic Emphasis

Plow~Pointing furrows for sowing the profane/common without strongly grabbing hold to restrain/support without causing to heal the profane/common without wrapping firmly/gov- erning/restraining braking through without pressing the dwelling~place compelling/withdrawing without searching for something/someone the door/opening to the dwelling~place/house strongly grabbing holding to restrain/support breaking apart headship through the opening.

It is our aim to show that the Atonement of Christ lays the foundation equally for deliverance from sin and for deliverance from disease.

That complete provision has been made for both; that in the exercise of faith under the conditions prescribed, we have the same reason to believe that the body may be delivered from sickness; that we have that the soul shall be delivered from sin; in short; that both branches of the deliverance stand on the same ground; and that it is necessary to include both in any true conception of what the Gospel offers to mankind.

The atoning sacrifice of Christ covers the physical as well as the spiritual needs of the race.

Healing of the body is NOT, therefore, a "*side-issue*," as some represent it.

It is no more this than the healing of the soul is a "*side-issue.*"

They are both but parts of the same Gospel, based equally upon the same great Atonement.

The healing of the body is an essential element of the Gospel, and must be preached and practiced.

God wills our health, that the Church, the "*Body of Christ*," has the same commission and the same power as "*The Head.*"

We, *as The Body of Christ* , with this true conception of God as Creative Love, must now give a suffering world this full Gospel of salvation from *Selfish~Independent~Nature* and its inevitable consequences.

He who waives away the healing power of Christ as belonging only to the New Testament times is not preaching the whole Gospel.

God was, and is, the Savior of the body as well as the soul.

By The Dominion Of Re~Natured Truth,
Reveal His Truth In The Grace
That Teaches Transcending Qualities
In Purpose Of Pursuing His Finished Work

Ezekiel 47:8
KJV+TVM

Then said[H559] [H8799] he unto me, These waters[H4325] issue out[H3318] [H8802] toward the east[H6930] country[H1552], and go down[H3381] [H8804] into the desert[H6160], and go[H935] [H8804] into the sea[H3220]: which being brought forth[H3318] [H8716] into the sea[H3220], the waters[H4325] shall be healed[H7495] [H8738]

Got Healing?

ORIGINAL THOUGHTS
...(47:8) By the Dominion of Re~natured Truth, reveal His Truth in the Grace that teaches transcending qualities in purpose of pursuing His Finished Work. Behold the quality of His Truth in contrast to His Faith transforming every portion of any issue perceived as teaching the experience of His Strength inhabiting His Grace. Within every addition finished, His Actions fashion every purpose through each journey maturing in His Perfection, revealing the Truth of His memory, and revealing the practices of His Spoken Word finishing each effort.

By the Dominion of Re~natured Truth, reveal His Truth in the Grace that teaches transcending qualities in purpose of pursuing His Finished Work.

Let yourself be silently drawn by the stronger pull of WHO you really love.

In the instance of our first breath, we are permeated with the single greatest force in the universe~~*the power of the Living God, Who translates the possibilities of our minds into the reality of our world by the strength and presence of His* .

To fully awaken our power, however, requires a subtle change in the way we think of ourselves in life, if you will, as a shift in our belief.

Just the way sound creates visible waves as it travels through a droplet of water, our *"belief waves"* ripple through the quantum fabric of the universe to become our bodies and the healing, abundance, and peace~~or disease, lack, and suffering~~that we experience in life.

And just the way we can tune a sound to change its patterns, we can tune our beliefs to preserve or destroy all that we cherish, including life itself.

Behold the quality of His Truth in contrast to His Faith transforming every portion of any issue perceived as teaching the experience of His Strength inhabiting His Grace.

In a malleable world, where everything from atoms to cells is changing to match our beliefs, we are limited only by the way we think of ourselves in that world.

Our acceptance of such an awesome power, knowing that we are never more than a belief away from our greatest LOVE, DEEPEST HEALING, and MOST PROFOUND MIRACLES, becomes a redeeming experience setting us free from those bondages that keep us less than whole!

Got Healing?

Within every addition finished, His Actions fashion every purpose through each journey maturing in His Perfection, revealing the Truth of His memory, and revealing the practices of His Spoken Word finishing each effort.

From the healing of disease, to the length of our lives, to the success of our careers and relationships, everything that we experience as *"life"* is directly linked to what we believe.

To change our lives and relationships, heal our bodies, and bring peace to our families and nations~~requires a simple yet precise shift in the way we use belief.

For those who accept what science has led us to believe for the last 300 years, even to consider that our inner experience can affect reality is nothing short of heresy.

The very idea blurs the safety zone that has traditionally separated science and spirituality~~and us~~from our world.

Rather than thinking of ourselves as *passive victims* in a place where, for example, things just *happen for no apparent reason*, such a consideration now places us squarely in the driver's seat of life.

In this position, we find ourselves faced with undeniable evidence confirming that we are the creators of our realities.

With this confirmation, we also see that we have the power to make disease obsolete and relegate war to a memory of our past.

Suddenly, the key to catapulting our greatest dreams into reality is within our reach.

The focus of our intentions changes reality itself and suggests that we live in an interactive universe; especially the universe that resides within our being/existence.

SEMITIC~ARAMAIC~HEBRAIC THESAURUS
Aramaic before first {
Semitic Root before first =
Lettering for ParaPhrase after second =

...(47:8), Then said[H559] אמר{ɯ ⴸ =carefully wrapped}=א Aleph-dominion ability confirm- Mem-renature challenge
remembered-Lamed-instruct truth provide- he unto[H413] אל{ɯ ⴸ =as looking toward something/some-one}=ה Hey-
fragrance reveal grace-Lamed-instruct truth provide- me, These[H428] אלה{ɯ ⴸ =being removed far away}=ה Hey[behold/the]-
quality reveal grace-Lamed[to/toward]-instruct acquire provide- waters[H4325] =working with unknown
chaos}=מ Mem[from/out of]-transform encounter remembrance- Hey[behold/the]-quality reveal grace- issue
out[H3318] יצא{ע =that comes out from}= Yud-purpose posture actions- Tsad-pursuit journey anticipate- Final-Aleph-ending
finish maturity- toward[H413] אל{ɯ ⴸ =being removed far away}=ה Hey[behold/the]-quality reveal grace-Lamed-instruct truth
provide- the east[H6930] קדמן{ɯ ⴸ =coming before in time/preceding}=ק Quph-contrast parallel structure- Dalet-

Got Healing?

faith establish presence-מ Mem[from/out of]-transform encounter remembrance-ו Vav-[and/in addition]increase degree assure-ן Final-Nun-issue perseverance progress-**country** H1552 הלילה{וּלָ=the door}=ג Gimal-experience understanding encounter-ל Lamed[to/toward]-instruct acquire provide-י Yud-purpose posture actions-ל Lamed[to/toward]-instruct acquire provide-ה Hey[behold/the]-quality reveal grace-**and go down** H3381 דרי{חָא=the man entering}=ד Dalet-faith establish presence-ה Yud-purpose posture actions-ר Resh-process beginning strength-**into the** H5921 עֶל{סֵצ=experience knowing}=ע Ayin-pierce perceive wisdom-ל Lamed-instruct truth provide-**the desert** H6160 עֲרָבָה{תָא=the decree/judgment}=ג Gimal-experience understanding encounter-ר Resh-process beginning strength-ב Beyt[within/in/inside]-pattern thought inhabit-ה Hey[behold/the]-quality reveal grace-**and go into** H935 בוֹא{עָא=entering}=ב Beyt[within/in/inside]-pattern thought inhabit-ו Vav-[and/in addition]increase degree assure-א Final-Aleph-ending finish maturity-**the sea:** H3220 יָם{=working with unknown chaos}=י Yud-purpose posture actions-ם Final-Mem-trial fashions prevail-**which being brought forth** H3318 יָצָא{ץא=that comes out from}=י Yud-purpose posture actions-צ Tsad-pursuit journey anticipate-א Final-Aleph-ending finish maturity-**into** H413 אֶל{לֶא=being removed far away}=ה Hey-fragrance reveal grace-ל Lamed-instruct truth provide-**the sea** H3220 **the waters** H4325 מימֵיהֶ{חמ=working with unknown chaos}=מ Mem[from/out of]-transform encounter remembrance-י Hey[behold/the]-quality reveal grace-**shall be healed** H7495 רפֵא{פֵר=causing to heal}=ר Resh-practice beginning strength-פ Pey-mouth SpokenWord speak-א Final-Aleph-ending finish maturity-

The Semitic Emphasis

<u>Carefully wrapped as looking toward something/someone being removed far away working with unknown chaos that comes out from being removed far away coming before in time/preceding the door the man entering experience knowing the decree/judgment entering working with unknown chaos that comes out from being removed far away working with unknown chaos causing to heal.</u>

Is it any wonder we often feel powerless to help loved ones and even ourselves in facing the turmoil and upsets of life?

Is it at all surprising that we frequently feel just as helpless, when our world changes so fast that we describe the calamities, and in justices of our day as though our lives are *"falling apart at the seams"*?

Suddenly, it seems that everything from personal potentials and restrictions to our realities, publically, as well as privately, are *"up~for~grabs"*?

It's as if the conditions of living appear to force us into new borderlines of awareness itself, driving us~~making us to rediscover/reinvent who we are *"in order just to survive what we haven't even created around us?"*

Healing is another part of who we are, and it is more often than not created in the manner through we belief or don't belief, embrace or deny, step toward or shrink back from!

Healing is not a new frontier, as some would call it; but it is a parallel of every human~being's livelihood that sooner or later will not be skirted as having or not!

We do not need to have physicians, doctors and the like telling us that WE CONTROL what we are, and how we look, and how we behave~~good or bad~~right or wrong.

Got Healing?

We need to return to the Creator of our making, giving God the place upon the throne of our heart, to <u>guide</u> and <u>direct</u> the controls of our living.

The Quality Of His Purpose
Reveals The Consent/Agreement With
Each Portion/Degree Of His Instruction

<u>EZEKIEL 47:9</u>
KJV+TVM

And it shall come to pass[H1961] that every[H3605] thing[H5315] that liveth[H2416] which[H834] moveth[H8317] whithersoever[H413 H3605 H834 H8033] the rivers[H5158] shall come[H935] shall live[H2421] and there shall be[H1961] a very[H3966] great[H7227] multitude of fish[H1710] because[H3588] these[H428] waters[H4325] shall come[H935] thither[H8033] for they shall be healed[H7495] and every thing[H3605] shall live[H2416] whither[H834 H8033] the river[H5158] cometh[H935]

ORIGINAL THOUGHTS

...(47:9) The quality of His Purpose reveals the consent/agreement with each portion/degree of His Instruction. The Seed of His Spoken Word enlarges the specifics of single~mindedness confirming each exchange of beginning for the next exchange of process out of purpose. The Fragrance of His Truth offers the increase of His Promise and conforms every compelling prevail to continue sharing His Teachings. His Pattern~of~Thought increases maturity that determines actions revealing the Grace of His Truth, while positioning to behold the transcending enabling/empowering each degree of His Faith. In each platform of His Dominion add the Confidence/Trust of His Faith experiencing the revelation of agreement, while single~mindedly beholding the teaching that transforms the Grace of His Truth inhabiting the addition of His Finished Work. Compelling Prevail practices the Spoken Word of His Finished Work, obtaining every assurance provided. Beyond the single~mindedness of His Dominion, exchanges through every process the seeding of the unseen providing the Pattern~of~His~Thoughts in addition to His Finished Work.

<u>The quality of His Purpose reveals the consent/agreement with each portion/degree of His Instruction.</u>

In everything said so far, we need to ask ourselves one soulful, insightful question: <u>Why would God want to heal us</u>?

Simple Answer: Because He LOVES US!

Such thoughts tells us the TRUTH of our convictions.

<u>Thinking</u> that He loves us gets us in the door, but how do we proceed in

scooching~up~to~the~table and partake of what He offers?

I continue practicing what got me here in the first place!

Realizing that questions are not the answer, but the solution can always be found in HIM; now THIS is the solution necessary in every parallel we see.

The Seed of His Spoken Word enlarges the specifics of single~mindedness confirming each exchange of beginning for the next exchange of process out of purpose.

The hard~won experiences of Healing should not be sacrificed to the pre~packaged definitions handed to us by those who fail at searching out every nugget for its individual value.

To settle for less than the Father God offers is the complacent shame of those who tire of each day's journey.

Yet, we must realize that each day's journey is but one moment closer to the eternal riches He has stored up for those who walk uprightly with a determined course of living in pursuit of HIM!

Each journey, beloved, is the continuance of an eternal existence IN HIM!

The Fragrance of His Truth offers the increase of His Promise and conforms every compelling prevail to continue sharing His Teachings.

The pure sweetness of His Smell invites and invigorates the soul to search farther, deeper, stronger into the folds and parallels of His Eternality!

If we agree the answers/solutions are only found in HIM, then why would we seek elsewhere for Who it is that we have right in ourselves?

Sometimes we use the word, *"healing or health"* in relation to *'dis~ease'*, sometimes in relation to *'ill~ness'*, and sometimes in relation to *'sick~ness'*.

Such use is ambiguous in response to the Word of God telling us the TRUTH!

His Pattern~of~Thought increases maturity that determines actions revealing the Grace of His Truth, while positioning to behold the transcending enabling/empowering each degree of His Faith.

When we proceed to uncover and discover more of HIM in us, we open doors yet unlocked because of being *"faint~at~heart"*!

Such action, or the lack thereof, offers no solution, and we blame our inconsistencies on His apparent lack of action on our behalf; when in reality, it is our LACK OF ACTION in discovering the fullness of His BE~ing!

Thinking the way He thinks leads us to but one road, and that is the same highway upon which the sick, the halt, the lame, the blind, the mute find the salvation for their souls.

"*Healing and Health*" must become about the restoration of appropriate functional wholeness to the organism of our soul, before it will ever manifest in the organism of our body!

In each platform of His Dominion add the Confidence/Trust of His Faith experiencing the revelation of agreement, while single~mindedly beholding the teaching that transforms the Grace of His Truth inhabiting the addition of His Finished Work.

By the platform of "*dis~ease*", we discover that the unsettle commitments of our FAITH IN HIS FAITH is a matter of the lack of our TRUST IN HIM!

By the platform of "*ill-ness*", we reveal to ourselves that the subjective perceiving of disorder in our living must be corrected out of our kneeling before Him in prayer, in agreement, and in action.

"*Healing*" then becomes the restoration of a person's sense of their own well-being.

By the platform of "*sick~ness*", we can mean a socially defined deviation from what is scripturally acceptable, or even tolerable.

Thusly, "*Healing and Health*" can be broad term, with apparent fuzzy edges.

However, the closer we are drawn to the Father, through the Word/Son, by the influence of the Spirit, the greater will be the finished product of a day~to~day relationship established FIRST upon one's surrender to the Creator of All!

Compelling Prevail practices the Spoken Word of His Finished Work, obtaining every assurance provided.

God's sheep may wander out of the fold for a time, but His Sheep KNOW His Voice; and they always return to the flock He places them in.

Whether we see what it is we think we need to see or not; there is no

God like our God; He will perform what others cannot!

If we say, *"what if we pray, and the healing does not come?"*; we pervade the atmosphere of our thinking with doubts that will sap Faith right out of you!

If we turn on an electric light and it fails to shine, we would not say, *"There is no electricity!"*

We would say, *"There is something wrong with this lamp."*

Being knowledgeable of always seeking from the simplest position FIRST, we must always then, seek His Kingdom and Righteousness from the outset of our query!

Beyond the single~mindedness of His Dominion, exchanges through every process the seeding of the unseen providing the Pattern~of~His~Thoughts in addition to His Finished Work.

Let us understand, then that if our experiment fails it is not due to a lack in God, but to a natural and understandable lack in ourselves.

What scientist would be discouraged if their first experiment failed?

Since we intend with His help to allow Him to heal our shortcomings, to repair our wiring, we need not fear to test His power by prayer.

SEMITIC~ARAMAIC~HEBRAIC THESAURUS

Aramaic before first {

Semitic Root before first =

Lettering for ParaPhrase after second =

(47:9) And it shall come to pass {=existing/having breath} =Hey[behold/the]-quality reveal grace-Yud purpose posture actions-Hey[behold/the]-quality reveal grace-*that every* {=the whole reason for this is} =Kaph-surrender obtains consent-Vav-[and/in addition]increase degree assure-Lamed[to/toward]-instruct acquire provide-*thing* {=The whole of a person/the body, breath and mind} =Nun-seed patience continue-Pey-mouth SpokenWord speak-Shin-pressure exchange disperse-*that liveth* {=a raw state/condition/fresh flowing/undiluted} =Hhet-specific share beyond-Yud-purpose single~mindedness actions-*which* {=pressing each beginning} =Aleph-authority ability confirm-Shin-pressure exchange disperse-Resh-process beginning strength-*moveth* {=increased in abundance} =Shin-pressure exchange disperse-Resh-process beginning strength-Yud-purpose single~mindedness actions-*whithersoever* [discovering/exposing truth] {=looking toward something} =Hey-fragrance reveal grace-Lamed-instruct truth provide-{=the whole reason for this is} =Kaph-surrender obtains consent-Vav-[and/in addition]increase degree assure-Lamed[to/toward]-instruct acquire provide-*beginning* {=pressing each beginning} =Aleph-authority ability confirm-Shin-pressure exchange disperse-Resh-process beginning strength-*fashions prevail* {=wind/breath/character of someone/something} =Shin-pressure exchange disperse-Final-Mem-trial beyond-*the rivers* {=to inherit/occupy/distribute} =Nun-seed patience continue-Hhet-specific share beyond-Lamed[to/toward]-instruct acquire provide-*shall come* {=filling an empty space} =Beyt[within/inside]-pattern thought inhabit-Vav-[and/in addition]increase degree assure-Final-Aleph-ending finish maturity-*shall live* {=a raw state/condition/fresh flowing/undiluted} =Hhet-specific share beyond-Yud-purpose single~mindedness actions-*and there shall be* {=existing or having breath} =Hey[behold/the]-quality reveal grace-Hey[behold/the]-

quality   reveal   grace-Yud-purpose   posture   actions-Hey[behold/the]-quality   reveal   grace-*a*

very H3966 צ{ע ◌◌}=enveloping}= מ Mem[from/out of]-transform encounter remembrance-Aleph-authority ability confirm-Vav- [and/in addition]increase degree assure-Dalet-faith establish presence- **great** H7227 {ע ◌◌}=enveloping}= מ Mem[from/out of]- transform encounter remembrance-Aleph-authority ability confirm-Vav-[and/in addition]increase degree assure-Dalet-faith establish presence-

multitude of fish H1710 {◌◌ ◌}=great concern}= Dalet-faith establish presence-Gimal-experience understanding encounter- Hey[behold/the]-quality reveal {grace}= **because** H3588 {◌ש}=because of}= Kaph-surrender obtains consent-Yud-purpose single~mindedness actions- **these** H428 {◌ת}=looking toward something/some-one}= Hey[behold/the]-quality reveal grace- Lamed[to/toward]-instruct acquire provide- **waters** H4325 {◌◌}= working with unknown chaos}= Mem[from/out of]- transform encounter remembrance-Hey[behold/the]-quality reveal grace- **shall come** H935 {◌◌}=filling an empty space}= Beyt[within/inside]-pattern thought inhabit-Vav-[and/in addition]increase degree assure-Final-Aleph-ending finish maturity- **thither** H8033 {◌◌}=with wind/breath/character of someone/something}= ש Shin-pressure exchange disperse- Final-Mem-trial fashions prevail- **for they shall be healed** H7495 {◌◌}=causing to heal}= Resh-practice beginning strength-Pey-mouth SpokenWord speak-Final-Aleph-ending finish maturity- **and every thing** H3605 {◌◌}=the whole reason for this is}= Kaph-surrender obtains consent-Vav-[and/in addition]increase degree assure-Lamed[to/toward]-instruct acquire provide- **shall live** H2416 {◌◌}=a raw state/condition/fresh flowing/undiluted}= Hhet-specific share beyond-Yud-purpose single~mindedness actions- **whither** H834 {◌◌}= pressing each beginning}= Aleph-authority ability confirm-Shin-pressure exchange disperse-Resh-process beginning strength- H8033 **the river** H5158 {◌◌}=to inherit/occupy/distribute}= Nun- seed patience continue-Hhet-specific share beyond-Lamed[to/toward]-instruct acquire provide- **cometh.** H935 {◌◌}=filling an empty space}= Beyt[within/inside]-pattern thought inhabit-Vav-[and/in addition]increase degree assure-Final-Aleph-ending finish maturity-

The Semitic Emphasis

Existing/having breath~~the whole reason for this is the whole of a person/the body, breath and mind~~a raw state/condition/fresh flowing/undiluted pressing each beginning increased in abundance looking toward something~~the whole reason for this is pressing each beginning wind/breath/character of someone/something to inherit/occupy/distribute filling an empty space~~a raw state/condition/fresh flowing/undiluted existing/ having breath enveloping~~enveloping great concern because of looking toward something/someone working with unknown chaos filling an empty space with wind/breath/character of someone/something causing to heal~~the whole reason for this is a raw state/condition/fresh flowing/undiluted pressing each beginning to inherit/occupy/distribute filling an empty space.

Existing/having breath conveys the thought of God's LIFE being exchanged in one's living after HIM.

Life is never about anyone else but HIM.

Our living is increased, enlarged, and enhanced~~when such living seeks the strategies of His Eternal Wisdom.

What is it that we miss, when we do not understand the volume of Wisdom He contains in Himself?

How is it that humanity is so full of themselves, when history glaringly discounts any thought of their being wise!

The whole reason for this is the whole of a person/the body, breath and mind, explains the workings of the inner being through the inward being having expression through the outward being of one's existence.

Once the heart embraces His Eternal Existence as being within our own, giving us the animation of living in this dimension; there is realized the beginnings of His Majesty that awaits our examining, investigating, and embracing all that is HIM!

_A_ _raw_ _state/condition/fresh_ _flowing/undiluted_ _pressing_ _each_ _beginning_ _increased_ _in_ _abundance_ _looking_ _toward_ _something,_ describes the unabashed/bold appearing of one's realizing that they are now, and forever have been, a child of the Almighty.

He is more than just Lord, more than just a King.

He is the Almighty; the Creator of all that we survey, throughout our living then, here, now, and there!

The _whole_ _reason_ _for_ _this_ _is_ _pressing_ _each_ _beginning_ _wind/breath/character_ _of_ _someone/something_ _to_ _inherit/occupy/distribute_ _filling_ _an_ _empty_ _space_; explaining the why and wherefore regarding each beginning discovered.

How strange it is that people who fear to do this do not hesitate to pray for the most difficult objectives of all, such as the peace of the world or the salvation of their souls!

If they have so little confidence in prayer that they do not dare to test their powers of contacting God by praying for an easy thing, it is probable that their cosmic intercessions are of little force.

If everyone who prayed for the peace of the world had enough prayer power to accomplish the healing of a head cold, this would be a different world within twenty-four hours.

_A_ _raw_ _state/condition/fresh_ _flowing/undiluted_ _existing/having_ _breath_ _enveloping,_ regards a person's acumen over accepting God's instructions in these matters, or not!

Let us not be afraid, then, to choose for a prayer-experiment an objective that is simple and personal.

This objective must of course be in accordance with God's will, for it is as difficult to make God's power operate contrary to His will, as it is to make water flow uphill.

A wise engineer studies the laws of flowing water, and builds his water system in accordance with those laws.

A wise scientist studies the laws of nature and adapts his experiments to those laws.

And a wise seeker after God studies the laws of God and adapt their prayers to those boundaries imposed by the Creator of ALL.

Got Healing?

Enveloping great concern because of looking toward something/someone working with unknown chaos filling an empty space with wind/breath/character of someone/something causing to heal; emanates the characteristics of God through an open forum that allows us to learn, as well as to experience the healing we seek.

There is no great mystery concerning the will of God, in so far as it applies to ourselves.

God's will is written into His nature, as well as written into the nature of His BE~ing within our own heart and mind; and the nature of God is love!

Therefore, when we pray in accordance with the law of love, we are praying in accordance with the will of God.

The whole reason for this is a raw state/condition/fresh flowing/undiluted pressing each beginning to inherit/occupy/distribute filling an empty space.

The simplest and most direct of all prayer-projects is the healing of the body.

The body is indeed a laboratory exquisitely adapted to the working out of the power of God.

And healing by many forms of prayer or faith is as natural and as instinctive as breathing.

It has been practiced, with or without understanding, by people of every age.

It is as old as history and as modern as computers of today.

Almost everyone in times of great stress cries out to someone—to something—even if they do so only by a blind, instinctive urge, while denying their own impulse immediately afterwards.

Much of this clamoring to Deity has failed to produce results.

Therefore a great many Christians, unwilling to believe that God *cannot* heal them, *have persuaded themselves that He will not.*

In so doing, they forget both the example and the words of Jesus Christ.

He told us that God is a loving Father, who delights to give good gifts to His children. *LUKE 11 KJV*

The Pattern~Thought Of Pursuit
Qualifies The Experience

Outlining His Finished Work

EZEKIEL 47:11
KJV+TVM

But the miry places[H1207] *thereof and the marishes*[H1360] *thereof shall not be healed*[H7495] *[H8735]; they shall be given*[H5414] *[H8738] to salt*[H4417].

ORIGINAL THOUGHTS
...(47:11)

The Pattern~Thought of pursuit qualifies the experience outlining His Finished Work.

The PATTERN for God's Will is outlined in a familiar passage that has been misdirected for so many years, by so many.

LUKE 4:18-19 KJV

The Spirit of the Lord is upon me, because He hath anointed me to preach the gospel to the poor; He hath sent me to heal the brokenhearted, To preach deliverance to the captives, and recovering of sight to the blind, to set at liberty them that are bruised, To preach the acceptable year of the Lord.

The Spirit of the Lord is upon me is the proclamation that sets the purpose for every action by the Spirit of the Lord, whether coming/manifesting through Jesus, or those who come after HIM, robed in the Power that IS HIM in the believer!

1st. Because He hath anointed me to preach the gospel to the poor;
- *a.* The GREATEST method of healing is found in ministering/serving~up UNDERLINE THE WORD OF GOD through our proclaiming, declaring, and agreeing with what God says about us~~and our healing!
- *b.* NOTHING brings more glory into the happening, as when we declare the beauties, and glories of His Person!
- *c.* Proclaiming is DECLARING / ANNOUNCING / TESTIFYING of His Word...which is about HIM!

2nd. He hath sent me to heal the brokenhearted,
- *a.* The HEALING OF THE HEART is necessary to expend the energies of the Spirit in making/creating the necessary pattern for healing to manifest, and appear throughout one's living.
- *b.* Except we learn to AGREE, we will never APPLY what He has already given us!

---

    c. BROKENHEARTED implies there is a breach in the boundaries of our thought~processes, which empties rather than embodying the FULLNESS OF HIM that is ours and US IN HIM!

3rd. _To preach deliverance to the captives,_
    a. <u>DELIVERANCE</u> = pardon; freedom~~~
    b. We have been made free therefore, when we agree with the TRUTH of His Word, about us, we are SET~FREE through the Glory of His Presence already resident within us...
    c. All we NEED to do is agree mentally, verbally, and thoughtfully!

4th. _And recovering of sight to the blind,_
    a. Recovering <u>SIGHT</u>~~
    b. In the Aramaic, the term <u>SIGHT</u> implies _to be victorious over; to be in the ascendant_~~~
    c. The Aramaic, the original language of the New Testament, indicates that the believer is to realize they are the triumphant as existing IN HIM, the Christ!

5th. _To set at liberty them that are bruised,_
    a. Setting at <u>LIBERTY</u>~~
    b. In the Aramaic, the term LIBERTY means _remission; exemption; forgivable; pardonable_~~~
    c. In the Aramaic, the term CAPTIVES denotes _that was taken; prisoners_~~~

6th. _To preach the acceptable year of the Lord._
    a. Proclaiming the <u>ACCEPTABLE</u> year~~~
    b. In the Aramaic, the term <u>YEAR</u> is noted as _a measure of time._
    c. In the Aramaic, the term <u>ACCEPTABLE</u> notes _one's facing towards, or opposite of something/someone._

<u>The Truth of His Counsel grows/matures through the practice of His Spoken Word, completing the establishing of His Evidence progressing to transform and provide the Unseen.</u>

The inside is bigger than the outside, when you have the eyes necessary to see!

Much of what we think HEALING is or is about is nothing more than the illusions that the world, the flesh, and the unrenewed mind have conjured to keep the soul away from the REAL TRUTH!

From our point of view, we might say that *'life"* happened to us: *big and little losses inside the everyday; the accumulation and embracing of lies and betrayals; the absence of parents when we needed them; the failure of systems; the choices to protect ourselves, which,* while keeping us alive, also inhibited our ability to be open to the very things that would heal our hearts, our lives, and our bodies!

From God's perspective, it was death not life, an unreality we were never designed for.

This illusion of living was un~love, un~light, un~truth, un~freedom.

Understand that a significant reason why we fear death is because of our atrophied and minuscule perception of <u>LIFE</u>.

The immensity and grandeur of God's Life within us, continually absorbs and eradicates death's power and presence.

We tend to believe death is the end, an event causing *a cessation of things that truly matter,* and therefore it becomes the great wall, the inevitable inhibitor of joy, love, and relationship.

SEMITIC~ARAMAIC~HEBRAIC THESAURUS
Aramaic before first {
Semitic Root before first =
Lettering for ParaPhrase after second =

...*(47:11) But the miry places* H1207 {to establish} =⊐/⊡ Beyt[within/inside]-pattern thought inhabit / Tsad-
pursuit journey anticipate- Hey[behold/the]-quality reveal grace- *thereof and the marishes* H1360 {into the
presence/possession of someone}=⍺/⌂/ Gimal-experience understanding encounter- Beyt[within/inside]-pattern thought inhabit-
/ Final-Aleph-ending finish maturity- *thereof shall not* H3808 {without}= Lamed-instruct truth provide- Vav-
intensify degree counsel- Final-Aleph-perfected finished matured- *be healed:* H7495 {causing to heal} = Resh-practice
beginning strength- Pey-mouth SpokenWord speak- Final-Aleph-ending finish maturity- *they shall be*
given H5414 {giving/considering}= Nun-seed patience continue- Taw-evidence prove sign- Final-Nun-issue
perseverance progress- *to salt.* H4417 {to have maintenance} = Mem[from/out of]-transform encounter
remembrance- Lamed[to/toward]-instruct acquire provide- Hhet-specific share beyond-

The Semitic Emphasis

<u>To establish into the presence/possession of someone without causing to heal~~giving/considering to have maintenance.</u>

The truth is death has only been a shadow of things uselessly defined.

What we call death is indeed a separation of sorts, but not anything like what we have imagined it as.

We have focused on self and defined existence with reference to the fear of that singular last~breath event rather than recognizing death's permeating presence all around us~~such within our words, our touch, our choices, our sorrows, our unbelief, our lies, our judgment, our unforgiveness, our prejudices, our power-seeking, our betrayals, our hiding.

The '*event*' of death is only one small expression of that presence, but we have made that expression everything, not realizing that we cause ourselves to swim in death's ocean every single day.

We were not designed for death, but neither was death intended for this universe.

Inherent in the event of death is a promise, a baptism in this ocean that rescues, not drowns.

Humanity as uncreated life has brought that un~life into our experience, so out of respect for us, God wove it from the beginning into the larger tapestry. We now experience this underlying tension between life and death every day until we are released through the event of death.

Yet, instead of death, we were designed to deal with its encroachment in community, inside relationship, not in a self~centered isolation like our tiny, limited, unforeseen mentalities!

The Practice Of Declaring His Finished Work Pervades Every Exchange Of Beginnings And Enables The Truth Of His Wisdom To Increase Every Portion Of Perseverance

HOSEA 7:1
KJV+TVM

When I would have healed$^{H7495\,[H8800]}$ Israel^{H3478}, then the iniquity^{H5771} of Ephraim^{H669} was discovered$^{H1540\,[H8738]}$, and the wickedness^{H7451} of Samaria^{H8111}; for they commit$^{H6466\,[H8804]}$ falsehood^{H8267}; and the thief^{H1590} cometh in$^{H935\,[H8799]}$, and the troop^{H1416} of robbers spoileth$^{H6584\,[H8804]}$ without^{H2351}.

ORIGINAL THOUGHTS

...(7:1) The practice of declaring His Finished Work pervades every exchange of beginnings, and enables the Truth of His Wisdom to increase every portion of perseverance, while the very dominion of speaking the strengths of His Single~Mindedness prevails. With perception, acquire the revelation of His Wisdom to process the enlarging and transforming that begins by adding the issue of surrender to the single~mindedness of His Spoken Word, when discerning His every Promise. Through the pressures

Got Healing?

of His Parallels, each process of experience seeds the very
pattern~of~His~thoughts abiding within His Finished Work. The encounter
of His Faith increases the fitting of His Spoken Word to exchange and
reveal the Unseen in assurance of anticipation.

<u>The practice of declaring His Finished Work pervades every exchange of beginnings, and enables the Truth of His Wisdom to increase every portion of perseverance, while the very dominion of speaking the strengths of His Single~Mindedness prevails.</u>

The comforting/pervading of each exchange within His Beginnings, extended the measure of His Faith, His Grace, with His Purposes to provide for every soul created through the LOVE of the Father, the Son, and the Spirit.

As They continue eternally in agreement for the sharing of Themselves with us Their Creation, so even do we eternally grow and mature beyond every moment we have with Them, in Them, and through Them!

As They continue eternally in agreement, so do we enlarge, expand, and enhance the fullness of WHO They are in us, and WHOSE we are in THEM!

The longer the Silence, the Greater the Breath!

The greater the bearing forth of Themselves through our living here, the larger the expanse of the Universe continues in its course to create even as His Word creates in us the fullness of His Expanse, stretching us beyond the limits of this flesh, this world, and this dimension.

By Their sharing of Who They are, there is enlarged and enhanced a greater completeness of WHOSE we become!

<u>With perception, acquire the revelation of His Wisdom to process the enlarging and transforming that begins by adding the issue of surrender to the single~mindedness of His Spoken Word, when discerning His every Promise.</u>

The blending of His Purpose through every Promise saturates and transfuses the eternal magnificence of His Spoken Word, producing in us and all that is around us to transform and transcend beyond any boundaries that anyone or anything has ever tried to place upon our living as believing believers!

It is when SURRENDER is added/blended with SINGLE~MINDEDNESS that His Intended Plan flourishes within the courts of our existence as HIM in this physical dimension; and as well,

His Plan succeeds in bringing to eternal fruition the unlimited, unconditional, unimaginable, unfathomable benefits of His Destiny intertwined with our humility, teachableness, and willingness to sacrifice all that we ARE, so that He may impart to us all that HE IS!

Through the pressures of His Parallels, each process of experience seeds the very pattern~of~His~thoughts abiding within His Finished Work.

The closer the parallels within every wheel of His Purpose, the greater the pressing to enable the stronger the tie between Creator and Creation.

As the parallels begin to become entwined within our experiences, we become aware to a greater dispensation and consciousness of WHY we are HIS, and HOW He makes us like Himself, as in the Image of HIMSELF!

The more intricate the patterns of His Purposes become, the stronger the resolve of our being in being drawn nearer to HIM!

The more we desire to embrace of HIM, the greater the drive to encompass and comprehend the fullness that makes Him Who He is to us, His Creation.

The encounter of His Faith increases the fitting of His Spoken Word to exchange and reveal the Unseen in assurance of anticipation.

The stronger His Faith intertwines our belief and conviction, the greater we are persuaded that His Ways, His Thoughts, His Ideals are surpassed by nothing other than the very Presence, Person, and Power that He eternally remains.

God, the Father, the Son, and the Spirit broke death's illusion of power and dominance, when Jesus, the God~Man rose from the grave, ascended to the heavens, and took His place with us as the Father's right~hand.

Heaven's halls, God's domain welcomed the returning prodigal of humanity, held safely within the bosom of the Son.

What we must realize is that every time we do choose to not continue in His Faith, as He IS NOW, we create a crisis of faith in ourselves.

More often it happens in the moment of one's physical death, but since there have never been formulas governing relationships and we who are alive now are not actually dead yet, something special and mysterious is happening.

As we LEARN HIM, and as He resides/abides IN US, we determine that nothing has, nor can, nor every will~~separate us from HIM!

Got Healing?

SEMITIC~ARAMAIC~HEBRAIC THESAURUS

Aramaic before first {
Semitic Root before first =
Lettering for ParaPhrase after second =

...(7:1) When I would have healed [H7495] {=causing to heal} = Resh-practice beginning strength- Pey-mouth SpokenWord speak- Final-Aleph-ending finish maturity- Israel [H3478] {=God prevails} = Yud-purpose posture actions- Shin-pressure exchange disperse- Resh-practice beginning strength- Aleph-dominion ability confirm- Lamed-instruct truth provide- then

the iniquity [H5771] {=inwardly/inside within} = Ayin-pierce perceive wisdom- Vav-[and/in addition]increase of degree assure- Vav-[and/in addition]increase degree assure- Final-Nun-issue perseverance progress-

Ephraim [H669] {=doubly fruitful} = Aleph-authority ability confirm- Pey-mouth SpokenWord speak- Resh-process beginning strength- Yud [of/through]-purpose single-mindedness actions- Final-Mem-trial fashions

prevail- was discovered [H1540] {=according to} = Ayin-pierce perceive wisdom- Lamed[to/toward]-instruct acquire provide- Hey[behold/the]-quality reveal grace- and the wickedness [H7451] {= direct consequence of one's action} = Ayin-pierce perceive wisdom- Resh-process beginning strength- of Samaria [H8111] {=to encounter remembrance-

hedge about/to protect} = Shin-pressure exchange disperse- Mem[from/out of]-transform encounter remembrance- Resh-process beginning strength- Vav-[and/in addition]increase degree assure- Final-Nun-issue perseverance progress-

for [H3588] {=in order that} = Kaph-surrender obtains consent- Yud [of/through]-purpose single-mindedness actions- they

commit [H6466] {=to practice/prepare} = Pey-mouth SpokenWord speak- Ayin-pierce perceive wisdom- Lamed[to/toward]-instruct acquire provide- Quph-contrast parallel structure- falsehood [H8267] {=violating an agreement} = Resh-process beginning strength- and the

thief [H1590] {=doing something in a secretive manner} = Beyt[within/inside]-pattern thought inhabit- Gimal-experience understanding encounter- Nun- seed patience continue- cometh in [H935] {= causes to come in} = Final-Aleph-ending finish maturity-

in} = Beyt[within/inside]-pattern thought inhabit- Vav-[and/in addition]increase degree assure- Gimal-experience understanding encounter- and the troop of robbers [H1416] {=a furrow cut for sowing} = Vav-[and/in addition]increase degree assure- Dalet-faith establish presence- Dalet-faith establish presence-

spoileth [H6584] {=to spread out/invade} = Pey-mouth SpokenWord speak- Shin-pressure exchange disperse- Hey[behold/the]-quality reveal grace- without [H2351] {=separating by a wall/outside} = Hhet- specific share beyond- Vav-[and/in addition]increase degree assure- Tsad-pursuit journey anticipate-

The Semitic Emphasis

Causing to heal~~God prevails inwardly/inside within doubly fruitful~~according to direct consequence of one's action to hedge about/to protect~~in order that to practice/prepare violating an agreement doing something in a secretive manner causes to come in a furrow cut for sowing to spread out/invade separating by a wall/outside.

The influences of this world, the flesh, and the unrenewed seek to create a separation by spreading a wall of influence away from everything that is GOD!

It is the thoughts of separation from the God of the Universe~~the God that created us in His Mentalities~~these thoughts of separation are the lies perpetuated by outside influences.

These are the lies of separation that need to be squashed and removed from every thought~provoking ideal ever conceived in our unrenewed minds.

The passion and enormity of the Universe dwelling in us is the awe~inspiring place wherein we discover the REST OF HIM!

While we look at the things which remain as UNSEEN, we dwell in our thoughts upon THEM, our God, our Savior, and our Mentor.

Herein, within His LOVE~~we find solace, peace, and contentment because we are in the bosom of the GODHEAD Who created us before ever the foundations of the world were laid.

The crux of the problems we have~~lay in the fact that we do not THINK in terms of relationship, in the manner of God does!

We tend to see everything through a grid of isolated experiences we call, our life!

There are so many answers to problems that would bewilder us, making no sense whatsoever, because we do NOT even have a frame of reference that would allow them to become understood within our limited regions of thought.

Part of the wonder of Jesus, being ALWAYS God, joining the human race~~ is that He was not some actor added to the cast of characters, but literally became fully human as a forever reality.

He never stopped being fully God, or fully the creator, or fully the partner.

It is true now and has been since the beginning of time that the entire cosmos exists inside HIM, and that He hold it all together, sustaining it, even now, right this moment, and that would include us along with every other created thing.

Leading With A Continued Determination
Strengthens One's Understanding
Learning To Enable His Spoken Word
Processes A Single~Minded Prevail

Hosea 11:3
KJV+TVM

I taught[H8637] Ephraim[H669] also to go[H8637] [H8809], taking[H3947] [H8800] them by their arms[H2220]; but they knew[H3045] [H8804] not that I healed[H7495] [H8804] them.

Original Thoughts
...(11:3) Leading with a continued determination strengthens one's

---

understanding, learning to enable His Spoken Word processes a single~minded prevail. Strengthening understanding acquires the abilities of His Spoken Word to process single~mindedly through the triumphs providing the parallels of the Unseen. Perceiving His Truth alters the beginnings of increasing His Wisdom. The purpose of His Faith perceiving/discerning His Truth identifies the counsel of His Influence. Obtaining single~mindedness strengthens the speaking/declaring of His Finished Work.

Leading with a continued determination strengthens one's understanding, learning to enable His Spoken Word processes a single~minded prevail.

"If ye be willing and obedient, ye shall eat the good of the land:" ISAIAH 1:19 KJV

It seems so many are faltering asking, "Why" that they forget to TRUST!

If God's plan requires that we know, then just such an answer will appear.

However, we are always asked by the Spirit TO TRUST the leadings of the Father's Will by remaining *willing and obedient!*

Strengthening understanding acquires the abilities of His Spoken Word to process single~mindedly through the triumphs providing the parallels of the Unseen.

Being a believing believer is an activity; it's not a category for filing away what cannot be explained to the flesh!

Understanding is an action of TRUST, wherein we discover God's leading, not necessarily the answers to every question we think upon!

The journey of healing is about learning, examining, and proving what it is we know the Father through.

Jesus came to show us the Father!

The Spirit came to show us Jesus!

In these three, we find the summation and totality of everything!

Perceiving His Truth alters the beginnings of increasing His Wisdom.

Healing is NOT an action of God's submission to our begging, pleading, or whining.

Praying is NOT an action done only when we think we will get what we want.

He is the Potter, we are clay; stop reversing roles.

Some, it appears, do not get their healing; the reasons for us are

---

unknown.

Suspicion, suspense, and intrigue are the commodities of a dime~store novel; not the characteristics of an all~knowing Creator!

THE TRUTH is what He is about; yet, His LOVE is WHO HE IS!

The purpose of His Faith perceiving/discerning His Truth identifies the counsel of His Influence.

Invitations are not cause for an expectation.

God has no *agenda*, except that of loving His children!

Many of us are unwilling to completely surrender for fear that God will ask us to do something we don't want to do!

Realize this: God forgives us even for those things we don't understand!

Often, it is that we ISOLATE ourselves without even knowing why!

God's invitations must become an expectation of His Love, His Goodness, and His Kindness.

This is the sharing of His Eternal **BE**~ing!

Obtaining single~mindedness strengthens the speaking/declaring of His Finished Work.

Realizing that God accepts us the WAY we are causes a consternation in a lot of people's thinking.

They think because they are poor, or without certain accoutrements in life, they are unworthy, or unfit to offer God anything they have!

WHAT A CROCK of B.S.! You know, bologna~sausage!

God will accept residence in the tiniest, smallest place of our heart or mind, just for the opportunity to show us what He can do with the smallest of nothing!

Our failure is found in not realizing all the grandeur of what untold things He has imparted to us, and we know nothing about them at all!

SEMITIC~ARAMAIC~HEBRAIC THESAURUS

Aramaic before first {
Semitic Root before first =
Lettering for ParaPhrase after second =

...(11:3) I^{H595} אָנֹכִי {=as for me}= ...Aleph-authority ability confirm- ...Nun-seed patience continue- ...Hhet-specific share beyond- encounter- taught ^{H8637} {=causing to walk}= ...Resh-process beginning strength- ...Gimal-experience understanding Lamed[to/toward]-instruct acquire provide- Ephraim ^{H669} {=doubly fruitful}= ...Aleph-authority ability confirm- Pey-mouth SpokenWord speak- ...Resh-process beginning strength- Yud

Got Healing?

[of/through]-purpose single~mindedness actions- /Final-Mem-trial fashions prevail- **also to go** H8637 =causing to **walk**} / Resh-process beginning strength- /Gimal-experience understanding encounter- Lamed[to/toward]-instruct acquire provide- H669 =**doubly fruitful**} / Aleph-authority ability confirm- Pey-mouth SpokenWord speak- / Resh-process beginning strength- /Yud [of/through]-purpose single~mindedness actions- /Final-Mem-trial fashions prevail- **taking** H3947 =**to remove/take away**} / Lamed[to/toward]-instruct acquire provide- /Quph-contrast parallel structure- Hhet-specific share beyond- **them by** H592 =**on behalf of**} Ayin-pierce perceive wisdom- Lamed- instruct truth provide- **their arms** H2220 =**strengthening**} / Zayin-skill alter instrument- /Resh-process beginning strength- /Vav-[and/in addition]increase degree assure- /Ayin-pierce perceive wisdom- **but they knew** H3045 =**the door to the eye/insight**} / Yud [of/through]-purpose single~mindedness actions- /Dalet-faith establish presence- /Ayin- pierce perceive wisdom- **not** H3808 =**without**} /Lamed-instruct truth provide- Vav-intensify degree counsel- Final-Aleph- perfected finished matured- **that** H3588 =**because/for**} /Kaph-surrender obtains consent- /Yud [of/through]-purpose single~mindedness actions- **I healed** H7495 =**causing to heal**} Resh-practice beginning strength- Pey-mouth SpokenWord speak- Final-Aleph-ending finish maturity- **them**

The Semitic Emphasis

As for me~~causing to walk doubly fruitful~~causing to walk doubly fruitful to remove/take away on behalf of strengthening the door to the eye/insight~~without~~because/for causing to heal.

Often, we tell ourselves we are trying to understand, and yet we resist everything internally.

This is where absolute surrender comes into play.

We use the term, "*Surrender*" to express a desire; and yet, sometimes it is only just that, a desire!

We never continue to act on the desire by actually picking up a book, or a concordance, or the Bible for that matter; and investigate just what it is that we are dealing with.

"*If any of you lack wisdom, let him ask of God, that giveth to all men liberally, and upbraideth not; and it shall be given him.*" JAMES 1:5 KJV

25 verses examined...

NEW TESTAMENT PARADIGMS

Revealing In Addition To His Faith
Every Purpose Of Issue Perceives
The Seed Of His Finished Work

MATTHEW 4:4
KJV+TVM
But[G1161] he answered[G611] [G5679] and said[G2036] [G5627], It is written[G1125] [G5769],

Got Healing?

Man^{G444} shall^{G2198} not^{G3756} live^{G2198} $^{[G5695]}$ by^{G1909} bread^{G740} alone^{G3441}, but^{G235} by^{G1909} every^{G3956} word^{G4487} that proceedeth^{G1607} $^{[G5740]}$ out of^{G1223} the mouth^{G4750} of God^{G2316}.

Original Thoughts

...(4:4) Revealing in addition to His Faith, every purpose of issue perceives the Seed of His Finished Work. In addition to enabling the encountering of His Strength, agree with the Evidence of His Purpose within His Faith, teaching/learning the qualities that increase His Finished Work. Behold every addition of His Efforts Finished, within the instruction beyond each encountering through His Finished Work. Within every instruction of the Unseen Increase of His Faith, share the positioning of His Finished Work. The Pattern~Thoughts of beginnings continue to enlarge His Finished Work, and enable the provisions of His Finished Work. Within each consent toward remembrance, allow the Influence of Completed Efforts establishing the Seed of His Spoken Word to parallel that of His Finished Work. Transforming every issue of His Spoken Word assures the encountering of every grace of His Presence to enable/empower the teaching that beholds His Finished Work.

Revealing in addition to His Faith, every purpose of issue perceives the Seed of His Finished Work.

It is important to recognize in thought, as in any science or court of law, the nature of the questions we ask determines the kind of answers we give or receive.

It is in allowing the Spirit to have the liberty wherewith to reveal the hidden mysteries of God's unconditional love that we find our circumspection of the world's ideals, attitudes, and demeanor as not to our judging, but we are to bow in obedience to His decisions in the seeing of those around us.

"So then every one of us shall give account of themselves to God." ROMANS 14:12 KJV

How much better to defer to His Wisdom, than to be caught in the intrigue of our beguiling of another's responsibilities.

In addition to enabling the encountering of His Strength, agree with the Evidence of His Purpose within His Faith, teaching/learning the qualities that increase His Finished Work.

We instead, need to seek after and secure a total baptism in beauty, glory, and delight, a baptism that would flow over into every nook and cranny of our humanity.

God is Father, Son and Spirit, existing in a passionate and joyous fellowship.

The Trinity is not three highly committed religious types sitting around some room in heaven.

The Trinity is a circle of shared life, and the life shared is full, not empty, abounding and rich and beautiful, not lonely and sad and boring.

The river begins right there, in the fellowship of the Trinity.

The great dance is all about the abounding life shared by the Father, Son and Spirit.

It all boils down to three things: *First,* there is the Trinity and the great dance of life and glory and joy shared by the Father, Son and Spirit.

Second, there is the incarnation as the act of the Father, Son and Spirit reaching down, extending the circle, their great dance of life, TO US.

Third, there is our humanity, which is the theatre in which the great dance is played out through the Spirit.

Behold every addition of His Efforts Finished within the instruction beyond each encountering through His Finished Work.

God is not an isolated sovereign, a self-centered king who demands that everything revolve around Him and be done for His glory.

God is not a legalist, a divine bookkeeper, who watches us like a hawk to see if we keep His little rules, nor is He some boring old religious type, a cosmic killjoy who sits in heaven thinking up ways to stifle everything that is good.

On the other hand, neither is God like some goofy Santa Claus, who doles out goodies without regard to what we are capable of receiving and enjoying.

The truth is: God is a circle of passion and life and fellowship.

Within every instruction of the Unseen Increase of His Faith, share the positioning of His Finished Work.

What the doctrine of the Trinity is telling us is that God is fundamentally a relational being.

We are saying that there has never been a moment in all eternity when God was alone.

We are saying that God has always been Father, Son and Spirit.

We are saying that there was never a time when the Father was not

Father, when the Son and the Spirit were not there and there was just God, so to speak, just some abstract divinity.

God has always existed in relationship.

Fellowship, camaraderie, togetherness, communion have always been at the center of the very being of God, and always will be.

The Pattern~Thoughts of beginnings continue to enlarge His Finished Work, and enable the provisions of His Finished Work.

In the spiritual pattern of things, we only see it the things of the spiritual realm when we look for them and only experience them if we expect them.

In American history we use the term *"The Great Awakening"* to describe several periods of widespread revival and spiritual transformation.

It is interesting that they occurred in the generation that preceded a great national struggle.

The term *"awakening"* implies that people were spiritually asleep and needed to be awakened to God's very real presence and purpose.

We would suggest that the awakening was a shift within the hearts of the people to search for the reality of God and His will above the everyday desires of life.

It has always been interesting to many that some who believe in a God who is all-powerful~~as well as in angels, heaven, and biblical miracles~~have difficulty believing that this same God would manifest His power through signs and wonders in our day.

Heaven is a real place and God's miraculous manifestation is available to the spiritually awake.

The miraculous is real, but we often need to be awakened to its nearness and its reality.

Our dreams, whatever they may be, remain only dreams until they are in some way manifested in the earth.

Within each consent toward remembrance, allow the Influence of Completed Efforts establishing the Seed of His Spoken Word to parallel that of His Finished Work.

The spiritual manifestation accompanying an open portal always points to God and His greater purpose.

So if God has provided for you in some significant way, that blessing or miraculous manifestation should also be accompanied by understanding, direction, and, most of all, a greater sense of who and what God is to you.

Self-examination and expectation are keys that allow you to access the miraculous, like the people in Elijah's day, who had to be awakened to the reality of God.

Doubt and fear block an expectant faith.

The Scriptures are replete and repetitious with examples of God's people turning their hearts toward HIM, and HIS answering prayers that sought only HIM, and not just His Benefits!

The Seed of His Spoken Word regales the very nature of God Himself in pouring out blessing upon the people that call after His NAME!

It is by Divine Pursuit and expectation that we are awaken to greater spiritual possibilities.

Transforming every issue of His Spoken Word assures the encountering of every grace of His Presence to enable/empower the teaching that beholds His Finished Work.

Transforming, or Converting the Spoken Word of God into the language of our surrendered heart and mind, continues the Presence of the Spirit to remain in charge of every outcome sought.

As we consciously speak the words He has spoken regarding any situation at hand, the Spirit is being allowed to move and intersect and interact within our living to produce the greatest of God's benefits withheld until we surrender completely to Her, and Him!

SEMITIC~ARAMAIC~HEBRAIC THESAURUS
Aramaic before first {
Semitic Root before first =
Lettering for ParaPhrase after second =

(‸:4) He)הוֹא $S5005$ {הוֹא=he is the one}= Hey[behold/the]-quality reveal grace- Vav-[and/in addition]increase degree assure-
(but)וַיַּ $S4405$ {וייִ=on the other hand}= Dalet-faith establish presence- Yud-purpose posture actions- Final-Nun-issue perseverance
progress- (answered)עֲנֵי $S15985$ {ענה=to respond}= Ayin-pierce perceive wisdom- Nun-seed patience continue- Final-Aleph-ending
finish maturity- (& said)אֲמַר $S1290$ {אמר=making a legal declaration}= Vav-[and/in addition]increase degree assure- Aleph-
authority ability confirm- Mem[from/out of]-transform encounter remembrance- Resh-process beginning strength- (it was
written)כְּתִיב $S10732$ {כתב=to enscribe/compose/enroll}= Kaph-surrender obtains consent- Taw-evidence prove sign- Yud-
purpose posture actions- Beyt[within/in/inside]pattern thought inhabit- (that not)לָא $S10863$ {לא=perceiving/desiring
without}= Dalet-faith establish presence- Lamed[to/toward]-instruct acquire provide- Final-Aleph-ending finish maturity- (it
was)הוָא $S5144$ {אוה=to endure/exist/becom~}= Hey[behold/the]-quality reveal grace- Vav-[and/in addition]increase degree
assure- Final-Aleph-ending finish maturity- (by bread)בְּלַחְמָא $S11171$ {לחם=in exchange for
feeding}= Beyt[within/in/inside]-pattern thought inhabit- Lamed[to/toward]-instruct acquire provide- Hhet-specific share beyond-
Mem[from/out of]-transform encounter remembrance- Final-Aleph-ending finish maturity- (only)בִּלְחוֹד $S11149$ {חוד=on the sole

condition that}=⊐ Beyt[within/in/inside]-pattern thought inhabit-⅃ Lamed[to/toward]-instruct acquire provide-⊓ Hhet-specific share beyond-⅂ Vav-[and/in addition]increase degree assure-⅂ Dalet-faith establish presence-⊓⅃⊓=to be (lives) S6912 {⅃⊓=to be healed/sustained}=⊓ Hhet-specific share beyond-⅄ Yud-purpose posture actions-⅄ Final-Aleph-ending finish maturity-(a son of man) ⅁⅃⅄⅂⊐ S1441 {⅁⅄⅃ =inhabitant/household}=⊐ Beyt[within/in/inside]-pattern thought inhabit-⅃ Resh-process beginning strength-⅃ Nun-seed patience continue-⅄ Shin-pressure exchange disperse-⅄ Final-Aleph-ending finish maturity-((but) ⅃⅂⅃⅁ S892 {⅃⅃⅁=except/unless}=⅁ Aleph-authority ability confirm-⅃ Lamed[to/toward]-instruct acquire provide-⅄ Final-Aleph-ending finish maturity-(by every) ⅃⅂⅃⅁ S1007 {⅃⊐⅁=in exchange for all}=⅁ Beyt[within/in/inside]-pattern thought inhabit-⅁ Kaph-surrender obtains consent-⅃ Lamed[to/toward]-instruct acquire provide-⅃ Lamed[to/toward]-instruct acquire provide-⅄ Final-Aleph-ending finish maturity-(that encounter remembrance-⅃ Mem[from/out of]-transform word) ⅃⅂⅃⅁ S12109 {⅃⅂⅃⅁=promises}=⅁ (that proceeds) ⅁⅃⊐⅄⅃ S3356 {⅁⅃⊐⅄⅃=perceiving/desiring coming out/being translated}=⅃ Dalet-faith establish presence-⅁ Nun-seed patience continue-⅄ Pey-mouth SpokenWord speak-⅄ Quph-contrast parallel structure-⅄ Final-Aleph-ending finish maturity-(from) ⅁⅃ S12182 {⅁⅃=indicating the origin of movement through time}=⅁ Mem[from/out of]-transform encounter remembrance-⅄ Final-Nun-issue perseverance progress-(the mouth) ⅁⅁⅃⅄ S6475 {⅁⅁⅃⅄=the opening of a body of water/heart}=⊐ Pey-mouth SpokenWord speak-⅂ Vav-[and/in addition]increase degree assure-⅁ Mem[from/out of]-transform encounter remembrance-⅃ Hey[behold/the]-quality reveal grace-(of God) ⅁⅃⅃⅁ S914 {⅁⅃⅃⅁=behaving like God}=⅃ Dalet-faith establish presence-⅁ Aleph-authority ability confirm-⅃ Lamed[to/toward]-instruct acquire provide-⅃ Hey[behold/the]-quality reveal grace-⅄ Final-Aleph-ending finish maturity-

The Semitic Emphasis

He is the one on the other hand to respond making a legal declaration~~to inscribe/compose/enroll while perceiving/desiring without~~to endure/exist/become in exchange for feeding on the sole condition that to be healed/sustained as an inhabitant/household~~ except/unless in exchange for all promises perceiving/desiring coming out/being translated and indicating the origin of movement through time~~the opening of a body of water/heart behaving like God.

The word of God that is contained in the Bible has the power to do many marvelous things.

Its most powerful attribute, perhaps, is its ability to mold God's nature in us so that we begin to see as He sees and think as He thinks and act as He acts.

It molds us into His image and empowers us spiritually in our world!

God's Word is powerful.

His Word, as Jesus is the Word~~formed the universe and everything in it, brought forth all life, and can reach down into the deepest part of our hearts to change despair into hope and want into fulfillment.

God is doing notable miracles in every place that He abides, and those there with Him give Him place to accomplish His Will!

The Ability Of His Exchange
Proves The Transforming Wisdom Of His Balance
Within Every Pattern~Of~His~Thought

MATTHEW 4:24

Got Healing?

KJV+TVM

And[G2532] his[G846] fame[G189] went[G565] [G5627] throughout[G1519] all[G3650] Syria[G4947]: and[G2532] they brought[G4374] [G5656] unto him[G846] all[G3956] sick[G2560] people[G2192] [G5723] that were taken with[G4912] [G5746] divers[G4164] diseases[G3554] and[G2532] torments[G931], and[G2532] those which were possessed with devils[G1139] [G5740], and[G2532] those which were lunatick[G4583] [G5740], and[G2532] those that had the palsy[G3885]; and[G2532] he healed[G2323] [G5656] them[G846].

ORIGINAL THOUGHTS

...(4:24) The ability of His Exchange proves the transforming Wisdom of His Balance within every Pattern~of~His~Thought to reveal within the surrender acquiring the Grace of His Truth. Adjusting to every increase begins each purpose of His Finished Work, insuring through the parallels of His Strength within each degree of building the processing of His Pattern~of~Thought assured. To gaze through surrender, the instruction of the Grace of His Truth, each increase issues the abilities of His Motive/Reason to teach each purpose through progress. Faith in His Pattern~of~Thought exercises the Exchange within His Purpose to pressure perceiving inhabiting positions of His Faithfulness dealing with every issue. Abide through surrender to increase the process of His Grace/Truth to continue His Finished Work. Transcending each pressure determines the acquiring of His Spoken Word to finish with influence every increase of His Ability to create the provision of His Promises offered. Faith in His Abilities acquires the intent of His Wisdom to focus on each issue within His Evidence that exchanges while perpetuating His Purpose in parallel of His Finished Work. In addition to His Faith, His Motive/Reason increases to continue the Influence of Finished Efforts confirming with understanding, each beginning of His Finished Work. The addition of His Faith within each process increases the memories of His Exchange strengthening each exercise of His Finished Work. The Seed of His Ability apprehends the purpose identical to the Seed's increase and perseverance.

The ability of His Exchange proves the transforming Wisdom of His Balance within every Pattern~of~His~Thought to reveal within the surrender acquiring the Grace of His Truth.

In order to receive, we must surrender to accept.

Without surrender on our part, the Spirit remains hindered in Her giving of purpose through His Wisdom.

Hereby, confession of our Selfish~Independent~Nature is not the action in which we tell God about our problem; but it becomes the actions in which we tell our Selfish~Independent~Nature about our God's redemption!

Adjusting to every increase begins each purpose of His Finished Work, *insuring through the parallels of His Strength within each degree of building the processing of His Pattern~of~Thought assured.*

The Gospel is truth, not potential.

The good news unveils reality, the way God sees it.

The Gospel is truth, not potential. The good news unveils reality, the way God sees it.

What if some did not believe and were without faith? Does their lack of faith and their faithlessness nullify and make ineffective and void the faithfulness of God and His fidelity to His Word?

No, must we say; a thousand times NO!

Our faith, or lack thereof, does not make the faithfulness of God ineffective.

His death at Calvary, was the death of our *S*elfish~*I*ndependent~*N*ature.

Our relationship to our *S*elfish~*I*ndependent~*N*ature is eternally severed.

What remains for us to do is ask for the assistance of the Holy Spirit in discovering/uncovering the very elements of His Resurrection as being ours eternally!

To gaze through surrender, the instruction of the Grace of His Truth, each increase issues the abilities of His Motive/Reason to teach each purpose through progress.

His resurrection is our resurrection~~the orginal, pure and blameless person HE IMAGINED was raised in newness of life IN HIM, as HIM!

His ascension is our ascension~~raised to a place of honor, seated at the right hand of God, fully alive, fully ourselves.

Jesus is more than a historc person which is of potential benefit to us~~He is become the secret of our living IN HIM!

In HIM ALL THINGS CONSIST!

He has done all the hard work~~work which we could not do ourselves.

All that is left for us to do is allow the Spirit to open our eyes, to realize we are seeing through HIS!

Faith in His Pattern~of~Thought exercises the Exchange within His Purpose to pressure perceiving inhabiting positions of His Faithfulness dealing with every issue.

Thinking upon the Word of His BE~ing in us provides the pathway/journey to discover that in His Faithfulness, He fulfills every need within our living for HIM!

Take a look at *JOHN 1:1-14*.

It is this ever present source of all that is, that John calls God.

This God is no separate entity that creates from a distance, but rather a God entangled in creation, for it is through this Word that all things are made and without him nothing exists.

John continues to describe this God, not only as Word, but as light, life and grace.

This has special significance when we come to verse 14~~one of the most memorable of all scriptures: "and the Word became flesh."

Of what value is a word unless it is heard?

Of what significance is grace unless it is given?

Does light have any meaning if it is never seen?

And so grace is given, the invisible becomes tangible and the word becomes flesh.

Flesh is the manifestation of this underlying potentiality called God. If we could restate this using the language of modern science and philosophy, we might say something like this: In the field of quantum possibilities, it is the act of conscious observation that realizes a specific possibility.

Potential becomes reality in a specific instant.

And so the God of infinite possibility manifests Him/Herself in all of creation.

Our act of observation is therefore part of the creative process.

Abide through surrender to increase the process of His Grace/Truth to continue His Finished Work.

Observation requires abiding.

John clearly wants to focus on the unique revelation that came through Jesus, but we often jump to that conclusion too quickly and in so doing lose the depth and significance of what is communicated.

"The Word became flesh" is then simply translated to mean *"God became human."*

But flesh is more elemental than body, just as water is more elemental than any particular river. It weaves far beyond any individual identity, connecting life with its source.

Yes, in Jesus there is a unique event of word-becoming-flesh, but not unique in that it does not happen anywhere else.

The event of Jesus is not the first time that God experiences what it means to be human.

Rather, it is the first time that we know, that God knows what it is like to be human.

Jesus is a unique incarnation in that we recognize in Him the divine manifestation of what is possible everywhere.

"And the Word became flesh and dwelt among/in us, and we gazed on his glory – glory as of the only/unique Son from the Father, full of grace and truth." JOHN 1:14

Transcending each pressure determines the acquiring of His Spoken Word to finish with influence every increase of His Ability to create the provision of His Promises offered.

The same Word that sustains all of creation, the grace that gives itself in the reality of all things,~~yet, although this light was in the world, we did not recognize it as such, *JOHN 1:10 KJV*

It is this same word that has always been present that becomes uniquely visible, audible and recognizable in the event of Jesus.

In other words, Jesus did not come to show us what we could never be, but rather what we have always been, but did not recognize.

The grace of our own existence, the reality/truth of God's self-giving into our creation~~our flesh~~is revealed through the message of Jesus.

And so *"of His fulness have we all received."* *JOHN 1:16 KJV*

Faith in His Abilities acquires the intent of His Wisdom to focus on each issue within His Evidence that exchanges while perpetuating His Purpose in parallel of His Finished Work.

It is easy to justify a dualistic view of flesh and spirit~~a view that sees flesh and spirit as opposed and irreconcilable; through verses such as *"that is born of the flesh is flesh, and that which is born of the Spirit is spirit"* *JOHN 3:6 KJV* **or** *"It is the Spirit that gives life; the flesh is no help at all."* *JOHN 6:63*

But such interpretations ignore the overwhelming sense of the transformation of flesh portrayed in John's gospel.

Flesh does not remain a physical lump of meat, but is transformed as it is given.

"*Whoever feeds on my flesh and drinks my blood has eternal life.*" *JOHN 6:54*

In this instance flesh has the same benefit as spirit.

Flesh becomes bread and water and wine.

It is continually transformed as it is given to be consumed.

Suddenly the whole social context in which our labors and relationships produce bread, wine and commerce, becomes part of the flesh of our existence.

Here as well, the Word, the logic of God wants to manifest in a way that will make our societies just and our sustenance satisfying.

In addition to His Faith, His Motive/Reason increases to continue the Influence of Finished Efforts confirming with understanding, each beginning of His Finished Work.

It is exactly those who are born of flesh~~who can be transformed by His Spirit.

Yes, if flesh simply remains flesh, if it is not given for the benefit of others, it is of no benefit at all.

But Jesus opens up a new possibility, one in which it is our very fleshly existence that gives us an opportunity to transform what is limited and earthly, into heavenly bliss as we follow His example of giving ourselves away.

It is The Word that has been so freely given into our fleshly fabric, and it comes full circle as flesh when transformed by the Word that is His *BE*~ing!

The addition of His Faith within each process, increases the memories of His Exchange strengthening each exercise of His Finished Work.

Are you open to something truly surprising or have past experiences conditioned you to expect nothing more than what you are already familiar with?

Obviously we are meant to learn from our experiences, but the wisdom we gain from them should not close us to the possibilities of tomorrow.

It would be a tragedy if past disappointments become the boundaries of tomorrow's expectations.

Got Healing?

This is important, for expectation is not simply our best effort to foresee tomorrow, but to a large extent it determines our experience of tomorrow, when it becomes today.

Our expectations are formed under the influence of many factors~~some conscious, some unconscious:

past experiences,
the reality of our present circumstances,
our beliefs.

Taking all these factors into account, it might seem that tomorrow is largely determined.

The logic of cause and effect narrows the options before us.

Yet a very significant factor is often left out of our calculations:

the possibility that our experiences have no knowledge of,
the possibility that our beliefs do not yet acknowledge,
the possibility that is by its very definition larger than the present reality.

This possibility is what I call God.

It is a possibility beyond our logic of cause and effect.

Jesus spoke about God when He said *"for God all things are possible"*, MATTHEW 19:26 KJV
.

Or another way of translating it is: *"God is the possibility of all things."*

This is the God of novelty; the God who beckons us moment by moment to transcend the boundaries of what is and what has been.

Something truly new and truly beautiful is possible for you.

If you experience the excitement of what this sentence means~~a meaning beyond the words~~then you are experiencing God.

The Seed of His Ability apprehends the purpose identical to the Seed's increase and perseverance.

Very often plans are made in order to reduce unpleasant surprises.

These plans are often motivated by a desire to be in control.

An unintended consequence of such plans is that they also exclude the possibility for pleasant surprises.

Being in absolute control can also be absolutely boring.

Yes, some plans are good and necessary, but we need to learn the art of leaving space for the unplanned, space, as it were for surprising creativity.

SEMITIC~ARAMAIC~HEBRAIC THESAURUS
Aramaic before first {

Got Healing?

Semitic Root before first =

Lettering for ParaPhrase after second =

...(4:24) (& was heard)וישתמע[S21724] {שמע=also hearing to respond}=א Aleph-authority ability confirm-שShin-pressure exchange disperse-Taw-evidence prove sign-Mem[from/out of]-transform encounter remembrance-עAyin-pierce perceive wisdom-

(His fame)טבה[S7927] {טב=report/nature/character}=מ Mem[from/out of]-transform encounter-Thet-contain mixture balance-Beyt[within/in/inside]-pattern thought inhabit-Hey[behold/the]-quality reveal grace-

(in all)בכלה[S10008] {כל=with regard to/in exchange for all}=ב Beyt[within/in/inside]-pattern thought inhabit-Kaph-surrender obtains consent-Lamed[to/toward]-instruct acquire provide-Hey[behold/the]-quality reveal grace-

(Syria)סוריא[S14168] {סור=a length of line without width}=ס Samech-adjust apprehend source-Vav-[and/in addition]increase degree assure-Resh-process beginning strength-Yud-purpose posture actions-Final-Aleph-ending finish maturity-

(& they brought)ויקרבו[S18979] {קרב=also to touch/to bring near}=ו Vav-[and/in addition]increase degree assure-Quph-contrast parallel structure-Resh-process beginning strength-Beyt[within/in/inside]-pattern thought inhabit-Vav-[and/in addition]increase degree assure-

(to Him)לה[S10842] {לה=beyond/above/outside of}=ל Lamed[to/toward]-instruct acquire provide-Hey[behold/the]-quality reveal grace-

(all of them)בכלה[S10082] {כל=the whole reason for this is}=כ Kaph-surrender obtains consent-Lamed[to/toward]-instruct acquire provide-Hey[behold/the]-quality reveal grace-Vav-[and/in addition]increase degree assure-Final-Nun-issue perseverance progress-

(those)אילין[S660] {אנ=to be affected in quality/to be prepared}=א Aleph-authority ability confirm-Yud-purpose posture actions-Lamed[to/toward]-instruct acquire provide-Yud-purpose posture actions-Final-Nun-issue perseverance progress-

(who ill)דביש[S2297] {ביש=belonging to/related to someone/something, i.e. the antithesis of good}=ד Dalet-faith establish presence-Beyt[within/in/inside]-pattern thought inhabit-Yud-purpose posture actions-שShin-pressure exchange disperse-

(ill)ביש[S2286] {ביש=the antithesis of good}=ב Beyt[within/in/inside]-pattern thought inhabit-Yud-purpose posture actions-שShin-pressure exchange disperse-

(had become)עבידין[S14998] {עבד=to make/create/write acting in a certain manner}=ע Ayin-pierce perceive wisdom-Beyt[within/in/inside]-pattern thought inhabit-Yud-purpose posture actions-Dalet-faith establish presence-Yud-purpose posture actions-Final-Nun-issue perseverance progress-

(with diseases)בכורהנא[S10508] {כרה=in exchange for}=ב Beyt[within/in/inside]-pattern thought inhabit-Kaph-surrender obtains consent-Vav-[and/in addition]increase degree assure-Resh-process beginning strength-Hey[behold/the]-quality reveal grace-Nun-seed patience continue-Final-Aleph-ending finish maturity-

(various)משתחלפא[S7204] {חלפ=diverse/different}=מ Mem[from/out of]-transform encounter remembrance-שShin-pressure exchange disperse-Hhet-specific share beyond-Lamed[to/toward]-instruct acquire provide-Pey-mouth SpokenWord speak-Final-Aleph-ending finish maturity-

(& those)ואיליי[S675] {אנ=also those which}=ו Vav-[and/in addition]increase degree assure-Aleph-authority ability confirm-Yud-purpose posture actions-Lamed[to/toward]-instruct acquire provide-Yud-purpose posture actions-Final-Nun-issue perseverance progress-

(who were afflicted)אליציין[S1038] {אלצ=perceiving narrow/troubled/constrained}=ד Dalet-faith establish presence-Aleph-authority ability confirm-Lamed[to/toward]-instruct acquire provide-Yud-purpose posture actions-Ayin-pierce perceive wisdom-Yud-purpose posture actions-Final-Nun-issue perseverance progress-

(with severe pain)בתשניקא[S21979] {שנק=with regard to affliction}=ב Beyt[within/in/inside]-pattern thought inhabit-Taw-evidence prove sign-שShin-pressure exchange disperse-Nun-seed patience continue-Yud-purpose posture actions-Quph-contrast parallel structure-Final-Aleph-ending finish maturity-

(& the demon possessed ones)ודיונא[S4376] {דין=the darkness of ink}=ו Vav-[and/in addition]increase degree assure-Dalet-faith establish presence-Yud-purpose posture actions-Vav-[and/in addition]increase degree assure-Nun-seed patience continue-Final-Aleph-ending finish maturity-

(& lunatics)אנברו[S3289] {ברא=to fashion/create always with God as subject}=א Aleph-authority ability confirm-Gimal-experience understanding encounter-Resh-process beginning strength-Final-Aleph-ending finish maturity-Vav-[and/in addition]increase degree assure-Dalet-faith establish presence-

(gather)שרדב[S204] {שרב=to repair/restore}=ש Resh-process beginning strength-Beyt[within/in/inside]-pattern thought inhabit-Vav-[and/in]addition increase degree assure-Dalet-faith establish presence-

(& paralytics)ומשריא[S22302] {שר=to loosen/abide/begin to dwell}=ו Mem[from/out of]-transform encounter remembrance-שShin-pressure exchange disperse-Resh-process beginning strength-Yud-purpose posture actions-Final-Aleph-ending finish maturity-

(& He healed)ואסי[S1596] {אס=to them}=א Aleph-authority ability confirm-Samech-adjust apprehend source-Yud-purpose posture actions-

(them)אנון[S4989] {חה=to heal}=א Aleph-authority ability confirm-Nun-seed patience continue-Vav-[and/in addition]increase degree assure-Final-Nun-issue perseverance progress-

The Semitic Emphasis

Also hearing to respond in report/nature/character with regard to/in exchange for all~~a length of line without width~~also to touch/to bring near beyond/above/outside of the whole reason~~for this is *to be affected in quality/to be prepared belonging to/related to someone/something, i.e. the antithesis of good~~the antithesis of good to make/create/write acting in a certain manner in exchange for diverse/different also those which perceiving narrow/troubled/constrained with regard to affliction the darkness of ink to fashion/create always with God as subject to gather to loosen/abide/begin to dwell to repair/restore to heal.*

In remembering what He has said to us at other times, we open ourselves to His voice, to hear His current word for us.

We cannot deal with this *S*elfish~*I*ndependent~*N*ature ourselves; therefore the Word came in flesh as humanity to deal with the question of its interference once and for all.

God did not make a mistake when He gave the Law, neither was He unaware that the Law would, in itself, not solve the problem of separation.

He knew and purposely designed the Law in such a way that it would intensify the conflict~~that it would reveal the problem for what it really was and reveal man's importance to solve the problem by himself.

He designed this environment of conflict~~a conflict that was working its way towards a climax.

Under the Law, humanity and their Creator God never meet face~to~face.

Instead of direct contact with God, the Law became the intermediary by which man related to God based on the knowledge of good and evil, right and wrong.

The Law maintained the distance between God and man and in so doing prolonged and intensified the conflict.

The Law was designed though, to reveal the very problem that kept humanity away from God.

""*For I delight in the law of God according to the inward man. But I see another law in my members, warring against the law of my mind, and bringing me into captivity to the law of sin which is in my members.*" ROMANS 7:21-22

The experience of humanity under the law is that there is a stronger influence in humanity that forces them to live contrary to what they knows is right.

Flesh became the domain of *S*elfish~*I*ndependent~*N*ature, and *lorded it over humanity* who remained helpless to change the situation of their living.

I
One sat alone beside the highway begging,

Got Healing?

His eyes were blind, the light he could not see;
He clutched his rags and shivered in the shadows,
Then Jesus came and bade his darkness flee.

Chorus
When Jesus comes the tempter's pow'r is broken;
When Jesus comes the tears are wiped away.
He takes the gloom and fills our lives with glory,
For all is changed when Jesus comes to stay.

2
From home and friends the evil spirits drove him,
Among the tombs he dwelt in misery;
He cut himself as demon pow'rs possessed him,
Then Jesus came and set the captive free.

3
"Unclean! unclean!" the leper cried in torment,
The deaf, the dumb, in helplessness stood near;
The fever raged, disease had gripped its victim,
Then Jesus came and cast out every fear.

4
Their hearts were sad as in the tomb they laid him,
For death had come and taken him away;
Their night was dark and bitter tears were falling,
Then Jesus came and night was turned to day.

5
So men today have found the Savior able,
They could not conquer passion, lust and sin;
Their broken hearts had left them sad and lonely,
Then Jesus came and dwelt, Himself, within.

Perceiving The Seed Of His Finished Work Parallels His Seed With The Balance Of His Strength And Perpetuates His Finished Work

MATTHEW 8:8
KJV+TVM

The centurion[G1543] answered[G611 [G5679]] and[G2532] said[G5346 [G5713]] Lord[G2962], I am[G1510 [G5748]] not[G3756] worthy[G2425] that[G2443] thou shouldest come[G1525 [G5632]] under[G5259] my[G3450] roof[G4721]: but[G235] speak[G2036 [G5628]] the word[G3056] only[G3440], and[G2532] my[G3450] servant[G3816] shall be healed[G2390 [G5701]].

ORIGINAL THOUGHTS
...(8:8) Perceiving the Seed of His Finished Work parallels His Seed with the balance of His Strength and perpetuates His Finished Work. Behold the increase assured by the Dominion of transcending each beginning to transform each of His Purpose providing His Finished Work. In exchange for the increase of His Finished Work the Seed of

Got Healing?

His completed efforts to establish the Intent of His Wsidom to assure each provision. By the evidence of His Purpose shown, encounter each mixture of instruction with learning to exercise the Abilities of acquiring His Finished Work. Within each instruction the Unseen increases His Faith enabling each remembrance to process each pattern~of~His~thought; while transforming the acquired evidence of His Finished Work. In addition to the Seed prove the Dominion/Authority apprehending His Finished Work as balancing each provision with every promise of His Purpose.

Perceiving the Seed of His Finished Work parallels His Seed with the balance of His Strength and perpetuates His Finished Work.

Thus, then, God the Word revealed Himself to men through His works.

We must next consider the end of His earthly life and the nature of His bodily death.

This is, indeed, the very center of our faith, and everywhere you hear men speak of it; by it, too, no less than by His other acts, Christ is revealed as God and Son of God.

We have seen that to change the corruptible to incorruption was proper to none other than the Savior Himself.

He it is, Who in the beginning made all things out of nothing; that only the Image of the Father could re-create the likeness of the Image in men, that none save our Lord Jesus Christ could give to mortals immortality, and that only the Word, Who orders all things and is alone the Father's true and sole~begotten Son could teach men about Him and abolish the worship of idols.

Here, then, is the second reason why the Word dwelt among us, namely that having proved His Godhead by His works, He might offer the sacrifice on behalf of all, surrendering His own temple to death in place of all, to settle humanity's account with death and free them from the primal transgression of a *S*elfish~*I*ndependent~*N*ature!

In the same act also He showed Himself mightier than death, displaying His own body incorruptible by becoming the first~fruits of the resurrection.

Behold the increase assured by the Dominion of transcending each beginning to transform each of His Purpose providing His Finished Work.

We are speaking of the good pleasure of God and of the things which

---

He in His loving wisdom thought fit to do, and it is better to put the same thing in several ways than to run the risk of leaving something out.

The body of the Word, then, being a real human body, in spite of its having been uniquely formed from a virgin, was of itself mortal and, like other bodies, liable to death.

However, *the indwelling of the Word* loosed it from this natural liability, so that corruption could not touch it.

Thus it happened that two opposite marvels took place at once: *the death of all was consummated in the Lord's body; yet, because the Word was in it, death and corruption were in the same act utterly abolished.*

In exchange for the increase of His Finished Work the Seed of His completed efforts to establish the Intent of His Wsidom to assure each provision.

Now that the common Savior of all has died on our behalf, we who believe in Christ no longer die, as men died aforetime, in fulfillment of the threat of the law.

That condemnation has come to an end; and now that, by the grace of the resurrection, corruption has been banished and done away, we are loosed from our mortal bodies in God's good time for each, so that we may obtain thereby a better resurrection.

Like seeds cast into the earth, we do not perish in our dissolution, but like them shall rise again, death having been brought to nought by the grace of the Savior.

That is why blessed Paul, through whom we all have surety of the resurrection, says: "*This corruptible must put on incorruption and this mortal must put on immortality; but when this corruptible shall have put on incorruption and this mortal shall have put on immortality, then shall be brought to pass the saying that is written, 'Death is swallowed up in victory. O Death, where is thy sting? O Grave, where is thy victory?*" FIRST CORINTHIANS 15:53 KJV

By the evidence of His Purpose shown, encounter each mixture of instruction with learning to exercise the Abilities of acquiring His Finished Work.

Just as it would not have been fitting for Him to give His body to death by His own hand, being Word and being Life, so also it was not consonant with Himself that He should avoid the death inflicted by others.

Rather, He pursued it to the uttermost, and in pursuance of His nature neither laid aside His body of His own accord nor escaped the plotting

Jews.

And this action showed no limitation or weakness in the Word; for He both waited for death in order to make an end of it, and hastened to accomplish it as an offering on behalf of all.

Moreover, as it was the death of all mankind that the Savior came to accomplish, not His own, He did not lay aside His body by an individual act of dying, for to Him, as Life, this simply did not belong.

However, He accepted death at the hands of men, thereby completely to destroy it in His own body.

Within each instruction, the Unseen increases His Faith enabling each remembrance to process each pattern~of~His~thought; while transforming the acquired evidence of His Finished Work.

Fitting indeed, then, and wholly consonant was the death on the cross for us; and we can see how reasonable it was, and why it is that the salvation of the world could be accomplished in no other way.

Even on the cross He did not hide Himself from sight; rather, He made all creation witness to the presence of its Maker.

Then, having once let it be seen that it was truly dead, He did not allow that temple of His body to linger long, but forthwith on the third day raised it up, impassable and incorruptible, the pledge and token of His victory.

It was, of course, within His power thus to have raised His body and displayed it as alive directly after death.

Nevertheless, the all-wise Savior did not do this, lest some should deny that it had really or completely died.

Besides this, had the interval between His death and resurrection been but two days, the glory of His incorruption might not have appeared.

He waited one whole day to show that His body was really dead, and then on the third day showed it incorruptible to all.

The interval was no longer, lest people should have forgotten about it and grown doubtful whether it were in truth the same body.

In addition to the Seed prove the Dominion/Authority apprehending His Finished Work as balancing each provision with every promise of His Purpose.

A very strong proof of this destruction of death and its conquest by the cross is supplied by a present fact, namely this.

Got Healing?

All the disciples of Christ despise death; they take the offensive against it and, instead of fearing it, by the sign of the cross and by faith in Christ trample on it as on something dead.

Before the divine sojourn of the Savior, even the holiest of men were afraid of death, and mourned the dead as those who perish.

But now that the Savior has raised His body, death is no longer terrible, but all those who believe in Christ tread it underfoot as nothing, and prefer to die rather than to deny their faith in Christ, knowing full well that when they die they do not perish, but live indeed, and have become incorruptible through His Faith as theirs, by believing in His Resurrection.

SEMITIC~ARAMAIC~HEBRAIC THESAURUS

Aramaic before first {

Semitic Root before first =

Lettering for ParaPhrase after second =

...(8:8) (answered)ויען S15985 ענא={to respond}=Ayin-pierce perceive wisdom-Nun-seed patience continue-Final-Aleph-ending finish maturity-

(the centurion)קנטרונא S16725 {קנטרונא=reigning to prevail}=Quph-contrast parallel structure-Nun-seed patience continue-Thet-contain mixture balance-Resh-process beginning strength-Vav-[and/in addition]increase degree assure-Nun-seed patience continue-Final-Aleph-ending finish maturity-

(that)הו S5044 {הו=he raises objection and solves it}=Hey[behold/the]-quality reveal grace-Vav-[and/in addition]increase degree assure-

(& he said)ואמר S1290 {אמר=making a legal declaration}=Vav-[and/in addition]increase degree assure-Aleph-authority ability confirm-Mem[from/out of]-transform encounter remembrance-Resh-process beginning strength-

(my Lord)מרי S12405 {מרי=the Master}=Mem[from/out of]-transform encounter remembrance-Resh-process beginning strength-Yud-purpose posture actions-

(not)לא S10878 {לא=without}=Lamed[to/toward]-instruct acquire provide-Final-Aleph-ending finish maturity-

(worthy)שוא S30200 {שוא=to be equal/to join together with someone}=Shin-pressure exchange disperse-Vav-[and/in addition]increase degree assure-Final-Aleph-ending finish maturity-

(I am)אנא S1378 {אנא=as for me}=Aleph-authority ability confirm-Nun-seed patience continue-Final-Aleph-ending finish maturity-

(that You should enter)דתעל S15607 {עלל=perceiving/desiring to enter into a place}=Dalet-faith establish presence-Taw-evidence prove sign-Ayin-pierce perceive wisdom-Vav-[and/in addition]increase degree assure-Lamed[to/toward]-instruct acquire provide-

(under)תחית S22770 {תחית=instead of}=Taw-evidence prove sign-Het-specific share beyond-Yud-purpose posture actions-Taw-evidence prove sign-

(my roof)מטללי S22006 {טלל=covering with pieces}=Mem[from/out of]-transform encounter remembrance-Thet-contain mixture balance-Lamed[to/toward]-instruct acquire provide-Lamed[to/toward]-instruct acquire provide-Yud-purpose posture actions-

(but)אלא S892 {אלא=except/unless}=Aleph-authority ability confirm-Lamed[to/toward]-instruct acquire provide-Final-Aleph-ending finish maturity-

(only)בלחוד S1149 {חור=on the sole condition that}=Beyt[within/in/inside]-pattern thought inhabit-Lamed[to/toward]-instruct acquire provide-Het-specific share beyond-Vav-[and/in addition]increase degree assure-Dalet-faith establish presence-

(say)אמר S1243 {אמר=making a legal declaration}=Aleph-authority ability confirm-Mem[from/out of]-transform encounter remembrance-Resh-process beginning strength-

(in a word)במלתא S12081 {מלל=with regard to promise}=Beyt[within/in/inside]-pattern thought inhabit-Mem[from/out of]-transform encounter remembrance-Lamed[to/toward]-instruct acquire provide-Taw-evidence prove sign-Final-Aleph-ending finish maturity-

(& will be healed)ונתאסא S1609 {אסא=to repair/restore}=Vav-[and/in addition]increase degree assure-Nun-seed patience continue-Taw-evidence prove sign-Aleph-authority ability confirm-Samech-adjust apprehend source-Final-Aleph-ending finish maturity-

(my boy)טלי S8154 {טליא=to lift up/to make dependent on hope}=Thet-contain mixture balance-Lamed[to/toward]-instruct acquire provide-Yud-purpose posture actions-Yud-purpose posture actions-

---

The Semitic Emphasis

<u>To respond reigning to prevail he raises objection and solves it making a legal declaration~~the Master</u>
<u>without to be equal/to join together with someone~~as for me perceiving/desiring to enter into a place</u>
<u>instead of covering with pieces~~except/unless on the sole condition that making a legal declaration</u>
<u>with regard to promise to repair/restore to lift up/to make dependent on hope.</u>

In a word, then, those who disbelieve in the resurrection have no support in facts, if their gods and evil spirits do not drive away the supposedly dead Christ.

Rather, it is He Who convicts them of being dead.

We are agreed that a dead person can do nothing: *yet the Savior works mightily every day, drawing men to relationship, persuading them to virtue, teaching them about immortality, quickening their thirst for heavenly things, revealing the knowledge of the Father, inspiring strength in face of death, manifesting Himself to each, and displacing the irreligion of idols; while the gods and evil spirits of the unbelievers can do none of these things, but rather become dead at Christ's presence, all their ostentation barren and void.*

By the sign of the cross, on the contrary, all magic is stayed, all sorcery confounded, all the idols are abandoned and deserted, and all senseless pleasure ceases, as the eye of faith looks up from earth to heaven.

Who then, are we to call dead?

Shall we call Christ dead, Who causes all of this?

Nevertheless, the dead have not the faculty to cause anything.

Or shall we call death dead, which causes nothing whatever, but lies as lifeless and ineffective as are the evil spirits and the idols?

The Son of God, *"living and effective,"* is active every day and effects the salvation of all.

However, death is daily proved to be stripped of all its strength, and it is the idols and the evil spirits who are dead, not He.

No room for doubt remains, therefore, concerning the resurrection of His body.

Surrender In Faith Of The Grace
He Insures Through His Finished Work

MATTHEW 8:16
KJV+TVM

When^{G1161} the even^{G3798} was come,^{G1096} they brought^{G4374} unto him^{G846} many^{G4183}

that were possessed with devils:[G1139] and[G2532] he cast out[G1544] the[G3588] spirits[G4151] with his word,[G3056] and[G2532] healed[G2323] all[G3956] that were sick:[G2192][G2560]

ORIGINAL THOUGHTS

...(8:16) Surrender in Faith of the Grace He insures through His Finished Work.

In faith position every issue of process to transform each exchange of His Finished Work, paralleling each beginning in the pattern~of~His~thoughts to increase the building of His Faith in the memories that insure/assure the qualities of every purpose. Establish each intent through the increase of every seed, finished and perfecting each adjusting with His Understanding working to confirm His Finished Work. In addition, the empowering of His Spoken Word builds and settles the focus of adding each position of His Grace to posture with increase, the actions of quality that insure progress. Within the memories of teaching that prove His Finished Work, enlarge and inspire agreement providing the Grace of His Truth to discover the outflow that confirms the purpose of teachings creating every development. With the presence of each Pattern~of~His~Thought, enable the exchange of His Dominion in purpose of proving the Wisdom of His Indwelling, and posturing His Faith so as to discern His Faith in purpose of each recovery. Behold every increase of His Design and enable the apprehending of His Purpose to confirm His Patience assuring each persistence.

<u>Surrender in Faith of the Grace He insures through His Finished Work.</u>

The stipulation of His Faith's operation is that we believe beyond the point of our reality, and claim His Word Spoken as be the real purpose of our living at this point of need.

Healing, though present in the Old Testament, was more of a stream when compared to the flood of healing we see in the New Testament.

REMEMBER: *It is NEVER about what we HAVE TO DO; it is ALWAYS about what the Father wants to do, and HAS FINISHED IN CHRIST JESUS!*

<u>In faith position every issue of process to transform each exchange of His Finished Work, paralleling each beginning in the pattern~of~His~thoughts to increase the building of His Faith in the memories that insure/assure the qualities of every purpose.</u>

The beginning of any prayer for healing must involve God!

It is *through the name of Jesus, by the power of the Spirit within us, and in the will of the Father* that His Healing Flow releases throughout the individual's body, for whom we are praying!

AGAIN: *it is never what we have to do; it is always what God wants to do!*

Got Healing?

Establish each intent through the increase of every seed, finished and perfecting each adjusting with His Understanding working to confirm His Finished Work.

Discover each motive/reason for the hidden intentions of being a part of the mindsets controlling our living.

It is FACT: the mindsets by which our living is controlled hinder or surrender to the Lord's desire to heal completely.

We must come to believe that a deficiency in love is at the heart of most of, if not in fact, all of our trouble.

The greatest longing of our hearts is to be in union, to love and to be loved.

God has created us in His Divine Image, and God desires union with us; therefore our hearts cannot be at rest until this desire for union with God is satisfied.

In addition, the empowering of His Spoken Word builds and settles the focus of adding each position of His Grace to posture with increase, the actions of quality that insure progress.

Our lives are shaped by those who love us, by those who refuse to love us, and by those who can't love us.

We need to be loved into being, first by God, then by others.

Those who are born into rigid, disengaged, emotionally unavailable families may need to experience the healing love of Jesus much more than those who are born into nurturing, loving families.

Acknowledging, and then accepting the LOVE OF GOD makes us more pliable and teachable, in order to acknowledge and accept another's love as well.

The wounded, inner child perceives the world and relationships with fear, suspicion, and mistrust.

And yet the opposite is often true~~we keep on reaching out for LOVE, affirmation, and deepened relationships.

What we find is the timeless, healing power of God's LOVE can reach that inner child and bring the wholeness and freedom that we all long for.

Within the memories of teaching that prove His Finished Work, enlarge and inspire agreement providing the Grace of His Truth to discover the outflow that confirms the purpose of teachings creating every development.

We need, through prayer and surrender, to ask God to HEAL the destructive aspects our past.

This method of *surrender/prayer* is also called, *inner healing, the healing of the heart, and the healing of all memories, past~present~future!*

His Faith in us must become a function within our will, as His thoughts become our thoughts as well.

Learn to rebuke/reprove/censure thoughts that accept sickness to operate in the body/physical.

Next, rebuke/reprove/censure thought accepting sickness, and accommodate such sicknesses~~by the *"grit~your~teeth"* exercise.

Daddy always said, *"it only takes two thinks to serve God and embrace healing: 1)-grit and 2)-grace: if you supply the grit, God will always supply the Grace"*!

Discover that our loving God has equipped us with enough *chutzpah/grit* to overcome the objections of mind, emotions, and symptoms.

If we willfully persist in using our authority to rebuke these things for a few minutes, over 98% of new symptoms disappear within hours.

When an illness is thoroughly entrenched, it usually takes longer.

Never continue to accept thoughts that project the undeniable and unopposable part of yourselves.

These type of thoughts must be *cast down*, through exalting the Majesty and Person of the Lord Jesus Christ above EVERYTHING ELSE!

With the presence of each Pattern~of~His~Thought, enable the exchange of His Dominion in purpose of proving the Wisdom of His Indwelling, and posturing His Faith so as to discern His Faith in purpose of each recovery.

We can willingly and willfully direct our thoughts to align with God's to see the moving of healing throughout our physical being, as well as our mental habitation.

"Finally, brethren, whatsoever things are true, whatsoever things are honest, whatsoever things are just, whatsoever things are pure, whatsoever things are lovely, whatsoever things are of good report; if there be any virtue, and if there be any praise, think on these things." PHILIPPIANS 4:8 KJV

Rebuke improper thoughts about yourselves, and refuse to let such thoughts to have any influence over you.

If a feeling of guilt accompanies such thought, rebuke those as well.

Take your authority, *THROUGH THE NAME OF JESUS*, knowing

that you have been given the very best of God's arsenal in being a winning~part to every battle and skirmish.

Behold every increase of His Design and enable the apprehending of His Purpose to confirm His Patience assuring each persistence.

Don't be a spiritual *"freeloader"*!

Don't just expect God to do everything in your living, when you are, in most instances, your own worst enemy!

Go ahead~~cuss, rant, rave, get angry, tell God off~~~By the way, how's that workin' for you?

No, you are responsible to fellowship with those of like precious faith; you're responsible to hold to God's promises, and speak the fresh manna from heaven out of your mouth consistently, contagiously, consciously, and continuously.

Our task, as believers, is bringing our thoughts/words/deeds/habits/mindsets into conformity and agreement with Jesus Christ, and the Word He has spoken for our benefit.

SEMITIC~ARAMAIC~HEBRAIC THESAURUS

Aramaic before first {

Semitic Root before first =

Lettering for ParaPhrase after second =

(8·16) (when) S9812 {ш=inasmuch as}= Kaph-surrender obtains consent- Dalet-faith establish presence- (it was) S5086 {=the Self~Same One}= Hey[behold/the]-quality reveal grace- Vav-[and/in addition]increase degree assure- Final-Aleph-ending finish maturity- (but) S4405 {=advocated}= Dalet-faith establish presence- Yud-purpose posture actions- Final-Nun-issue perseverance progress- (evening) S20086 {=at the close of the day}= Resh-process beginning strength- Mem[from/out of]-transform encounter remembrance- Shin-pressure exchange disperse- Final-Aleph-ending finish maturity- (they brought) S19007 {=to approach/be near}= Quph-contrast parallel structure- Resh-process beginning strength- Beyt[within/in/inside]-pattern thought inhabit- Vav-[and/in addition]increase degree assure- (before Him) S18102 {=in the presence of/reflecting close relationship to a king or God}= Quph-contrast parallel structure- Dalet-faith establish presence- Mem[from/out of]-transform encounter remembrance- Vav-[and/in addition]increase degree assure- Hey[behold/the]-quality reveal grace- Yud-purpose posture actions- (demon possessed) S4375 {=to invade/attack}= Dalet-faith establish presence- Yud-purpose posture actions- Vav-[and/in addition]increase degree assure- Nun-seed patience continue- Final-Aleph-ending finish maturity- (many) S13929 {=being multiplied}= Samech-adjust apprehend source- Gimal-experience understanding encounter- Yud-purpose posture actions- Aleph-authority ability confirm- Final-Aleph-ending finish maturity- (& He cast out) S13368 {=causing to come forth/to remove/expel}= Vav-[and/in addition]increase degree assure- Aleph-authority ability confirm- Pey-mouth SpokenWord speak- Quph-contrast parallel structure- (their demons) S4369 {=the efficient source of control/desire}= Dalet-faith establish presence- Yud-purpose posture actions- Vav-[and/in addition]increase degree assure- Yud-purpose posture actions- Hey[behold/the]-quality reveal grace- Vav-[and/in addition]increase degree assure- Final-Nun-issue perseverance progress- (with a word) S12081 {=with regard to/in exchange for a promise}= Beyt[within/in/inside]-pattern thought inhabit- Mem[from/out of]-transform encounter remembrance- Lamed[to/toward]-instruct acquire provide- Taw-evidence prove sign- Final-Aleph-ending finish maturity- (& all of them) S10069 {=the whole reason for this is}= Vav-[and/in addition]increase degree assure- Lamed[to/toward]-

Got Healing?

instruct acquire provide-₍Kaph-surrender obtains consent-₍Lamed[to/toward]-instruct acquire provide-₍Hey[behold/the]-quality reveal grace-₍Vav-[and/in addition]increase degree assure-₍Final-Nun-issue perseverance progress- (who) אילין *S660* ﹛ﬞﬞ=those which﹜=א Aleph-authority ability confirm-₍Yud-purpose posture actions- Lamed[to/toward]-instruct acquire provide-₍Yud-purpose posture actions-₍Final-Nun-issue perseverance progress- (ill) דבישאית *S2313* ﹛=perceived ruin/destruction﹜= Dalet-faith establish presence-₍Beyt[within/in/inside]-pattern thought inhabit-₍Yud-purpose posture actions-₍Shin-pressure exchange disperse-₍Aleph-authority ability confirm-₍Yud-purpose posture actions-₍Taw-evidence prove sign- (become) עבידין *S14998* ﹛=transferring ownership/remaking/repairing﹜= Ayin-pierce perceive wisdom-₍Beyt[within/in/inside]-pattern thought inhabit-₍Yud-purpose posture actions-₍Dalet-faith establish presence-₍Yud-purpose posture actions-₍Final-Nun-issue perseverance progress- (had) הוו *S5147* ﹛=the self-same one﹜- Hey[behold/the]-quality reveal grace-₍Vav-[and/in addition]increase degree assure-₍Vav-[and/in addition]increase degree assure- (He healed) אסי *S1582* ﹛=repairing/refuting﹜ Aleph-authority ability confirm-₍Samech-adjust apprehend source-₍Yud-purpose posture actions- (them) אנין *S4989* ﹛=these﹜ Aleph-authority ability confirm-₍Nun-seed patience continue-₍Vav-[and/in addition]increase degree assure-₍Final-Nun-issue perseverance progress-

The Semitic Emphasis

<u>Inasmuch as the Self~Same One advocated at the close of the day~~to approach/be near in the presence of/reflecting close relationship to a king or God~~to invade/attack being multiplied~~causing to come forth/to remove/expel the efficient source of control/desire~~with regard to/in exchange for a promise~~the whole reason for this is those which perceived ruin/destruction transferring ownership/remaking/repairing the self~same one repairing/refuting these.</u>

What kinds of thoughts bother you?

Thoughts related to temptation; thoughts designed to produce fear in you; thoughts of superiority over others; thoughts of self-condemnation; thoughts which counter the revealed Word of God; thoughts of lust; thoughts which promote dishonesty.

Take authority over them.

Don't be passive or fatalistic about them.

When you exercise your will against these things, God swings into action to augment your decision and His power is released against that which is attacking you.

Our God is addicted to incarnation.

Having created us in His image, He is determined to reveal His image in us, do His works through us, and speak His words through us.

He is not an exclusionist; however, He does reserve to Himself the managing of the galaxies, the seasons, genetic decisions, and the number of hairs on our heads, without our help.

Nevertheless, He places a very significant amount of humanity's interaction in humanity's hands, and He seems always eager to increase rather than decrease this mode of operation.

Specify The Purpose Of His Faith

To Position By Perseverance
The Parallels Of Strengthened Pattern~Thoughts
Increasing The Teachings Of His Grace/Truth

MATTHEW 12:22
KJV+TVM

Then[G5119] was brought[G4374] unto Him[G846] one possessed with a devil,[G1139] blind,[G5185] and[G2532] dumb:[G2974] and[G2532] He healed[G2323] him,[G846] insomuch that[G5620] the[G3588] blind[G5185] and[G2532] dumb[G2974] both[G2532] spake[G2980] and[G2532] saw.[G991]

ORIGINAL THOUGHTS

...(12:22) Specify the purpose of His Faith to position by perseverance the parallels of strengthened pattern~thoughts increasing the teachings of His Grace/Truth. Exhibit every intention by increasing the seed of His Finished Work, when specifying the proving of His Faith to share in beginnings that expand/stretch the additions of His Wisdom to assure the actions as strengthened. In addition, enable/empower/initiate apprehending every purpose of the Grace of His Truth by agreeing with actions that consent to the seeding of His Finished Work, to spread beyond beginnings that exchange with His Finished Work. Any degree of adjusting transforms the actions of His Finished Work, so continue restoring provision providing each increase of His Pattern~of~Thought determining the instrument of His Finished Work.

Specify the purpose of His Faith to position by perseverance the parallels of strengthened pattern~thoughts increasing the teachings of His Grace/Truth.

Many mainline churches focus primarily on Jesus' teaching and preaching ministries (*explanation of God's love*), while giving little attention to Jesus' healing ministry (*experience of God's love*).

This is puzzling, since 40% of the Gospels of Matthew and Mark, and about a third of

Luke and John, focus on healing.

The book of Acts exhibits a similar abundance of healing miracles. Jesus sent His disciples out to (1) *"preach the Gospel,"* (2) *"heal the sick,"* (3) *"raise the dead,"* and (4) *"cast out demons."* MATTHEW 10:1; LUKE 9:1, 10:1

This verse alone, presents a four~folded Gospel, which is a matter of ongoing process, from beginning to end, in the living of every believer following after the Lord Jesus!

These were *"signs"* of the Kingdom of God.

Got Healing?

All of these are part of His commission to *"teach them obey all things whatsoever I have commanded you."*

Many have emphasized true doctrine or *"explanation and proclamation,"* almost to the <u>exclusion</u> of an experience of God and His powerful Spirit.

Today's churches seem to have lost that connection between salvation and healing.

> *The ancient Christian communities, healing prayer and laying on of hands were commonplace and significant liturgical practices. But large-scale deaths, such as those caused by the Black Plague during the Middle Ages, led Christians to associate "salvation" with saving souls for the afterlife. From the Renaissance on, medicine dominated to the point where Christians started viewing it as a replacement for, rather than a complement to prayer. The Enlightenment tended to separate the physical from the spiritual (dualism). By the mid-20th century, mainline Christians were so committed to rationalism that they often felt a need to give "scientific" explanations for Biblical stories of healing—even if doing so distorted the stories.*

<u>Exhibit every intention by increasing the seed of His Finished Work, when specifying the proving of His Faith to share in beginnings that expand/stretch the additions of His Wisdom to assure the actions as strengthened.</u>

Healing is not about us, *but about giving Jesus the glory and serving others with God's power.*

God is always ready to heal our spiritual attitudes. This may be the most difficult healing of all, due to the imbedded nature of the physical within our psyche. Physical and emotional healing can, and will however, follow. *LUKE 5 KJV*

The more the Word of God invades the thoughts of our mindsets, the greater the implosion of His Will, His Way, through His Word!

The more we discover in His Word that which IS HIM, the greater the delivering of His Healing~Force that brings to the forefront all He promised.

<u>In addition, enable/empower/initiate apprehending every purpose of the Grace of His Truth by agreeing with actions that consent to the seeding of His Finished Work, to spread beyond beginnings that exchange with His Finished Work.</u>

The product of our choice is left to us.

If it is the *healing of body* that we seek, then that is available.

However, we must approach the Wisdom of God from the vantage point of His Thoughts, by embracing ALL THAT HE IS, so that we can

---

enjoy all that He is in all that is us!

Healing is the second of the four~folded process, wherein by the Presence of the Spirit we are RENEWED to RECLAIM and RESPOND to the splendor of His Grace and Mercy throughout our lifetime here, and in eternity.

Any degree of adjusting transforms the actions of His Finished Work, so continue restoring provision providing each increase of His Pattern~of~Thought determining the instrument of His Finished Work.

Even when the soul opens a little, the Spirit of God rushes in to fill the aching void of the heart, mind, and body with the Love, Grace, and Mercy of ALL THAT IS HIMSELF!

Just as some have viewed medicine as a replacement for (_rather than a complement to_) prayer, others have gone to the opposite extreme, endangering themselves or others by refusing medical intervention.

God as The Incarnate Presence works not only through prayer, but also through all practices that <u>honor</u> the body, including science and the medical arts.

All things HEALING, <u>MUST</u> begin in Him, with Him at the helm of our living.

SEMITIC~ARAMAIC~HEBRAIC THESAURUS
Aramaic before first {
Semitic Root before first =
Lettering for ParaPhrase after second =

...(12:22) (then) ‬יְדִי‪ S4405 {=then}= Hhet-specific share beyond- Yud-purpose posture actions- Dalet-faith establish presence- Yud-purpose posture actions- Final-Nun-issue perseverance progress- (they brought) ‬קְרְבוּ‪ S19007 {=to approach/be near}= Quph-contrast parallel structure- Resh-process beginning strength- Beyt[within/in/inside]-pattern thought inhabit- Vav-[and/in addition]increase degree assure- (to Him) ‬לֵהּ‪ S10842 {=it is necessary}= Lamed[to/toward]-instruct acquire provide- Hey[behold/the]-quality reveal grace- (demoniac) ‬דֵּיוָנָא‪ S4374 {=to subdue/rule}= Dalet-faith establish presence- Yud-purpose posture actions- Vav-[and/in addition]increase degree assure- Nun-seed patience continue- Final-Aleph-ending finish maturity- (a certain) ‬חַד‪ S6244 {=by how much more}= Hhet-specific share beyond- Dalet-faith establish presence- (mute) ‬חַרֵשׁ‪ S7636 {=perceiving/desiring/requesting without speech}= Dalet-faith establish presence- Hhet-specific share beyond- Resh-process beginning strength- Shin-pressure exchange disperse- (& blinded) ‬וּעֵוַר‪ S15414 {=to be laid bare/act in an aroused manner/to put out the eyes}= Vav-[and/in addition]increase degree assure- Ayin-pierce perceive wisdom- Vav-[and/in addition]increase degree assure- Yud-purpose posture actions- Resh-process beginning strength- (& He healed him) ‬וְאַסְיֵהּ‪ S1597 {=to repair}= Vav-[and/in addition]increase degree assure- Aleph-authority ability confirm- Samech-adjust apprehend source- Yud-purpose posture actions- Hey[behold/the]-quality reveal grace- (so that) ‬אַכְנָא‪ S638 {=in such a way that}= Aleph-authority ability confirm- Kaph-surrender obtains consent- Nun-seed patience continue- Final-Aleph-ending finish maturity- (the mute) ‬חַרְשָׁא‪ S7637 {=being silent}= Dalet-faith establish presence- Hhet-specific share beyond- Resh-process beginning strength- Shin-pressure exchange disperse- Final-Aleph-ending finish maturity- (& blind man) ‬וּסְמַיָא‪ S14527 {=losing sight}= Vav-[and/in addition]increase degree assure- Samech-adjust apprehend source-

Mem[from/out of]-transform encounter remembrance-Yud-purpose posture actions-Final-Aleph-ending finish maturity-(could speak) נמלל S12063 {U ᴍᴍ=enable someone to speak}=נ Nun-seed patience continue-Mem[from/out of]-transform encounter remembrance-Lamed[to/toward]-instruct acquire provide-Lamed[to/toward]-instruct acquire provide-(& could see)ביחזא S6666 {ח ⊏ᴍ=to understand/realize}=ו Vav-[and/in addition]increase degree assure-Beyt[within/in/inside]-pattern thought inhabit-Hhet-specific share beyond-Zayin-skill alter instrument-Final-Aleph-ending finish maturity-

The Semitic Emphasis

Then to approach/be near~~it is necessary to subdue/rule by how much more perceiving/desiring/requesting without speech to be laid bare/act in an aroused manner/to put out the eyes~~to repair in such a way that being silent~~losing sight~~enable someone to speak to understand/realize.

Things seemingly forgotten have the potential of becoming a great source of harm.

These secrets of the soul dwell in the darkness of our shame.

These crushing, painful memories can rise up to destroy us in body, mind, and spirit.

We may be able to survive with broken bodies, but not with broken spirits: _"The soul's attitude will endure sickness; but a broken spirit who can bear?"_ PROVERBS 18:14

In the process of inner healing, our wounded memories become a source of healing.

Once we identify the pain and bring it into the light, Jesus can transform it and free us from its crippling effects.

He doesn't erase the memory, but he does remove the devastating effect of the memory.

After prayer we can still remember what happened, but the memory no longer has its old power over us.

In Addition To Continuing His Spoken Word
By Building Every Purpose/Intent
By The Exchange Of Each Portion Of His Wisdom
Share The Skills Of His Finished Work

MATTHEW 14:14
KJV+TVM

And[G2532] Jesus[G2424] went forth[G1831] and saw[G1492] a great[G4183] multitude[G3793] and[G2532] was moved with compassion[G4697] toward[G1909] them[G846] and[G2532] he healed[G2323] their[G846] sick[G732]

Got Healing?

ORIGINAL THOUGHTS

...(14:14) In addition to continuing His Spoken Word, build every purpose/intent, by the exchange of each portion of His Wisdom, sharing the skills of His Finished Work. Obtain the patience of exchanging His Finished Work, and apprehend the understanding to act by agreement/consent toward His Finished Work. In addition, encourage the evidence of every beginning through unseen prevail that perceives the teachings focused upon discoveries assuring progress. In addition to His Dominion, adjust through actions that surrender to each process that positions you in the Grace of His Truth, while exercising the real portion of perseverance.

In addition to continuing His Spoken Word, build every purpose/intent, by the exchange of each portion of His Wisdom, sharing the skills of His Finished Work.

It is truly astounding that whenever the sick approach Jesus and ask for healing, Jesus responds by making them well.

We have no record of Jesus ever refusing to heal someone.

The extraordinary thing is that Jesus is never recorded as having told a sick person (*as we might be tempted to do*) that God was testing that person in order to teach him patience.

Instead, we always read that Jesus *healed the one who asked*.

Sickness is not seen as a blessing in disguise, but as a curse.

The gospels encourage us to pray for sickness to go away.

Biblical healing focuses on and gives glory to Jesus alone.

Obtain the patience of exchanging His Finished Work, and apprehend the understanding to act by agreement/consent toward His Finished Work.

Instead of just seeking "a healing", why not discover how to completely release the fullness of the God of our creation, within the midst of us, His Creation?

If we try turning on an electric iron and it does not work, we look to the wiring of the iron, the cord, or the house. We do not stand in dismay before the iron and cry, "Oh, electricity, please come into my iron and make it work!" We realize that while the whole world is full of that mysterious power we call electricity, only the amount that flows through the wiring of the iron will make the iron work for us.

The same principle is true of the creative energy of God. The whole universe is full of it, but only the amount of it that flows through our own being will work for us.

Got Healing?

Learn, in His Presence, how to allow the FLOW OF THE SPIRIT to operate within your living.

We doubt the *willingness* or the *ability* of God to actually produce within our lives and bodies the results that we desire.

We do not doubt our own ability to come into His presence and fill ourselves with Him, but we do doubt His willingness to be in us, filling us with Himself by His Indwelling.

In addition, encourage the evidence of every beginning through unseen prevail that perceives the teachings focused upon discoveries assuring progress.

If our minds and thoughts are filled with hesitancies, and indecisions; or perhaps there is bitterness and resolves of hatred spewing out distinctions that do not honor the God of the living; then, we must realize we are setting ourselves up for failure.

If instead, we could embrace the *joy that is on the inside of our being*, the joy that is HIM, we would find an inexplicable amount of REST in trusting that He is our God, and He knows how to remedy what ails us!

That which is available to ALL OF US is the *infinite LIFE OF GOD Himself!*

When we know we are safe within His Person, we KNOW we have *whatsoever we ask*, through Jesus' name!

In addition to His Dominion, adjust through actions that surrender to each process that positions you in the Grace of His Truth, while exercising the real portion of perseverance.

In addition to praying for others, realize that as you pray, those needs you may have personally can be met as well!

"Greater love hath no man than this that a man lay down his life for his friends." JOHN 15:13 KJV

Our prayers are the laying down of our needs in place of the needs of another.

This is the redeeming aspect of Calvary, as well as every part of Jesus' life and ministry upon this earth, and throughout eternity!

SEMITIC~ARAMAIC~HEBRAIC THESAURUS
Aramaic before first {
Semitic Root before first =
Lettering for ParaPhrase after second =

...(14:14) (& came down)וַיֵּצֵא S13381 {◌◌=and issuing forth}= Vav-[and/in addition]increase degree assure- Nun-seed patience continue- Pey-mouth SpokenWord speak- Quph-contrast parallel structure-

(Yeshua)יֵשׁוּעַ S9573 {◌◌=being saved}= Yud-purpose posture actions- Shin-pressure exchange disperse- Vav-[and/in addition]increase degree assure- Ayin-pierce perceive wisdom-

(seeing)רָאָה S6673 {◌◌=to see/understand/realize}= Hhet-specific share beyond- Zayin-skill alter instrument- Final-Aleph-ending finish maturity-

(the crowds)כְנֻשָׁא S10319 {◌◌=gathering}= Kaph-surrender obtains consent- Nun-seed patience continue- Shin-pressure exchange disperse- Final-Aleph-ending finish maturity-

(great)סַגִּיא S13929 {◌◌=in a manifold way}= Aleph-authority ability confirm- Yud-purpose posture actions- Gimal-experience understanding encounter- Samech-adjust apprehend source- Final-Aleph-ending finish maturity-

(& He was moved with pity)אֶתְרַחַם S19796 {◌◌=to desire/prefer/have mercy upon}= Aleph-authority ability confirm- Taw-evidence prove sign- Resh-process beginning strength- Hhet-specific share beyond- Final-Mem-trial fashions prevail-

(for them)עֲלֵיהוֹן S15705 {◌◌=in measure of}= Ayin-pierce perceive wisdom- Lamed[to/toward]-instruct acquire provide- Yud-purpose posture actions- Hey[behold/the]-quality reveal grace- Vav-[and/in addition]increase degree assure- Final-Nun-issue perseverance progress-

(& He healed)וְאַסִּי S1596 {◌◌=to repair/restore}= Vav-[and/in addition]increase degree assure- Aleph-authority ability confirm- Samech-adjust apprehend source- Yud-purpose posture actions-

(their sick)כְרִיהַיְהוֹן S10539 {◌◌=false weakness}= Kaph-surrender obtains consent- Resh-process beginning strength- Yud-purpose posture actions- Hey[behold/the]-quality reveal grace- Yud-purpose posture actions- Hey[behold/the]-quality reveal grace- Vav-[and/in addition]increase degree assure- Final-Nun-issue perseverance progress-

The Semitic Emphasis

And issuing forth being saved~~to see/understand/realize gathering in a manifold way~~to desire/prefer/have mercy upon in measure of to repair/restore false weakness.

God is both within us and without us.

He is the Source of all life; the Creator of universe behind universe; and of unimaginable depths of inter-stellar space and of light-years without end.

However, He is also *The Indwelling Life* of our own little selves.

And just as a whole world full of electricity will not light a house unless the house itself is prepared to receive that electricity; even so the infinite and eternal life of God cannot help us, unless we are prepared to receive that life within ourselves.

Only the amount of God that we release by TRUSTING HIM COMPLETELY, will work for us.

"The Kingdom of God is within you," said Jesus.

It is *the Indwelling Light, the secret Place of our Consciousness of the Most High* that is the Kingdom of God in its present manifestation in our earthen vessel.

Learning to live IN the Kingdom of God is learning to turn on the light of God within.

Adding Each Parallel Of Beginning Pattern~Thoughts Increases The Teachings That Insure

Got Healing?

The Evidence In The Grace Of His Truth

MATTHEW 15:30
KJV+TVM

And^{G2532} great^{G4183} multitudes^{G3793} came^{G4334} unto him,^{G846} having^{G2192} with^{G3326} them^{G1438} those that were lame,^{G5560} blind,^{G5185} dumb,^{G2974} maimed,^{G2948} and^{G2532} many^{G4183} others,^{G2087} and^{G2532} cast them down^{G4496} ^{G846} at^{G3844} Jesus^{G2424} feet;^{G4228} and^{G2532} he healed^{G2323} them:^{G846}

ORIGINAL THOUGHTS

...(15:30) *Adding each parallel of beginning pattern~thoughts, increases the teachings that insure the evidence in the Grace of His Truth, and obtain the resources enlarging His Finished Work. Adjusting to experiences of every purpose we enable His Finished Work to establish and confirm actions that prove the quality of every portion assured through His Wisdom, while transforming each discovery of increased progress. The Unseen encounters that process His Finished Work, assures the apprehending of each remembrance that exercises the perfected completion of each portion His Spoken Word enhances through the positionings of His Finished Work. Increase then, the determination of handling the pressings/compellings of His Finished Work, by increasing His Spoken Word for the exchange of actions that only encounter His Finished Work. Adjusting each experience to locate the abilities of completed influences, assures the agreement in process of encountering the workings that increase toward each portion of evidence.*

Adding each parallel of beginning pattern~thoughts, increases the teachings that insure the evidence in the Grace of His Truth, and obtain the resources enlarging His Finished Work.

His parallels of pattern~thoughts coincide with everything His Will and Design have planned for all of humanity.

If we are patient enough to allow the seasons designed by His Wisdom, and Understanding, there is provided to us a virtual myriad of multiplicities, whereby any believer remains in blessings personified.

If we patiently await His Season, and timing, we never fail at attaining to the goals and imaginations that we prophetically see as coming, through our prayer~lives, our study~lives, and through ourselves as individuals.

Adjusting to experiences of every purpose we enable His Finished Work to establish and confirm actions that prove the quality of every portion assured through His Wisdom, while transforming each discovery of increased progress.

Some day we will understand the scientific principles that underlie the miracle-working powers of God, and we will accept His intervention as simply and naturally as we do the radio.

We must begin to realize that everything that is around us, and flowing through us is a marvel of God's Creative Majesty.

It is always when two atoms of Hydrogen join with one atom of Oxygen that water indeed is made.

A REMARKABLE DISCOVERY LINKING the biblical alphabets of Hebrew and Arabic to modern chemistry reveals that a lost code—a translatable alphabet—and a clue to the mystery of our origins, has lived within us all along. Applying this discovery to the language of life, the familiar elements of **hydrogen, nitrogen, oxygen, and carbon** that form our DNA may now be replaced with key letters of the ancient languages.

In doing so, the code of all life is transformed into the words of a timeless message.

Translated, the message reveals that the precise letters of God's ancient name are encoded as the genetic information in every cell, of every life.

The message reads: "*God/Eternal within the body.*"

The meaning: *Humankind is one family, united through a common heritage, and the result of an intentional act of creation!*

The discovery of God's name within the essence of all life demonstrates that we are related not only to one another, but also to life itself, in the most intimate way imaginable.

By the command of His Faith, through our dominion given of Him, the God; the Word of God become a super~imposition/demand/request of the higher law of His Life over a lower law of biology, anthropology, and/or faith~filled words and thoughts; where then is the conflict except in our unwillingness to surrender to His Ultimate Plan of Health and Eternal Life!

The Unseen encounters that process His Finished Work, assures the apprehending of each remembrance that exercises the perfected completion of each portion His Spoken Word enhances through the positionings of His Finished Work.

God does nothing except by the limitations of boundaries He has placed upon the world, the humanity He created, and Himself.

Nonetheless, He has provided enough power within His the limitations of His boundaries to do anything that is in accordance with His will.

His Will includes unlimited miracles.

It is for us to learn His will, and to seek the simplicity and the beauty of the limitations of boundaries that set free His power.

This is almost as great a miracle as the miracle of the frost, weaving ever-changing patterns on the window-pane.

It is almost as great a miracle as the miracle of day and night, of sunrise and sunset, caused by the never-ceasing swing of the earth and the sun and the moon in a pattern of motion controlled and adjusted by cosmic forces beyond the knowledge of the astronomer.

Learning His Will, which has always been right at our fingertips, is the greatness of His WILL performed in the smallness of our living in this expanse we call Universe.

Increase then, the determination of handling the pressings/compellings of His Finished Work, by increasing His Spoken Word for the exchange of actions that only encounter His Finished Work.

Happy are those people who know that their spirituality is small, and that their creeds are imperfect, and that their instruction concerning God and humanity is incomplete.

Happy are those who know that they do not know all that is of His Truth.

However, only those who admit their spiritual need for more of HIM are willing to learn that which is evermore ONLY HIM!

Our bodies have been super-imposed through the D.N.A. of God applied, with all the power and abilities of an everlastingly, ETERNAL GOD, and there is nothing that He, through Faith in His Word, His Way, and His Will cannot, and will not allow to happen~~as is according to His Plan, Design, and Strategy.

He SHARES with us all that He is, so that humanity can become all that He intended for us to become IN HIM!

We are not *rubber~stamped idealists*, having our living *robotisized*, while removing our individualities He made by His Thoughts within our own.

NO, A THOUSAND TIMES AND MORE~~NO!

We are the evidence of the God of the Universe, God of Creation, God of Humanity; and we are not soon, nor every, destroyed or reduced to inactivity, so long as the Breath of the Eternal, Immortal, and Only Wise God be GLORY FOREVER AND EVER, AMEN!

Adjusting each experience to locate the abilities of completed influences, assures the agreement in process of encountering the workings that increase toward each portion of evidence.

Our attitude must be the attitude of perfect teachableness!

Having an unshakable Faith in the boundaries of nature combined with perfect humility toward those boundaries, joined with a patient determination to learn them at whatever cost, humanity will exercise the Will of their Creator above and beyond their own, being forevermore involved in the Creativity and Bliss of knowing the Almighty is the God they serve with praise, worship, and communion.

Through the same teachableness those who seek God can produce results by learning to conform to limitations of boundaries through His Faith and love.

SEMITIC~ARAMAIC~HEBRAIC THESAURUS

Aramaic before first {

Semitic Root before first =

Lettering for ParaPhrase after second =

...(15:30) (& they came near)וְקָרְבוּ^{S18978} {ᴑꞁ-ᴏ-=*approaching/exhibiting*}=ꞁ Vav-[and/in addition]increase degree assure-Ꞁ Quph-contrast parallel structure-Ꞁ Resh-process beginning strength-Ꞁ Beyt[within/in/inside]-pattern thought inhabit-Ꞁ Vav-[and/in addition]increase degree assure-

(to Him)לְוָתֵהּ^{S1II37} {ꞇ>Ꞁꟿ=*towards as regards/compared to*}=ꞁ Lamed[to/toward]-instruct acquire provide-Ꞁ Vav-[and/in addition]increase degree assure-Ꞁ Taw-evidence prove sign-Ꞁ Hey[behold/the]-quality reveal grace-

(the crowds)כִּנְשָׁא^{S10319} {ꞁꟿꟿ=*in groups*}=ꟾ Kaph-surrender obtains consent-Ꞁ Nun-seed patience continue-Ꞁ Shin-pressure exchange disperse-Ꞁ Final-Aleph-ending finish maturity-

(many)סַגִּיאָא^{S13929} {ꞁꟿꞲ= *manifold/many~folded*}=ꞁ Samech-adjust apprehend source-Ꞁ Gimal-experience understanding encounter-Ꞁ Yud-purpose posture actions-Ꞁ Aleph-authority ability confirm-Ꞁ Final-Aleph-ending finish maturity-

(that)דְּאִיתָ^{S732} {ꞇ>ꟿꟿ=*perceive/desire as necessary to do*}=ꞁ Dalet-faith establish presence-Ꞁ Aleph-authority ability confirm-Ꞁ Yud-purpose posture actions-Ꞁ Taw-evidence prove sign-

(were)הֲווֹ^{S5147} {ꞁꟿꞲ=*enduring/existing*}= Ꞁ Hey[behold/the]-quality reveal grace-Ꞁ Vav-[and/in addition]increase degree assure-Ꞁ Vav-[and/in addition]increase degree assure-

(with them)עַמְּהוֹן^{S15788} {ᴑꟿᴏ=*in the presence of/in possession of*}=ꞁ Ayin-pierce perceive wisdom-Ꞁ Mem[from/out of]-transform encounter remembrance-Ꞁ Hey[behold/the]-quality reveal grace-Ꞁ Vav-[and/in addition]increase degree assure-Ꞁ Final-Nun-issue perseverance progress-

(the lame)חֲגִירֵא^{S6220} {ꞁꟿꞲ=*weak~voiced*}= Ꞁ Hhet-specific share beyond-Ꞁ Gimal-experience understanding encounter-Ꞁ Yud-purpose posture actions-Ꞁ Resh-process beginning strength-Ꞁ Final-Aleph-ending finish maturity-

(& blind)וּסְמַיָּא^{S14528} {ꞁꟿꞲ=*and to lose light*}=ꞁ Vav-[and/in addition]increase degree assure-Ꞁ Samech-adjust apprehend source-Ꞁ Mem[from/out of]-transform encounter remembrance-Ꞁ Yud-purpose posture actions-Ꞁ Final-Aleph-ending finish maturity-

(& dumb)וְחַרְשָׁא^{S7638} {ꞁꟿꞲ=*creating without speech*}=ꞁ Vav-[and/in addition]increase degree assure-Ꞁ Hhet-specific share beyond-Ꞁ Resh-process beginning strength-Ꞁ Shin-pressure exchange disperse-Ꞁ Final-Aleph-ending finish maturity-

(& crippled)וּפְשִׁיגֵא^{S17363} {ᴑꟿꞁꞲ=*weakness in walking*}=ꞁ Vav-[and/in addition]increase degree assure-Ꞁ Pey-mouth SpokenWord speak-Ꞁ Shin-pressure exchange disperse-Ꞁ Yud-purpose posture actions-Ꞁ Gimal-experience understanding encounter-Ꞁ Final-Aleph-ending finish maturity-

(& others)וְאַחֲרָנֵא^{S7688} {ꞁꟿꞲꞲ=*besides*}=ꞁ Vav-[and/in addition]increase degree assure-Ꞁ Aleph-authority ability confirm-Ꞁ Hhet-specific share beyond-Ꞁ Resh-process beginning strength-Ꞁ Nun-seed patience continue-Ꞁ Final-Aleph-ending finish maturity-

Got Healing?

(many)סֻבָּאִ S13929 {ל־Y=־ = **manifold/many~folded**} = ס Samech-adjust apprehend source-ꜰGimal-experience understanding
encounter-ꜰYud-purpose posture actions-ꜰAleph-authority ability confirm-ꜰFinal-Aleph-ending finish maturity-ꜰ(& they

laid)יַאֲרֻמֵי S20045 {ꜱ=**throwing oneself into something**} = ꜰVav-[and/in addition]increase degree assure-ꜰAleph-
authority ability confirm-ꜰResh-process beginning strength-ꜰMem[from/out of]-transform encounter remembrance-ꜰYud-purpose posture actions-ꜰVav-
[and/in addition]increase degree assure-(at)לִוָת S1136 {t־YU=**towards**}= ꜰLamed[to/toward]-instruct acquire provide-ꜰVav-[and/in
addition]increase degree assure-ꜰTaw-evidence prove sign-(them)וִוָאֻן S15788 {ꜱ=**in the presence of/in possession

of**}= ꜰAleph-authority ability confirm-ꜰNun-seed patience continue-ꜰVav-[and/in addition]increase degree assure-ꜰFinal-Nun-issue perseverance
progress-(His feet)דִרַגְלוֹהִי S19405 {Uꜱꜱ=**as a measure**}= ꜰResh-process beginning strength-ꜰGimal-experience understanding
encounter-ꜰLamed[to/toward]-instruct acquire provide-ꜰVav-[and/in addition]increase degree assure-ꜰHey[behold/the]-quality reveal grace-ꜰYud-
purpose posture actions-(of Yeshua)דִישׁוּעַ S9568 {ꜱYꜱꜱ=**being saved**}= ꜰDalet[of]-faith establish presence-ꜰYud-purpose
posture actions-ꜰShin-pressure exchange disperse-ꜰVav-[and/in addition]increase degree assure-ꜰAyin-pierce perceive wisdom-(& He

healed)וַאֲסִי S1596 {ꜰꜱꜱ=**to repair/refute**}= ꜰVav-[and/in addition]increase degree assure-ꜰAleph-authority ability confirm-
ꜰSamech-adjust apprehend source-ꜰYud-purpose posture actions-(them)אֻנוּן S4989 {ꜱ=**that one**}= ꜰAleph-authority ability confirm-
ꜰNun-seed patience continue-ꜰVav-[and/in addition]increase degree assure-ꜰFinal-Nun-issue perseverance progress-

The Semitic Emphasis

Approaching/Exhibiting towards as regards/compared to in groups manifold/many~folded~~perceive/desire as necessary to do enduring/existing in the presence of/in possession of weak~voiced and to lose light~~creating without speech~~weakness in walking besides the manifold/many~folded throwing oneself into something towardsas a measure being saved to repair/refute that one.

We must <u>learn</u> that God is not an unreasonable; nor is He an impulsive sovereign who breaks His own laws/teachings at will.

As soon as we learn that God does things ***through us*** (*not for us*), the matter becomes as simple as breathing, as inevitable as the sunrise or sunset.

"But God is omnipotent!" some people say. *"He can do anything He likes!"*

Certainly, nonetheless, He has made a world that runs within certain boundaries, and He does not break such boundaries.

Few of us in the north would ask God to produce a full-blown rose out of doors in January.

Yet, He can do this very thing, if we adapt our greenhouses to the boundaries of heat and light, so as to provide necessities that meet the needs of the rose.

And, He can produce a full-blown answer to prayer, ***if*** we adapt our earthly tabernacles to the certain boundaries of His Love and His Faith; so as to provide the necessities of *Answered Prayer*.

Someday the world will come to understand this fact, as it now understands the miracle of sound waves.

For one generation's miracles are the commonplaces of another generations living.

Surrendering Through The Assurance Of His Dominion Proves Every Portion Of His Pattern~Of~Thought Signifying His Process As Revealed/Discovered

MATTHEW 19:2
KJV+TVM

And^{G2532} great^{G4183} multitudes^{G3793} followed^{G190} Him;^{G846} and^{G2532} He healed^{G2323} them^{G846} there.^{G1563}

ORIGINAL THOUGHTS

...(19:2) Surrendering through the assurance of His Dominion, proves every portion of His Pattern~of~Thought signifying His Process as revealed/discovered. Adjust each experience to position by the abilities of His Finished Work, and confirm such adjusting through actions that enable the Seed of His Increase to issue the evidence that transforms one's progress.

Surrendering through the assurance of His Dominion, proves every portion of His Pattern~of~Thought signifying His Process as revealed/discovered.

Surrendering through the assurance of His Dominion, literally activates and operates the will of God throughout our living.

It is when we surrender that the Spirit offers the smell of God's savor; the beauty of God's flavor; and the grandeur of God's design, purpose, and plan.

It is when we seek HIM that *proves every portion of His Pattern~of~Thought* working in our living, portrays the elemental, fundamental foundations of all that He is.

Whether we are enthralled with His LOVE, or His GRACE, or whatever takes our breath away, or overwhelms us His realities~~He is STILL THE ONE that shapes our destiny, forms our priorities, and fashions the mysteries that make us HIS!

Even when *signifying His Process as revealed/discovered*, we become the direct LINK for God to operate all that He is, through all that we give Him of ourselves.

Adjust each experience to position by the abilities of His Finished Work, and confirm such adjusting through actions that enable the Seed of His Increase to issue the evidence that transforms one's progress.

Adjust each experience to position by the abilities of His Finished Work, and teach us to learn to covet/desire the BEST of His Gifts and Giftings.

How we are used depends upon how open we are to His flow through everything we are to become throughout eternity.

Confirm such adjusting through actions that enable the Seed of His Increase, because it is in friendship we discover the things that please HIM~~~the secret things of His heart.

We need to realize that the instinct of the true believer is to search for and find that which brings pleasure to THEM, the THREE~AS~ONE *to issue the evidence that transforms one's progress.*

SEMITIC~ARAMAIC~HEBRAIC THESAURUS

Aramaic before first {
Semitic Root before first =
Lettering for ParaPhrase after second =

...(19:2) (& came)וּבֹאֵתֶם S2135 {ﬡﬨﬠ =to reach the point that}=ﬢ Kaph-surrender obtains consent-ﬡVav-[and/in addition]increase degree assure-ﬡAleph-authority ability confirm-ﬡTaw-evidence prove sign-ﬡVav-[and/in addition]increase degree assure-ﬡ(after him)בָּתְרַהּ S2220 {ﬡﬨﬠ =gradually/successively}=ﬢ Beyt[within/in/inside]-pattern thought inhabit-ﬡTaw-evidence prove sign-ﬡResh-process reveal grace-ﬡHey[behold/the]-quality (crowds)נְשַׁיָּא S10319 {ﬡﬡﬠ=gathering/assembling}=ﬢ Nun-seed patience continue-ﬡShin-pressure exchange disperse-ﬡFinal-Aleph-ending finish maturity-ﬡ(great)סַגִּיאָא S13929 {ﬡﬡﬠ=in a manifold way}=ﬢ Samech-adjust apprehend source-ﬡGimal-experience understanding encounter-ﬡYud-purpose posture actions-ﬡAleph-authority ability confirm-ﬡFinal-Aleph-ending finish maturity-ﬡ(& He healed)וַאֵסִי S1596 {ﬡﬡﬠ=to repair/refute}=ﬢ Vav-[and/in addition]increase degree assure-ﬡAleph-authority ability confirm-ﬡSamech-adjust apprehend source-ﬡYud-purpose posture actions-ﬡauthority ability confirm-ﬡNun-seed patience continue-ﬡVav-[and/in addition]increase degree assure-ﬡFinal-Nun-issue perseverance progress-ﬡ(them)הֶתְמָן S4989 {ﬡﬡﬠ=a violent period of time}=ﬡAleph- (there)תַּמָּן S22880 {ﬡﬡﬨ=as a chronological indication}=ﬢ Taw-evidence prove sign-ﬡMem[from/out of]-transform encounter remembrance-ﬡFinal-Nun-issue perseverance progress-

The Semitic Emphasis

To reach the point that gradually/successively gathering/assembling in a manifold way~~repairs/refutes a violent period of time as a chronological indication.

The first step in seeking to produce results by any power is to contact that power.

The first step then, in seeking help from God is to contact God.

"Be still and know that I am God." PSALMS 46:10 KJV

Let us then lay aside our worries and cares, quiet our minds and concentrate upon **the reality of God**.

We may not know who God is or what God is, but we know that there is something/someone that sustains this universe, and that something is not ourselves.

So another part of **the first step** is to relax and to remind ourselves that there is a source of life outside of ourselves.

The second step is to turn the power on, by some such prayer as this: "*Heavenly Father, I thank you that You increase in me at this time Your life~giving power.*"

We are seldom taught that this journey, of which so many about, is an eternal walk, and needs an awareness built~up in knowing WHO we walk with, and WHO abides within us, since before the foundations of the worlds were laid!

The third step is to believe that this power, *His Power*, is coming into use and to accept it by faith.

No matter how much we ask for something <u>it</u> <u>becomes</u> <u>ours</u> <u>only</u> <u>as</u> <u>we</u> <u>accept</u> <u>it</u> <u>and</u> <u>give</u> <u>thanks</u> <u>for</u> <u>it</u>.

"*Thank You,*" we can say, "*that Your LIFE is in me forevermore, and increasing Your LIFE in my spirit and mind and body.*"

And *the fourth step* is to observe the operations of His Light and Life.

In order to do so, we must decide on some tangible thing that we wish accomplished by His Power, so that we can know without question whether our investigation/research/provings succeeded or failed.

How strange it is that people who fear to do this do not hesitate to pray for the most difficult objectives of all, such as the peace of the world or the salvation of their souls!

If they have so little confidence in prayer that they do not dare to test their powers of contacting God by praying for an easy thing, it is probable that their cosmic intercessions are of little force.

If everyone who prayed for the peace of the world had enough prayer power to accomplish the healing of a head cold, this would be a different world within twenty-four hours.

In Addition To Building Strong Understanding
Reveal The Pattern~Of~His~Thoughts
By Discovering The Purpose That Obtains
The Instruction Of His Finished Work

MATTHEW 21:14

Got Healing?

And^{G2532} the blind^{G5185} and^{G2532} the lame^{G5560} came^{G4334} to Him^{G846} in^{G1722} the^{G3588}
temple^{G2411} and^{G2532} He healed^{G2323} them^{G846}

ORIGINAL THOUGHTS

...(21:14) In addition to building strong understanding, reveal the
Pattern~of~His~Thoughts by discovering the purpose that obtains the
instruction of His Finished Work. Adjust each remembrance by positioning
the finish of each portion beyond experience through actions that access
His Finished Work. Assured of His Abilities adjusting each posture/position,
enable the Seed to increase one's progress.

In addition to building strong understanding, reveal the Pattern~of~His~Thoughts by discovering the purpose that obtains the instruction of His Finished Work.

It was never about our inviting Him to come to us; but of our becoming aware that He sent Jesus, the Son, as well as, She, the Spirit~~to come an make their abode within us, so that He might be welcomed to come as well and walk with us throughout the days of our living in this dimension.

You see, we are two~thirds SPIRITUAL!

We are SOUL, and we have His SPIRIT, as the Animator of our existence in HIM!

God, as being/existing in everything; He has never left us, nor forsaken us, because of His Plan given to us within our destiny!

Adjust each remembrance by positioning the finish of each portion beyond experience through actions that access His Finished Work.

God's intent is not to robotisize our existence, but rather to continue calling to the unknown depths of our living, so that He may be invited to reign in LIFE THROUGH ONE, JESUS CHRIST IN US, AS US, and THROUGH US!

If, through HIM, we are to become the light unto the world, then we must endure the burning of what is us, in order for to embrace the ALL that is only HIM!

Assured of His Abilities adjusting each posture/position, enable the Seed to increase one's progress.

We were never created or designed to die.

This is why at this life's conclusion, we fight so hard to stay in this "earth~suit"!

Got Healing?

What we are not taught, and what we have yet to recognize is that there is a drive in each of us to give ourselves to something, or SOMEONE bigger than ourselves, something out of or beyond our control that will save and deliver us from our sense of shame and guilt.

Love will never condemn us for being lost, but love will not let us stay there alone, even though it will never force us to come out of our hiding places.

Love is His invitation to, *"Come and dine"*!

SEMITIC~ARAMAIC~HEBRAIC THESAURUS

Aramaic before first {
Semitic Root before first =
Lettering for ParaPhrase after second =

...(21:14) (& they brought)קרבו S18979 {קרב = to approach/be near} = ו Vav-[and/in addition]increase degree assure- Quph-contrast parallel structure- Resh-process beginning strength- (to Him)ליה S10842 {ע = it is necessary to} = ל Lamed[to/toward]- instruct acquire provide- Hey[behold/the]-quality reveal grace- (in the temple)בהיכלא S5167 {שב = with regard to/in exchange for a dwelling place} = ב Beyt[within/inside]-pattern thought inhabit- Hey[behold/the]-quality reveal grace- Yud-purpose posture actions- Kaph-surrender obtains consent- Lamed[to/toward]-instruct acquire provide- Final-Aleph-ending finish maturity- (the blind)סמיא S14532 {סמ = to lose light} = ס Samech-adjust apprehend source- Mem[from/out of]-transform encounter remembrance- Yud-purpose posture actions- Final-Aleph-ending finish maturity- (& the lame)וחגיסא S6213 {חג = weak~walking} = ו Vav-[and/in addition]increase degree assure- Hhet-specific share beyond- Gimal-experience understanding encounter- Yud-purpose posture actions- Samech-adjust apprehend source- Final-Aleph-ending finish maturity- (& He healed)ואסי S1596 {אס = to repair/refute} = ו Vav-[and/in addition]increase degree assure- Aleph-authority ability confirm- Samech-adjust apprehend source- Yud-purpose posture actions- (them)אנון S4989 {אנ = the self~same one} = א Aleph-authority ability confirm- Nun-seed patience continue- Vav-[and/in addition]increase degree assure- Final-Nun-issue perseverance progress-

The Semitic Emphasis

To approach/be near it is necessary to with regard to/in exchange for a dwelling place weak~walking to repair/refute the self~same one.

Healing in never about just the experience.

Healing is a force that not only changes lives, but weaves the threads of God's character in and out of one's living.

While Experience is a force not easily discounted; Healing is a force to be reckoned with and realized most. It is when we REST IN HIM that Healing is able to do the best in exercising the elements of God's *Divine~Nature~Applied* to our being, exciting the senses of all three areas of our living.

You see, the humanity we seem to look at is only the physical, because we are taught all our lives to give attention to it.

The **BE**~ing of Humanity is actually made up of THREE PARTS:

Got Healing?

Spirit, *Soul*, and *Body*.

Each part of our <u>BE</u>~ing has in itself five major senses.

It is never about OUR performance, as much as it is about our KNOWING HIM!

As He is our Creator, KNOWING HIM provides the wrapping that includes all that is HIM, in all that becomes us!

As the God of the Ages, our Lord and King, is never sick, even so has He created humanity to not be sick as well.

We should not die sick, we should not live sick; however, KNOWING HIM is the same in context as taking Vitamin "C" in the flesh.

He is the resistance to every attack, whether physical, mental, spiritual, financial, or social.

His D.N.A. is the stability of our foundation, but it is only in KNOWING HIM that we discover the FULLNESS that is HIM in US!

In Addition To His Dominion Apprehended The Motive/Reason Of His Instruction Adjusts Each Experience By Actions That Conform To His Finished Work

MARK 1:34
KJV+TVM

And^{G2532} he healed^{G2323} many^{G4183} that were sick$^{G2192\ G2560}$ of divers^{G4164} diseases,^{G3554} and^{G2532} cast out^{G1544} many^{G4183} devils;^{G1140} and^{G2532} suffered^{G863} not^{G3756} the^{G3588} devils^{G1140} to speak,^{G2980} because^{G3754} they knew^{G1492} him.^{G846}

ORIGINAL THOUGHTS

...(1:34) In addition to His Dominion apprehended, the motive/reason of His Instruction adjusts each experience by actions that conform to His Finished Work. In presence of His Pattern~of~Thoughts exercise the Faith of His Purpose in persevering/persisting to discover the addition of each increase of His Indwelling, surrendering to insure one's strengthening by the Grace of His Truth perpetuating His Finished Work. Out of every exchange, determine to acquire the Spoken Word of His Finished Work, and increase by His Faith, every intention supporting His Finished Work. Adjusting each experience of His Purpose enables the maturing that confirms His Spoken Word in parallel of each degree of the teachings of His Finished Work. The exchange of His Pattern~Thoughts parallels specifically

Got Healing?

every increase of His Finished Work. Acquired by the Grace of His Increase, proceed toward His Faith in positioning the assurances of His Finished Work. Through Faith, patiently transcend the teachings of His Promises to increase the progress of remembering the blendings of His Provisions. Establish each purpose through the presence of His Wisdom, by actions that persist in revealing each portion that assures the acquiring of the Grace of His Truth.

<u>In addition to His Dominion apprehended, the motive/reason of His Instruction adjusts each experience by actions that conform to His Finished Work.</u>

From the beginnings of His Word over humanity, God teaches that He has given ONLY to humanity the abilities and power of His Dominion, in order to prove, not that humanity rules, but that God rules THROUGH humanity's efforts in glorifying HIM!

Power corrupts; and Absolute Power absolutely corrupts.

Therefore, we are in error if we think, or teach, that God has given us ALL authority, even though we point to the Scriptures as our proof.

If God gives His Creation ALL authority wherein does His Authority then lay?

God gives WHO HE IS to WHOM HE CREATED!

Humanity's God~Given Authority is the dominion by which we rule over this world, and its causes that are involved with our living FOR HIM, IN HIM, and THROUGH HIM!

To rule over anything, as does God, there must be an ACTIVE participation through one's living after Him!

<u>In presence of His Pattern~of~Thoughts exercise the Faith of His Purpose in persevering/persisting to discover the addition of each increase of His Indwelling, surrendering to insure one's strengthening by the Grace of His Truth perpetuating His Finished Work.</u>

There is a necessary portion in one's living that must contain the idea embraced, regarding the fullness of God's existence within our own living.

We cannot exist apart from HIM, and yet, we fail to recognize that such living is hindered when we are away from HIM in our mentalities, or our actions, and/or our presuppositions!

Supposing God will answer prayer is not a requirement for answers; but, there is a need for believing!

The greater the awareness of His Person and Presence, the greater He

---

extends and enlarges the consciousness of His Power at work within our living.

Without Him, apart from Him or not knowing Him places any soul in the same position of disparagement, when God is not honored by our every breath, step, and at every turn we make!

Out of every exchange, determine to acquire the Spoken Word of His Finished Work, and increase by His Faith, every intention supporting His Finished Work.

With every "*thank you for the day*", and every "*I need you always*"; find/discover the fullness awaiting the initiative of your choice and follow~through.

God HAS ALREADY DONE EVERYTHING we will EVER NEED!

Our waiting is on US, not on HIM!

We command the skies, the atmosphere, the throes of nature by the command and dominion of our God~Given Authority.

If Jesus healed all that came to HIM; why should it be any different when those having needs come to our church, or fellowship, or enter into a relationship with The MOST HIGH GOD?

Adjusting each experience of His Purpose, enables the maturing that confirms His Spoken Word in parallel of each degree of the teachings of His Finished Work.

How can we ADJUST to His Purpose when we fail at the point of knowing what, or Who His purposes are about?

Never picking up a bible; never taking the time to pray, and then listen to what the Spirit within would teach; these are failures that we initiate, not God!

The all~encompassing LOVE OF GOD will overwhelm all our self~ish desires, when we acknowledge HIM IN ALL OUR WAYS!

The exchange of His Pattern~Thoughts parallels specifically every increase of His Finished Work.

We see from every conceivable angle, throughout the Scriptures, there is no doctrine more clearly taught than God's will to heal ALL who have need of healing.

Jesus is not only the testator, who died; He was resurrected and is also the Mediator of the will.

He is our lawyer, so to speak.

He will not cheat us out of His Will.

He is our Representative at the right hand of God.

"And he cried unto the LORD; and the LORD shewed him a tree, which when he had cast into the waters, the waters were made sweet: there he made for them a statute and an ordinance, and there he proved them, And said, If thou wilt diligently hearken to the voice of the LORD thy God, and wilt do that which is right in His sight, and wilt give ear to His commandments, and keep all His statutes, I will put none of these diseases upon thee, which have come upon the Egyptians: for I am the LORD that healeth thee." EXODUS 15:25-26 KJV

There is literally, and absolutely nothing else for God to do, but honor the words we agree with **IN HIM**!

Acquired by the Grace of His Increase, proceed toward His Faith in positioning the assurances of His Finished Work.

All that encompasses the needs of humanity, individually, have been interlocked and made available since BEFORE the foundations of the worlds were laid!

The fact that remains yet untapped completely is the TRUTH of such a fact mentioned is in fact the reality of all that God CREATED!

As His Grace increases our awareness, and we begin to consciously assess that which is ours by the Divine Decree of His Eternal Majesty~~the enlarging of His Benefits becomes the overwhelming FACT of His Existence, Abiding, and Eternal Presence within our living.

So long as we draw breath, His Word is at our beckon~calling to perform the magnificence of His Will having begun before Creation occurred!

Through Faith, patiently transcend the teachings of His Promises to increase the progress of remembering the blendings of His Provisions.

"For all the promises of God IN HIM are yea, and IN HIM Amen, unto the glory of God by us. SECOND CORINTHIANS 1:20 KJV

God's Healing is about our understanding HOW He has made us, and HOW we must learn to cooperate and function in harmony with the multi~universe of His Design within our own.

Getting along with ourselves is about learning to TRUST Him through seeing His Creation from His Vantage~Point!

The teachings contained in His Word are not about do's and don'ts;

they are about recognizing HIM wherever, and whomever He presents Himself through.

He transcends, or goes beyond what He teaches in order to prove to us His LOVE for us as His OWN!

Herein, then is the HEALING that humanity has ascribed incorrectly all these centuries of existence on this planet.

He is the GOD OF ALL THINGS, visible and invisible, temporal and spiritual, limited and unlimited, conditionally and unconditionally.

Establish each purpose through the presence of His Wisdom, by actions that persist in revealing each portion that assures the acquiring of the Grace of His Truth.

Selfish~Independent~Nature ceases when we discover the One who LOVES us more than anything He ever created.

The apostle tells us that *"God is love"*; and therefore, seeing He is an infinite being, it follows that He is an infinite fountain of love.

Seeing He is an all-sufficient being, it follows that He is a full and overflowing, and inexhaustible fountain of love.

And in that He is an unchangeable and eternal being, He is an unchangeable and eternal fountain of love.

SEMITIC~ARAMAIC~HEBRAIC THESAURUS

Aramaic before first {

Semitic Root before first =

Lettering for ParaPhrase after second =

...(1:34) (& He healed)יאסי S1596 {ﬤﬤﬥ=to repair/refute/negate/proved false} = degree assure-Aleph-authority ability confirm-Samech-adjust apprehend source-Yud-purpose posture actions-

(multitudes)לסניאא S13926 {ﬡﬤ=in the direction to/that which belongs to} = Lamed[to/toward]-instruct acquire provide-Samech-adjust apprehend source-Gimal-experience understanding encounter-Yud-purpose posture actions-Aleph-authority ability confirm-Final-Aleph-ending finish maturity-(who ill)בישאית S2313 {שﬠﬨ=perceiving hurtfully} = Dalet-faith establish presence-Beyt[within/inside]-pattern thought inhabit-Yud-purpose posture actions-Shin-pressure exchange disperse-Aleph-authority ability confirm-Yud-purpose posture actions-Taw-evidence prove sign-(become)עבידין S14998 {טﬡﬠ=making/effecting/persuading} = Ayin-pierce perceive wisdom-Beyt[within/inside]-pattern thought inhabit-Yud-purpose posture actions-Dalet-faith establish presence-Yud-purpose posture actions-Final-Nun-issue perseverance progress-(had)הוו S5147 {ﬡﬠﬠ=to endure/exist} = Hey[behold/the]-quality reveal grace-Vav-[and/in addition]increase degree assure-Vav-[and/in addition]increase degree assure-(with diseases)בכורהנא S10508 {ﬡﬤ=with regard to/in exchange for weakness} = Beyt[within/inside]-pattern thought inhabit-Kaph-surrender obtains consent-Vav-[and/in addition]increase degree assure-Resh-process beginning strength-Hey[behold/the]-quality reveal grace-Nun-seed patience continue-Final-Aleph-ending finish maturity-(various)משחלפא S7204 {ﬥדּﬧהּﬨ=diverse/in a variety of ways} = Mem[from/out of]-transform encounter remembrance-Shin-pressure exchange disperse-Hhet-specific share beyond-Lamed[to/toward]-instruct acquire provide-Pey-mouth SpokenWord speak-Final-Aleph-ending finish maturity-(& evil spirits)דיוי S4371 {ﬡﬠ=an invasion/attack} = Vav-[and/in addition]increase degree assure-Dalet-faith establish presence-Yud-purpose posture actions-Vav-[and/in addition]increase degree assure-Final-

Got Healing?

Aleph-ending finish maturity-(many)םיבר S13929 {א=in a manifold/many~folded way}=ם Samech-adjust apprehend source-ג Gimal-experience understanding encounter-י Yud-purpose posture actions-א Aleph-authority ability confirm-ן Final-Aleph-ending finish maturity-

(He cast out)אפכ S13332 {=to experience successfully}=א Aleph-authority ability confirm-ן Pey-mouth SpokenWord speak-ם Quph-contrast parallel structure-(& not)אלו S10871 {=without}= ן Vav-[and/in addition]increase degree assure-ל Lamed[to/toward]-instruct acquire provide-ן Final-Aleph-ending finish maturity-(allow)שרש S2072

{=condoning/forgiving a debt}=ש Shin-pressure exchange disperse-ב Beyt[within/inside]-pattern thought inhabit-ם Quph-contrast parallel structure-(He did)אוה S144 {=coming into being}=ח Hhet-specific share beyond-ו Vav-[and/in addition]increase degree assure-ן Final-Aleph-ending finish maturity-(them)םהל S10844 {=to such a degree}=ל Lamed[to/toward]-instruct acquire provide-ה Hey[behold/the]-quality reveal grade-ו Vav-[and/in addition]increase degree assure-ן Final-Nun-issue perseverance progress-(the evil spirits)אידיל S4372 {=an invasion/attack}=ל Lamed[to/toward]-instruct acquire provide-ד Dalet-faith establish presence-י Yud-purpose posture actions-ו Vav-[and/in addition]increase degree assure-ן Final-Aleph-ending finish maturity-(to speak)וללמנה S12031 {=to console/to enable someone to speak}= ם Mem[from/out of]-transform encounter remembrance-ל Lamed[to/toward]-instruct acquire provide-ל Lamed[to/toward]-instruct acquire provide-ו Vav-[and/in addition]increase degree assure-ן Final-Nun-issue perseverance progress-(because)םטלמ S11636 {=on account of/concerning}=ם Mem[from/out of]-transform encounter remembrance-ט Thet-contain mixture balance-ל Lamed[to/toward]-instruct acquire provide-(know)ידיעיד S8638 {=becoming acquainted with}=ד Dalet-faith establish presence- י Yud-purpose posture actions-ד Dalet-faith establish presence-ע Ayin-pierce perceive wisdom-י Yud-purpose posture actions-ן Final-Nun-issue perseverance progress-(they did)ווח S5147 {=coming into being}=ה Hey[behold/the]-quality reveal grace-ו Vav-[and/in addition]increase degree assure-ו Vav-[and/in addition]increase degree assure-(Him)הל S10842 {=as regards a time frame}=ל Lamed[to/toward]-instruct acquire provide-ה Hey[behold/the]-quality reveal grace-

The Semitic Emphasis

Repaired/Refuted/Negated/Proven False in the direction to/that which belongs to perceiving hurtfully~ ~making/effecting/persuading to endure/to exist with regard to/in exchange for weakness diversely/in a variety of ways~~an invasion/attack in a many~folded way to experience successfully without condoning coming into being to such a degree an invasion/attack to console/to enable someone to speak on account of/concerning becoming acquainted with as regards a time frame.

The more we TAKE IN THE JOY OF THE LORD, the more He becomes our strength! *NEHEMIAH 8:10 KJV*

The greater the download, the larger the uptake.

The larger the uptake, the greater the expanse of the Spiritual Realm that takes over the indications and movements in time, while revealing and discovering the fullness that unveils the Person, Presence, and Power of Almighty God IN US!

Moving in the parallels of the spiritual that command the indications of living in the physical becomes the greater outcome of our RESTING IN HIM!

Apprehend Understanding By Enabling His Influence Encountered Through Purposes

That Strengthen Actions Within Beginnings Out Of His Dominion That Adjust To His Finished Work

MARK 3:10
KJV+TVM

For [G1063] He had healed [G2323] many [G4183] insomuch that [G5620] they pressed upon [G1968] Him [G846] for to [G2443] touch [G680] Him [G846] as many as [G3745] had [G2192] plagues. [G3148]

ORIGINAL THOUGHTS

...(3:10) Apprehend understanding by enabling His Influence encountered through purposes that strengthen actions within beginnings out of His Dominion that adjusts to His Finished Work. The qualities of each increase by His Finished Work, discerns/knows the Presence that transforms finish to maturity, and establishes patience to reveal the addition of every potion of progress. The Seed of His Spoken Word educates through the purposes issuing from His Wisdom, while providing the increase of His Grace through the single~mindedness that transforms each blending provided. His Faith spreads the evidence of each parallel in process of each Pattern~of~His~Thought, in addition to the progress that reveals the Grace of His Truth.

Apprehend understanding by enabling His Influence encountered through purposes that strengthen actions within beginnings out of His Dominion that adjusts to His Finished Work.

Every score found within the pages of God's Holy Writ contain a fragment of His Will, His Purpose, His Design, and/or His Promise.

Deciding whether or not His Word is a promise or just the sharing of an intimate design featuring the character of His Person in describing the actions produced, the sundry comments of each story throughout the Gospels captures pictures of God's undeniable, unfathomable Love for His Creation.

Understanding can sometimes form the premises for a new and brighter tomorrow.

Understanding can sometimes form the elements that when stretched and joined together provide the accompanying wonders of a building so magnificent that words pale in their ability to describe its substance.

Here, in reader's digest form, the translators of this Gospel portray the undefinable features of God's own expression of LOVE through Jesus through the healing of multitudes that pressed in to touch Him, out of their need.

The qualities of each increase by His Finished Work, discerns/knows the Presence that transforms finish to maturity, and establishes patience to reveal the addition of every potion of progress.

The myriad of qualities that come from the abundance of His Personage contained with the phrase, **His Finished Work**, mystifies humanity who only stoops to reason that these happenings created by Jesus' presence were mere "*chances*".

His Finished Work carries the design of the Eternal Godhead, Who together formed and fashioned the blueprint of every soul ever created, defining the purpose of God through that which imparted and hidden within the Spirit of His being in their existence.

Humanity themselves were not created to be the ungodly, defiled creatures that the world and the flesh have brought forth.

Humanity is the "*crown*" of God's Creation, and through His Love He returns humanity to the original design He made all of us to radiate.

Learning to allow the Spirit to lead, guide, and direct our steps to live within the outlines and patterns of His Finished Work, brings out the very best in spiritual substance that sustains the physical dimension of our existence.

The Seed of His Spoken Word educates through the purposes issuing from His Wisdom, while providing the increase of His Grace through the single~mindedness that transforms each blending provided.

Incredibly, few believers live each day as if the God of the universe has great affection for them.

This is because two thousand years of religious tradition have indoctrinated in us the mistaken notion that God's love is something we earn.

If we do what pleases Him, He loves us; if not, He doesn't.

Giving that up isn't easy.

Moving from a performance-based religious ethic to a relationship deeply rooted in the Father's affection is no small transition.

It is the most significant one to ever be made in our spiritual journey, and it will change anyone's life in Christ from a frustrating drudgery in the face of enticing temptations to a vital, fulfilling adventure that continues to transform them with each passing day.

It is through the eternal harvest of His Spoken Word having found a place in our everyday, moment~to~moment living IN HIM that causes the soul to discover why the First Commandment is the most necessary of all.

"Jesus said unto him, Thou shalt love the Lord thy God with all thy heart, and with all thy soul, and with all thy mind." MATTHEW 22:37 KJV

"And thou shalt love the Lord thy God with all thy heart, and with all thy soul, and with all thy mind, and with all thy strength: this is the first commandment." MARK 12:30 KJV

"And He answering said, Thou shalt love the Lord thy God with all thy heart, and with all thy soul, and with all thy strength, and with all thy mind; and thy neighbour as thyself." LUKE 10:27 KJV

His Faith spreads the evidence of each parallel in process of each Pattern~of~His~Thought, in addition to the progress that reveals the Grace of His Truth.

The real teachings of His Faith, and the impact of the Cross creates an initiative so great in the heart of the average church~goer that most mainline churches feel such teachings undermine the very fabric of their reason for being in church.

However, what many refuse to acknowledge is that in the Body of Christ we have forgotten, and many have never known what the reality of a person's DEEPER~LIFE IN GOD is truly all about.

Their unspoken thoughts tell them they need to have a steady dose of *"hell~fire and damnation"* in order to stay straight on the path of righteousness and heaven~bound desires.

What a shame that we have held of an incorrect~doctrine scraped together since the Council of Nicea in 345 A.D.; thinking that people need to be bludgeoned by fear and guilt and shame, instead of offering the real reason for Heaven's existence is that the Creator of ALL LOVES THE CREATION HE CREATED BEST!

SEMITIC~ARAMAIC~HEBRAIC THESAURUS
Aramaic before first {
Semitic Root before first =

Got Healing?

Lettering for ParaPhrase after second =

...(3:10) (many)אֲרֻכָּה S13929 {=in a manifold way} = Samech-adjust apprehend source- Gimal-experience understanding encounter- Yud [of/through]-purpose single-mindedness actions- Aleph-authority ability confirm- Final-Aleph-ending finish maturity- (for) S3714 {=in direct consequence of one's action} = Gimal-experience understanding encounter- Yud [of/through]-purpose single-mindedness actions- Resh-process beginning strength- (healing) אֲרֻכָה S1613 {=to repair/refute} = Samech-adjust apprehend source- Mem[from/out of]-transform encounter remembrance- Aleph-authority ability confirm- Final-Aleph-ending finish maturity- (He was) S5144 {=coming into being} = Hey[behold/the]-quality reveal grace- Vav-[and/in addition]increase degree assure- Final-Aleph-ending finish maturity- (until) S5208 {=as far as} = Ayin-pierce perceive wisdom- Dalet-faith establish presence- Mem[from/out of]-transform encounter remembrance- Final-Aleph-ending finish maturity- (they would be) S5080 {=perceiving/desiring coming into being} = Dalet-faith establish presence- Nun-seed patience continue- Hey[behold/the]-quality reveal grace- Vav-[and/in addition]increase degree assure- Vav-[and/in addition]increase degree assure- Final-Nun-issue perseverance progress- Nun-seed patience continue- (falling) S13301 {=given an opportunity} = Pey-mouth SpokenWord speak- Lamed[to/toward]-instruct acquire provide- Yud [of/through]-purpose single-mindedness actions- Final-Nun-issue perseverance progress- (upon Him) S15702 {=according to the opinion of} = Ayin-pierce perceive wisdom- Lamed[to/toward]-instruct acquire provide- Vav-[and/in addition]increase degree assure- Hey[behold/the]-quality reveal grace- Yud [of/through]-purpose single-mindedness actions- (so that) S11636 {=because of} = Mem[from/out of]-transform encounter remembrance- Thet-contain mixture- Lamed[to/toward]-instruct acquire provide- (they might touch) S18958 {=perceiving/desiring to approach} = Taw-evidence prove sign- Quph-contrast parallel structure- Dalet-faith establish presence- Nun-seed patience continue- Beyt[within/inside]-pattern thought inhabit- Vav-[and/in addition]increase degree assure- Resh-process beginning strength- Final-Nun-issue perseverance progress- (Him) S10842 {=outside of} = Lamed[to/toward]-instruct acquire provide- Hey[behold/the]-quality reveal grace-

The Semitic Emphasis

In a manifold way~~in direct consequence of one's action to repair/refute coming into being~~as far as perceiving/desiring coming into being~~given an opportunity according to the opinion of~~because of perceiving/desiring to approach outside of.

The dynamic pull of Religion and a False~System of Works/Performance can be, and for the most part always is stronger than the FREEDOM OF RELATIONSHIP IN GOD!

What a shame we miss the teachings of Jesus throughout the Gospels and subsequent Epistles because of the erroneous doctrines of men who seek to control the will of others to soothe their swelling conscience.

Healing is not a DOCTRINE; it is a way of life ONLY FOUND in the bosom of the Father, through the immaculate conception of the Word in our being, having moment~by~moment experiences in the leading/teaching/guiding of the Spirit's directing.

Those who are willing to substitute the demand of obligation for the power of affection have never tasted the LOVE OF GOD in any significant measure.

Instead of congregations full of indentured servitude, the Father shows us His UNCONDITIONAL LOVE through the offering of His ONLY SON on our behalf; and in turn, continually, constantly, consistently, and consciously seeks to PROVE that HIS LOVE FOR HIS CREATION is the single greatest gift every given to Humanity as a whole!

In Addition To His Pattern~Of~Thought
Perceive The Influence Of His Efforts
In Beholding The Increase Of His Purpose
Out Of The Seed Revealed In Apprehending
The Experience In Single~Mindedness

MARK 5:23
KJV+TVM

And^{G2532} besought^{G3870} Him^{G846} greatly,^{G4183} saying^{G3004} My^{G3450} little daughter^{G2365} lieth at the point of death^{G2192} ^{G2079} I pray$^{(G2443)}$ Thee come^{G2064} and lay^{G2007} Thy hands^{G5495} on her^{G846} that^{G3704} she may be healed^{G4982} and^{G2532} she shall live.^{G2198}

ORIGINAL THOUGHTS

...(5:23) In addition to His Pattern~of~Thought perceive the Influence of His Efforts in beholding the increase of His Purpose out of the Seed Revealed in apprehending the experience in single~mindedness. Increasing the abilities that transform each process acquire the revelation of His Pattern~Thought strengthening each wonder through the single~minded pattern that purposes each pressure in focus of evidence perceiving within a single~minded presenting of His Finished Work. Prove each finish as apprehended in purpose of prevail enabling the function of His Faith to acknowledge the Wisdom of His Promises through the qualities of the Grace of His Truth. In addition prove through His Evidence beyond His Teachings that fashions every increase proving the specifics of His Finished Work.

In addition to His Pattern~of~Thought perceive the Influence of His Efforts~~in beholding the increase of His Purpose out of the Seed Revealed~~in apprehending the experience in single~mindedness.

When we walk and serve and share the Word of the Living God, there is added a Pattern~of~Thought that can only be identified as HIM!

In these revealed patterns know beyond any shadow of doubt that as He reveals Himself through His Word, even so does He reveal Himself through each healing promised, and then provided through Faith In His Word!

It is from out of the Word of God that we discover His Purpose revealed; and then, He shows Himself through the Promise of His Word to perform what He promised He would provide, *not by might, nor by power, but by HIS SPIRIT!* ZECHARIAH 4:6 KJV

When His Finished Work provides the mature, finished, and completed promise brought forth, such actions carry as well the unforgettable, undeniable experiences of seeing His Word unfold through His Promises shown as provided.

Increasing the abilities that transform each process~~acquire the revelation of His Pattern~Thought strengthening each wonder~~through the single~minded pattern that purposes~~each pressure in focus of evidence~~perceiving within a single~minded presenting of His Finished Work.

Like exercising any weakened area of the body, exercise the abilities given by God to your living, and show forth the mercies of His Great LOVE, as He transforms each vessel into a culpable, responsible happening through the Presence of His Spirit unfolding the wealth and strength of His Right Hand.

"And ye shall seek Me, and find Me, <u>when ye shall search for Me with all your heart</u>." JEREMIAH 29:13 KJV

He gives nothing less than His BEST when we seek Him with all of our BEST!

Those who believe the Word, understand the hope of His Calling on their lives, and know that God will move through them to accomplish the miraculous.

Out of the same single~minded efforts that Christ exemplified, even so must every believer surrender all that is themselves, in order to embrace on other's behalf all that is HIM!

<u>Prove each finish as apprehended in purpose of prevail</u>~~enabling the function of His Faith to acknowledge~~the Wisdom of His Promises through the qualities of the Grace of His Truth.

Living LIFE in this realm is a series of endings and beginnings; much like <u>GENESIS 1</u> records each day~~*the evening and the morning were.*

But in the scheme of living in this physical dimension, we need to realize the very fact: *if we take the time to think about an offense committed against us, and we wonder if God ever judged that person or not; then, the desires of vindication and retaliation will stir up our heart!*

Prove each finish as apprehended in purpose of prevail, knowing that because we see the victory of the triumph clearly, we realize that we could not have accomplished such if God were not with us, helping us, directing us, and leading us according to His WILL!

If it is a situation that did not go as we planned, then we need realize that God knows better, and through our willingness to remain obedient, giving all things into His hands; herein, is where we discover that His Purposes do not involve *hurt, pain, suffering, or sorrow!*

It is when are *enabling the function of His Faith to acknowledge* the extension of His influence, dominion, or strategy~~we realize that our journey is not only escorted by the Presence of the Spirit with ours, we recognize that when we turn to our own ways, there is an enfolding of darkness becoming visible in our turning from HIM as we, at that moment cease walking in The LIGHT!

"But seek ye first the kingdom of God, and His righteousness; and all these things shall be added unto you." MATTHEW 6:33 KJV

In *the Wisdom of His Promises through the qualities of the Grace of His Truth,* the soul, heart, and mind discover the faultless efforts that He transcends even beyond our wants bringing to us the better things He KNOWS we deserve!

In *addition* prove *through* His *Evidence* beyond His *Teachings~~that fashions every increase proving~~the specifics of* His *Finished Work.*

In addition prove through His Evidence beyond His Teachings, because those things wherein He leads us according to His WILL always reveal the perfection of His PLAN as the blessings never cease to emanate out of His Design for us!

It is the eternal LOVE of God *that fashions every increase proving the specifics of His Finished Work,* and determining to show forth the elemental, fundamental, foundational workings of His GRACE through our following the beginning theories of His TRUTH to which we TRUST every portion of our living to His leading and blessing!

SEMITIC~ARAMAIC~HEBRAIC THESAURUS

Got Healing?

Aramaic before first {

Semitic Root before first =

Lettering for ParaPhrase after second =

...(5:23) (& begging)וּבָעֵי S3007 {יוֹעֵבְוּ=and seeking for someone/something} =Y/ן Vav-[and/in addition]increase degree assure-ן/Beyt[within/inside]-pattern thought inhabit-ע/Ayin-pierce perceive wisdom-ב/ן Final-Aleph-ending

finish maturity-(he was)הֲוָה S5144 {הֲוָה=coming into being} =ﬡ/ן Hey[behold/the]-quality reveal grace-Y/ן Vav-[and/in addition]increase degree assure-ן/Yud [of/through]-purpose single~mindedness actions-(from Him)מִנֵּהּ S12183 {מִנֵּהּ=indicating the

origin of directional movement/movement of time}-ﬡ/ן Mem[from/out of]-transform encounter remembrance-ן/Nun-seed patience continue-ן/Hey[behold/the]-quality reveal grace-(greatly)סַגִּי S13927 {סַגִּי=in a long while} =ﬡ/ם Samech-adjust

apprehend source-ן/Gimal-experience understanding encounter-ן/Yud [of/through]-purpose single~mindedness actions-(& he

said)וַאֲמַר S1292 {וַאֲמַר=and/also making a legal declaration} =Y/ן Vav-[and/in addition]increase degree assure-/Aleph-authority ability confirm-ן/Mem[from/out of]-transform encounter remembrance-ן/Resh-process beginning strength-(to

Him)לֵהּ S10842 {=beyond/above/outside of} =U/ן Lamed[to/toward]-instruct acquire provide-ن/Hey[behold/the]-quality reveal grace-(my daughter)בְּרַתִּי S3319 {=a small part of something} =ם/ב Beyt[within/inside]-pattern thought inhabit-ן/Resh-process beginning strength-ن/Taw-evidence prove sign-ن/Yud [of/through]-purpose single~mindedness actions-(very

sick)בִּישָׁא S2312 {=in ruin/desolation} =ם/ב Beyt[within/inside]-pattern thought inhabit-ן/Yud [of/through]-purpose single~mindedness actions-(very)ن/Taw-evidence prove sign-ن/Shin-pressure exchange disperse-ن/Yud [of/through]-purpose single~mindedness actions-

evidence prove sign-(has been made)S14997 {=creating/transferring ownership/making

into} =ﬡ/ן Ayin-pierce perceive wisdom-ن/Beyt[within/inside]-pattern thought inhabit-ن/Yud [of/through]-purpose single~mindedness

actions-ن/Dalet-faith establish presence-ן/Final-Aleph-ending finish maturity-(come)S2164 {=coming to

mind} =ﬡ/ן Taw-evidence prove sign-ن/Final-Aleph-ending finish maturity-(lay)S14268 {=place things in

order} =ﬡ/ם Samech-adjust apprehend source-ن/Yud [of/through]-purpose single~mindedness actions-ن/Final-Mem-trial fashions

prevail-(Your hand)S574 {=to be able to do} =ﬡ/ﬡ Aleph-authority ability confirm-ن/Yud [of/through]-purpose

single~mindedness actions-ن/Dalet-faith establish presence-ن/Final-Kaph-acknowledge offer allow-(upon

her)עֲלַהּ S15704 {=on behalf of} =ﬡ/ע Ayin-pierce perceive wisdom-U/ל Lamed[to/toward]-instruct acquire provide-ن/Yud [of/through]-purpose single~mindedness actions-ن/Hey[behold/the]-quality reveal grace-(& she will be

healed)וְתִתְחַלַם S7143 {= recovering one's health} =Y/ן Vav-[and/in addition]increase degree assure-ن/Taw-

evidence prove sign-ن/Taw-evidence prove sign-ن/Hhet-specific share beyond-ن/Lamed[to/toward]-instruct acquire provide-

ﬡﬡ/Final-Mem-trial fashions prevail-(& she will live)וְתֵחֵא S6908 {=to revive/sustain/be

nourished/make live} =Y/ן Vav-[and/in addition]increase degree assure-ن/Taw-evidence prove sign-ن/Hhet-specific share beyond-

/Final-Aleph-ending finish maturity-

The Semitic Emphasis

And seeking for someone/something coming into being~~indicating the origin of directional movement/movement of time in a long while~~and/also making a legal declaration beyond/above/outside of a small part of something in ruin/desolation creating/trans-ferring ownership/making into coming to mind place~~things in order to be able to do on behalf of recovering one's health to revive/sustain/be nourished/make live.

It could be interpreted as those who believe that God will actually use them, those who believe God's Word is for them personally, and those who believe that God will move through them as they obey His Word.

And seeking for someone/something coming into being, we can clearly discern whether what we seek for is according to His Plan, or ours!

When we embrace His Insights as _indicating the origin of directional_ *movement/movement of time in a long while*, we tend to discover more out the developing assistance the Spirit works through in our everyday living.

And/Also making a legal declaration beyond/above/outside of a small part of something in ruin/desolation creating/transferring ownership/making into coming to mind, begins the process of Divine Directions that steadies the heart, clarifies the thoughts, and levels every playing field to the advantage of the KING of KINGS Who knows all things before they have happened.

You see, it is the intent of the word, *desire* is found in breaking down the syllables to note the original thought of God.

DE means "*of*". SIRE means "*father*".

The questions appearing at every crossroad, or intersection in our lives would be better explained when we ask, "*with what, with whom have I been in communion*"?

By *place things in order to be able to do on behalf of recovering one's health to revive/sustain/be nourished/make live*, we discover that God is, or is not, the priority of our living and livelihood.

If we spends more time analyzing whether this is God's Will or ours, we probably can learn to rest easy, knowing it is probably the *old~man~of~the~flesh* acting out *trying to be LIKE God!*

Whomever we have been fellowshipping with, it will be their influence that leads us to the choices we make; whether is in fellowshipping with thoughts of the past we have not relinquished to HIM; or it is the produce of our fellowshipping with God Who creates His desires in us as the *children/evidence* formed in our heart.

The Increase Of Face~To~Face
Shares The Faith Of His Efforts
Influencing Every Purpose
Through His Pattern~Of~Thought
Exchanging Evidence With The Memories That Wisely
Motivate The Patterns Of His Finished Work

MARK 5:29

Got Healing?

KJV+TVM

And[G2532] straightway[G2112] the[G3588] fountain[G4077] of her[G846] blood[G129] was dried up;[G3583] and[G2532] she felt[G1097] in her body[G4983] that[G3754] she was healed[G2390] of[G575] that plague.[G3148]

ORIGINAL THOUGHTS

...(5:29) *The increase of face~to~face shares the Faith of His Efforts influencing every purpose through His Pattern~of~Thought exchanging evidence with the memories that wisely motivates the Patterns of His Finished Work. Dignify His Faith out of the qualities that increase and enable the substance of things hoped for experiencing the enlarging of His Evidence. Inside of His Spoken Word intersect the strength of His Grace within the Faith of His Dominion and signify His Authority adjusting through every signal/sign of the Unseen Issues going beyond specifics of single~minded evidence revealed.*

The increase of face~to~face shares the Faith of His Efforts influencing every purpose through His Pattern~of~Thought exchanging evidence with the memories that wisely motivates the Patterns of His Finished Work.

The increase of face~to~face shares the Faith of His Efforts while distinguishing to us, the facts between *entering into the Kingdom of God*, and *living within the Kingdom of God*!

Through God's will reveal, we see His *influencing every purpose through His Pattern~of~Thought* not by those things He controls, but through the inter~personal relationships He forms, addresses, cultivates, and produces through our living with HIM, IN HIM!

It is within the Kingdom of God, by the *exchanging evidence with the memories* that we discover we longer are *servants, but friends* of the Most High God.

In the same manner, by which the Cross proclaims the resurrection, so our abandonment to His Will must not only precede God attending to ours, it must be the forthright announcing of His First~Right Priorities that we willingly follow!

When He is seen in the primary role of every choice we make, it is the Spirit of God *that wisely motivates the Patterns of His Finished Work*, thereby establishing the clarity of His Will within our living THROUGH HIM!

Dignify His Faith out of the qualities that increase and enable the substance of things hoped for experiencing the enlarging of His Evidence.

Dignify His Faith out of the qualities we learn to regard and care for as though being our own; because they are, as we recognize and maintain our awareness that He is the Author and Finisher of our Faith.

For these thoughts be the very initiatives *that increase and enable the substance of things hoped for* when as responding to Who we hear, we obey willingly and follow Their leading as God!

Experiencing the enlarging of His Evidence reveals through discovery that nothing of Himself does He withhold, from them *that walk uprightly!*

<u>Inside of His Spoken Word intersect the strength of His Grace within the Faith of His Dominion and signify His Authority adjusting through every signal/sign of the Unseen Issues going beyond specifics of single~minded evidence revealed.</u>

Inside of His Spoken Word intersect the strength of His Grace; for it is within the Seed of His every thought that there implodes the revealings that stir the heart and mind and soul with the very fabric and power of God maintaining all that we are IN HIM, and all that He has given of Himself as being HIM THROUGH US TO OTHERS!

Realize that *within the Faith of His Dominion* we actually embrace the strengths of His Provision, the steadfastness of His Promises, and the inalienable Spiritual right to wield the sword of His Word in establishing all that is Heaven upon all of that which is Earth.

Could it be that when we recognize and realize that through His Dominion given us, we exalt and magnify *and signify His Authority adjusting through every signal/sign of the Unseen Issues*, whereby the matchless beauties of Christ portray the unchallenged dulcet memories we find in God Themselves?

going beyond specifics of single~minded evidence revealed

SEMITIC~ARAMAIC~HEBRAIC THESAURUS

Aramaic before first {

Semitic Root before first =

Lettering for ParaPhrase after second =

...(5:29) (& at once)ומחדא S6243 {ᚷ⊔⊓⊞ᛘ=immediately}=Ɣ/ı Vav-[and/in addition]increase degree assure- ᛘ/מ Mem[from/out of]-transform encounter remembrance- ⊞/ח Hhet-specific share beyond- ⊔/ד Dalet-faith establish presence- Ɣ/ı Final-Aleph-ending finish maturity- (dried up)יבשת S8528 {ᰚᱚᱜᛁ=extinguished/hard to hear}=ᰚ/ı Yud [of/through]-purpose single~mindedness actions- ᱚ/ב Beyt[within/inside]-pattern thought inhabit- ᱜᱜ/ש Shin-pressure exchange disperse- ✝/ת Taw-evidence prove sign- ᛘ/מ Mem[from/out of]-transform encounter (the fount)מעינא S15506 {ᰚᱚᱜᛁ=shame/confusion/ /disappointment}=ᛘ/מ Mem[from/out of]-transform encounter remembrance- ◉/ע Ayin-pierce perceive wisdom- ᛁ/ı Yud [of/through]-purpose single~mindedness actions- ᱚ/ב Beyt[within/inside]-pattern thought inhabit- Ɣ/א Final-Aleph-ending finish maturity- (of blood) דדמה S4675 {ᛘ⊓ᛁ⊓=belonging/related to someone/something even unto congestion/pain/death}=⊓/ד Dalet-faith establish presence- ⊓/ד Dalet-faith establish presence- ᛘ/מ Mem[from/out of]-transform encounter remembrance- ᚷ/ה Hey[behold/the]-quality reveal grace- (& she

Got Healing?

sensed)וארגשת S19443 {ᛁᛁᛚᛉ=being aware of someone/something} =Y/ו Vav-[and/in addition]increase degree assure-
/א Aleph-authority ability confirm-ד/ד Dalet-faith establish presence-ᛌ/ᒐ Gimal-experience understanding encounter-ש/ש Shin-pressure
exchange disperse-ת/ת Taw-evidence prove sign-(in her body)בפגרה S16396 {ᕕᒪ◠=in the flesh}=ם/ב Beyt[within/inside]-
pattern thought inhabit-פ/פ Pey-mouth SpokenWord speak-ᒐ/ᒐ Gimal-experience understanding encounter-ᑭ/ר Resh-process beginning
strength-ᑫ/ה Hey[behold/the]-quality reveal grace-(that she was
healed)דתתאסיה S1590 {◠ᓬᛁᛁᛃ=perceiving/desiring to heal/repair/refute}=ד/ד Dalet-faith establish
presence-ᓬ/א Aleph-authority ability confirm-ת/ת Taw-evidence prove sign-ᓬ/א Aleph-authority ability confirm-ᛞ/ס Samech-adjust
apprehend source-ᒐ/י Yud [of/through]-purpose single~mindedness actions-ת/ת Taw-evidence prove sign-
(from)מן S12182 {ᛉᛉ=indicating the origin of directional movement/movement of
time}-ᛉᛉ/מ Mem[from/out of]-transform encounter remembrance-ᒐ/ן Final-Nun-issue perseverance progress-(her
plague)מחותה S11571 {ᛉᎩᎥᛉᛉ=}=ᛉᛉ/מ Mem[from/out of]-transform encounter remembrance-ᎣᎣ/ח Hhet-specific share beyond-
ᒐ/י Yud [of/through]-purpose single~mindedness actions-ת/ת Taw-evidence prove sign-ᛩ/ה Hey[behold/the]-quality reveal grace-

The Semitic Emphasis

Immediately extinguished/hard to hear shame/confusion/disappointment belonging/related to someone/some-thing even unto congestion/pain/death~~being aware of someone/something in the flesh perceiving/desiring to heal/repair/refute indicating the origin of directional movement/movement of time.

Immediately extinguished/hard to hear shame/confusion/disappointment belonging/related to someone/something even unto congestion/pain/death becomes the very places of one's living that deceive one's heart away from the Word of God's HEALING FLOW!

It is in _being aware of someone/something in the flesh_ that there is made conscious the movings of the Spirit within our living IN HIM; and here it is that we struggle in ourselves in finding the fullness He has given to each of us, continually.

Understand this: ~~that _perceiving/desiring to heal/repair/refute indicating the origin of directional movement/movement of time_ tells us that all things work together for good; and as this is God's promise, so even it is God's Work within our living to prove every evidence of what it is HE HAS PROMISED IS OURS THROUGH HIM!

_And Every Degree Of Teaching Influences By His Efforts
The Transforming Of Each Pressure Surrendered
Specifically To The Revelation
Assuring His Finished Work_

MARK 6:5

Got Healing?

KJV+TVM

And^{G2532} he could^{G1410} there^{G1563} do^{G4160} no^{G3756} mighty work,^{G1411} save that^{G1508} he laid his hands upon$^{G2007\ G5495}$ a few^{G3641} sick folk,^{G732} and healed^{G2323} them.

ORIGINAL THOUGHTS

...(6:5) And every degree of teaching influences by His efforts the transforming of each pressure surrendered specifically to the revelation assuring His Finished Work. Through the Faith of His Patient Wisdom, His Pattern~of~Thought establishes the significance of transfiguring the progress by Dominion of His Sound Advantage. The provisions of His Finished Work share in the Presence of the Unseen Single~Mindedness that is provided by His Finished Work. The parallels of His Teaching single~mindedness provide the adjusting that fashions each ability through Faith in the revelation of each portion of His Authority apprehending His Single~Mindedness.

And every degree of teaching influences by His efforts the transforming of each pressure surrendered specifically to the revelation assuring His Finished Work.

It is through His Word *and every degree of teaching influences by His efforts,* so that the heart/soul/mind and will come into AGREEMENT, while aligning such AGREEMENT with the will of God alone.

Confirming AGREEMENT not only defends the position of His HEALING, but deals with every conflicting condition of speech that would seek to contradict what God has said from the beginning!

Not until every member of the Body, whether physical or spiritual, comes into the AGREEMENT His LOVE provides, will there be the worldwide occurrences of manifestation He promised, and continues to promise as His Finished Work.

It is in *the transforming of each pressure surrendered* that the heart/soul/mind and will becomes the vessels, and then the channels necessary to influence the changing of the world around us, and the world in which we live.

Specifically to the revelation assuring His Finished Work, take heart to realize as He does it to the least of those we know and observe, regardless of what we think about others, He will do the same for us!

Through the Faith of His Patient Wisdom, His Pattern~of~Thought establishes the significance of transfiguring the progress by Dominion of His Sound Advantage.

Through the Faith of His Patient Wisdom, comes the undeniable abilities to embrace ALL THAT THEY ARE IN US, as the Godhead moves in THEIR WAYS, not necessarily ours.

His Pattern~of~Thought establishes the significance of transfiguring every portion of our living, and while transcending our imaginations through RESTING IN HIM, we discover the multitudes of paradigms and parallels configuring every portion of our living THROUGH HIM!

Throughout *the progress by Dominion of His Sound Advantage,* there is fashioned the eternal mindset that God is still GOD, and always will be GOD; therefore, to struggle with WHO HE IS, becomes a course no longer pursued due to the reality that HE DOES WHAT HE SAID HAS FINISHED!

Healing flows from the very nature of God, THEMSELVES!

And yet, HEALING is not the characteristic of THEIR NATURE being LIFE ETERNAL!

Because the Godhead is WHO THEY SAY THEY ARE, LIFE flows unhindered, unaltered, and undefiled by anything THEY HAVE CREATED!

The very name *JEHOVAH~RAPHA* signifies THEY ARE~~*the Lord Who HEALS you!*

If the character of THEIR very nature is LIFE, there is no need of healing, when THEIR LIFE sustains the quality of THEIR LIFE to begin with!

THEY are the "I" in the "*I AM*"; and we are the "AM" as THEY reveal the realities of the spiritual dimension created out of the wholeness that THEY ARE and REMAIN AS FOREVERMORE!

The provisions of His Finished Work share in the Presence of the Unseen Single~Mindedness that is provided by His Finished Work.

The provisions of His Finished Work share in the Presence of the Unseen Single~Mindedness bringing about the clarity of WHO THE GODHEAD actually remains as!

Everything provided through His Finished Work is sustained out of the ETERNAL PRESENCE of WHO the GODHEAD remains in being through THEIR eternal existence.

AS THEY have been, ALWAYS shall THEY BE and REMAIN AS THEY ARE!

These are the TRUTHS of His REVELATION IN US, as well as the understanding we are offered *that is provided by His Finished Work.*

Out of the very insights He reveals to us of WHO THE FATHER IS, the Spirit carries is further by revealing WHO THE ENTIRETY OF THE GODHEAD REMAINS!

That THEY are the GOD OF HEALING refers back again and again to the FACT THAT THEY ARE THE VERY LIFE OF OUR EXISTENCE IN THEMSELVES!

His PROPER LIFE provides our proper health, healing, and realities of experiencing ALL THEY PROVIDED ETERNALLY!

When confirming the influence of His Steadfastness confirming through perseverance the Faith of His Wisdom provide agreement through process in purpose of revelation out of His Finished Work.

When confirming the influence of His Steadfastness the TRUTH of our TRUSTING in Him AS THEM, provides the stability of knowing that THEIR LIFE continues through ours!

Look at Elijah and Elisha: they are the examples of what God will do through one generation into and including the next!

Elijah performed SEVEN MIRACLES, while Elisha performed FOURTEEN.

AS God is our first generation of inheritance, when we walk in the FULLNESS OF WHO THEY ARE, we operate our living through the *double portion THEY GIVE CONTINUALLY and ETERNALLY!*

Confirming through perseverance the Faith of His Wisdom becomes the apprehending of all THEY provide to us AS WE BELIEVE THEM.

To *provide agreement through process* there must be the actualities of clarifying WHOSE WE ARE; for in so doing we discover WHO WE ARE IN THEM, the THREE~AS~ONE!

It is through and *in purpose of revelation out of His Finished Work* that we discover the fullness of WHOSE WE HAVE ALWAYS BEEN; knowing that before the foundations of the worlds were laid, WE WERE AS A THOUGHT CONCEIVED IN THE MIND OF GOD THEMSELVES!

The parallels of His Teaching single~mindedness provide the adjusting that fashions each ability through Faith in the revelation of each portion of His

Got Healing?

Authority _apprehending_ His _Single~Mindedness._

The _parallels_ of _His Teaching single~mindedness_ enhance in us the understandings that triangulate the premises of humanity included in the DIAMOND of His PERFECTION!

PAPA

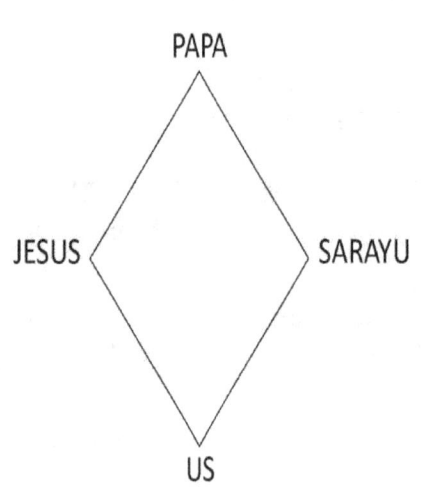

The illustration is the imagination/portrayal that shows the provisions that _provide the adjusting that fashions each ability_ in us as being in the LIKENESS OF THEM, AS THEY ARE THE THREE~AS~ONE!

Through Faith in the revelation of each portion of His Authority, we discover not only our place in THEM, but our position as well.

As we _face~to~face_ with THEM, we discover everything about THEM resides, abides, and dwells within everything there is about us!

This is the thoughts _apprehending His Single~Mindedness;_ for wherein we discover THEM, we discover the FULLNESS OF THEM IN US!

SEMITIC~ARAMAIC~HEBRAIC THESAURUS

Aramaic before first {

Semitic Root before first =

Lettering for ParaPhrase after second =

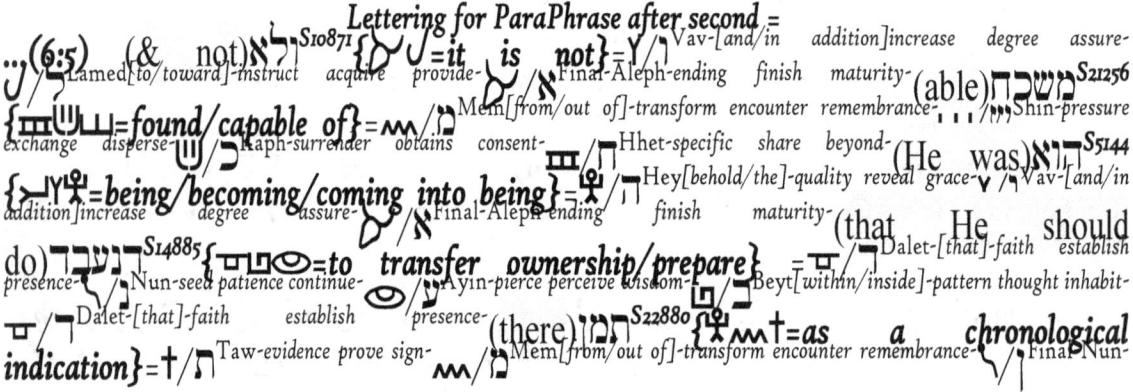

Got Healing?

issue perseverance progress- (even) ~ᴺᴬ *S1743* { } = ~ ¹little more/nothing at all} = -ability confirm- /Final-Pey-declare sound advantage- (not) Final-Aleph-ending *S10878* =it is not} = finish -instruct acquire provide- Hhet-specific share beyond- Dalet-[that]-faith establish

(one) *S6244* { someone/certain} = / Hhet-specific share beyond- presence- (powerful work) *S7043* { =heavenly host/intrinsic potency/innate Yud [of/through]-purpose single~mindedness- actions- force} = / Hhet-specific share beyond- Final-Aleph-ending finish maturity- (except) ᴺᴸᴬ *S892* Lamed[to/toward]-instruct acquire provide- Aleph-authority ability confirm- Lamed[to/toward]-instruct acquire provide-

{ =except/unless} = / ᴺᴬ Aleph-authority ability Final-Aleph-ending finish maturity- (only) *S1356* { =either/or} = / ᴺᴬ Aleph-authority ability confirm- Final-Nun-issue perseverance progress- (upon) *S15688* =in measure of} = Dalet-[that]-faith establish presence- Ayin-pierce perceive wisdom- Lamed[to/toward]-instruct acquire provide- (sick ones) ᴺᴬ *S10537* { =cutting to covenant} = / Kaph-surrender obtains consent- Resh-process beginning strength- Yud [of/through]-purpose single~mindedness actions- Hey[behold/ /the]-quality reveal grace- / Final-Aleph-ending finish maturity- (a few) *S18614* { = little by little} = / Quph-contrast parallel structure- Lamed[to/toward]-instruct acquire provide- Yud [of/through]- purpose single~mindedness actions- Lamed[to/toward]-instruct acquire provide- (He laid) *S14276* { =lay a foundation/ /indicate position} = / Samech-adjust apprehend source- Final-Mem-trial fashions prevail (His hand) *S561* { =to be able to do/come under the supervision or control of} = / Aleph-authority ability confirm- Yud [of/through]-purpose single~mindedness actions- Dalet-[that]- faith establish presence- Hey[behold/the]-quality reveal grace- (& healed) ᴺᴬ *S1596* { =to repair/restore} = / Vav-[and/in addition]increase degree assure- / Aleph-authority ability confirm- Samech- adjust apprehend source- Yud [of/through]-purpose single~mindedness actions-

The Semitic Emphasis

It is not found/capable of being/becoming/coming into being to transfer ownership/prepare as a chronological indication a little more/nothing at all~~it is not someone/certain heavenly host/intrinsic potency/innate force except/unless either/or in measure of cutting to covenant little by little lay a foundation/indicated position to be able to do/under the supervision or control of to repair/restore.

It is not found/capable of being/becoming/coming into being without the attention and agreement of what God already placed in motion, since before He created Adam, as a race of humanity through which He sought relationship eternally.

It has always been THEIR DESIRE to transfer ownership/prepare as a chronological indication a little more/nothing at all in persuading humanity to see what it is about the Godhead having provided in the fullness of Him Who was offered in their stead completely, without compromise!

It is not someone/certain of the heavenly host/intrinsic potency/innate force except/unless either/or in measure of cutting to covenant; it is therefore by that

---

which the Godhead eternally honors and respects, wherein THEY have decided to offer to this THEIR CREATION the right and the privilege being, living, and existing eternally even as THEY, the THREE~AS~ONE live THEMSELVES!

In that it is *little by little* to *lay a foundation/indicate position to be able to do/come under the supervision or control of repair/restore* that the Eternal Godhead that THEY ARE and REMAIN AS, offer to the humanity created the very same platform of privilege that THEY, the GODHEAD have always experienced.

Now, THEY offer to humanity the understanding of every revelation revealed in the circumstances that humanity must weather, and be a part in, THEY offer WHO THEY ARE, and WHAT THEY HAVE at THEIR DISPOSAL, in providing humanity not only with a WAY OF ESCAPE, but the ability while in the EYE OF EVERY STORM to remain secure, peaceful, and at REST IN THE FULLNESS OF WHO HE IS IN THEM COMPLETELY!

In Addition~~Exchanging His Authority To Establish The Influences Of His Efforts By Adjustings That Encounter The Single~Minded Abilities Of His Finished Work

MARK 6:13

KJV+TVM

And^{G2532} they cast out^{G1544} many^{G4183} devils,^{G1140} and^{G2532} anointed^{G218} with oil^{G1637} many^{G4183} that were sick,^{G732} and^{G2532} healed^{G2323} them.

ORIGINAL THOUGHTS

...(6:13) In addition exchanging His Authority to establish the influences of His Efforts by adjustings that encounter the single~minded abilities of His Finished Work. Out of every Spoken Word building the single~mindedness of His Perseverance it is the quality within every degree of increase that assures each remembrance of exchange beyond the purpose of each issue. Behold in addition to increase the Pattern~of~His~Thoughts to transfigure the spreading beyond His Finished Work, the obtaining of His Beginnings that purpose His Finished Work. Apprehend each experience as focused upon the Authority of His Finished Work and enable with the adjusting of a single~minded persistence, the qualities that add each degree of *assurance.*

In addition exchanging His Authority to establish the influences of His Efforts by adjustings that encounter the single~minded abilities of His Finished Work.

In addition exchanging His Authority for the confidence of calling those things that though they appear as being not, are of the spiritual substance given humanity since before the earth's foundations were laid.

If such substance is held in store for those knowing their righteousness abides ever more in HIM; then, such actions as calling what is not in this physical realm as though it is in the spiritual dimension, becomes but the agreement with those things God has provided since before humanity was born!

It is through such agreement *to establish the influences of His Efforts* that the believer's mental condition becomes the stable, peaceful realm of His Pattern~of~Thoughts.

it is *by adjustings that encounter the single~minded abilities of His Finished Work* that the stability and steadfastness of God's confidence and persuasive assurances fortify every element within the believer's outlook and own state~of~mind that provides the stable effect of TRUSTING INHIM!

Out of every Spoken Word building the single~mindedness of His Perseverance it is the quality within every degree of increase that assures each remembrance of exchange beyond the purpose of each issue.

Out of every Spoken Word the faithful believer in turn TRUSTS the outcome of their living to the workings and movings of the Spirit's direction and guidance as it is with the assurances that His Finished Work has covered every base of responsibility.

It is in *building the single~mindedness of His Perseverance* that the heart/soul/mind and will of believers transcends beyond the limited degrees of thought in this dimension, and continually entrusts every outcome to the simplicity of that which is HIS OWN THOUGHTS included within the DIMENSION OF HIS WILL PERSONIFIED within every believer!

It is the quality within every degree of increase that proves the indwelling by the Spirit, of His Person and Presence out of the Word; so that the believer begins realizing and recognizing that because of THEIR indwelling, the believer has a *face~to~face* experience waiting within every moment they remain at REST IN HIM!

It is when we, as believers, attain to understanding that we are ALREADY AT REST IN HIM, there is then found the REST OF HIM.

It is in knowing the Presence of the Spirit from within *that assures each remembrance of exchange* and thereby allows the smooth transitions by the Spirit's direction and guidance, into the fullness of WHO the Godhead is within every believer themselves!

While it is *beyond the purpose of each issue* that the Spirit seeks to take the believer beyond where they are currently residing; there must be a consistent, constant, conscious, and continual awareness that as a believer there is NO ONE ELSE but GOD that can lead them to where they want, and need, to be!

Behold in addition to increase the Pattern~of~His~Thoughts to transfigure the spreading beyond His Finished Work, the obtaining of His Beginnings that purpose His Finished Work.

Behold, in addition to increase the Pattern~of~His~Thoughts there is an ever available source in the Spirit to access those thoughts of God that enlarge and enhance the living of any believer who is willing to be obedient and yielded to the Will of the Father.

What we have before called, *tests or trials*, we now recognize that these are moments when the Spirit PROVES to us, as believers that under Her guidance, leadership, and tutelage, the soul/mind/heart and will discover a new course, and a new journey available causing the manifold discoveries of His Person, Presence, and Power.

To transfigure the spreading beyond His Finished Work, simply continually YIELD yourselves to Her leading, and as She is the TEACHER, She will guide your living into the many~folded parallels of eternal existence to be found in the Presence of the Most High!

It is in *the obtaining of His Beginnings that purpose His Finished Work*; and it is out of such obtaining that new horizons, new opportunities, and new insights begin occurring at a mind~boggling rate of increase!

Learn to continually seek HIS REST, and you will discover that not only is HEALING the option of LIFE IN GOD, but as an OPTION there is far more to discover in the FULLNESS OF HIS PRESENCE than we could have before found in the mere shallow agreements with the printed page of His Word.

NOW, we discover the WORD in it viability, when accessing the many~folded aspects of RELATIONSHIP through a *FACE~TO~FACE* experience IN HIM!

<u>*Apprehend each experience as focused upon the Authority of His Finished Work and enable with the adjusting of a single~minded persistence, the qualities that add each degree of assurance.*</u>

Apprehend each experience as focused upon the Authority of His Finished Work; for in doing this one simple excursion, there is opened to the believer, to you, an abundance of living never thought available before, much less possible to enjoy!

Learn to TRUST Who it is you believe, *and enable the adjusting of a single~minded persistence* to capture your desires, thoughts, and even your apprehensions.

It is through *the qualities that add each degree of assurance* that the security and peacefulness of GOD'S Presence, Person, and Power add to one's living.

SEMITIC~ARAMAIC~HEBRAIC THESAURUS
Aramaic before first {
Semitic Root before first =
Lettering for ParaPhrase after second =

...(6:13) (& evil spirits)שידרא ^{S20345} {ㅠﾉﾉﾑﾑ=disturbing}=Y/ר Vav-[and/in addition]increase degree assure- ﾑﾑ/ש Shin-pressure exchange disperse-ﾉﾉ/ﾉ Aleph-authority ability confirm-ㅠ/ㄱ Dalet-[that]-faith establish presence-ﾉ /ﾑ Final-Aleph-ending finish maturity-(many)סיניאב ^{S13929} {ﾉﾑﾑ=in a manifold way}=ﾉﾉ/ﾉ Samech-adjust apprehend source-ﾉ/ﾑ Gimal-experience understanding encounter-ﾉ/ﾉ Yud [of/through]-purpose single~mindedness actions-ﾉ/ﾑ Aleph-authority ability confirm-ﾉﾉ/ﾑ Final-Aleph-ending finish maturity-(casting out)ןיקפמ ^{S13399} {ﾉﾑﾑ=causing to come forth}=ﾑﾑ/ﾑ Mem[from/out of]-transform encounter remembrance-ﾉ/פ Pey-mouth SpokenWord speak-ﾉ/ﾑ Quph-contrast parallel structure-ﾉ/ﾉ Yud [of/through]-purpose single~mindedness actions-ﾉ/ﾉ Final-Nun-issue perseverance progress-(they were)ווה ^{S5147} {ﾉﾉﾉ=to come into being/coming to one's senses}=ﾉ/ﾉ Hey[behold/the]-quality reveal grace-ﾉ/ﾉ Vav-[and/in addition]increase degree assure-ﾉ/ﾉ Vav-[and/in addition]increase degree assure-(& anointing)ןיחשמו ^{S12489} {ﾑﾑﾑ=spreading with oil}=Y/ﾉ Vav-[and/in addition]increase degree assure-ﾑﾑ/ש Shin-pressure exchange disperse-ﾑﾑ/ﾑ Hhet-specific share beyond-ﾉ/ﾉ Yud [of/through]-purpose single~mindedness actions-ﾉ/ﾉ Final-Nun-issue perseverance progress-(they were)ווה ^{S5147} {ﾉﾉﾉ=to come into being/coming to one's senses}=ﾉ/ﾉ Hey[behold/the]-quality reveal grace-ﾉ/ﾉ Vav-[and/in addition]increase degree assure-ﾉ/ﾉ Vav-[and/in addition]increase degree assure-(with oil) אחשמב ^{S12505} {ﾉﾑﾑ=firm in resources}=ﾑ/ﾑ Beyt[within/inside]-pattern thought inhabit-ﾉﾉ/ﾑ Mem[from/out of]-transform encounter remembrance-ﾑﾑ/ש Shin-pressure exchange disperse-ﾑﾑ/ﾑ Hhet-specific share beyond-ﾉ/ﾑ Final-Aleph-ending finish maturity-(the sick)אירכ ^{S10537} {ﾑﾉﾉﾉﾉ=the impotent}=ﾉ/ש Kaph-surrender obtains consent-ﾉ/ﾑ Resh-process beginning strength-ﾉ/ﾉ Yud [of/through]-purpose single~mindedness actions-ﾉ/ﾑ Hey[behold/the]-quality reveal grace-ﾉ/ﾑ Final-Aleph-ending finish maturity-(many)אינס ^{S13929} {ﾉﾑﾑ=in a manifold way} =ﾉﾉ/ﾑ Samech-adjust

Got Healing?

apprehend source-ℵ /L/ Gimal-experience understanding encounter- _╮_ / Yud [of/through]-purpose single~mindedness actions- ⅄ /ℵ Aleph-authority
ability   confirm-ﬡ /ﬡ Final-Aleph-ending   finish   maturity-(&   healing)ﬢﬡﬣﬤ S1606 {ﬢﬣ}=to Samech-adjust
repair/restore/refute}= ⅄ /╮ Vav-[and/in addition]increase degree assure- ⅄ /ℵ Aleph-authority ability confirm-ﬡ /ﬤ
apprehend   source- _╮_ / Yud [of/through]-purpose   single~mindedness   actions- ⅄ /ℵ Final-Nun-issue   perseverance   progress-(they
were)ﬢﬣﬤ S5147 {ﬣﬤ}=to come into being/coming to one's senses} = ﬢ /ﬣ Hey[behold/the]-quality reveal grace- ⅄ /╮ Vav-
[and/in addition]increase degree assure- ⅄ /╮ Vav-[and/in addition]increase degree assure-

The Semitic Emphasis

<u>Disturbing in a manifold way~~causing to come forth coming into being/coming to one's senses~~spreading with oil coming into being/coming to one's senses firm in resources the impotent in a manifold way~~to repair/restore/refute coming into being/coming to one's senses.</u>

Disturbing in a manifold way is the apprehension that builds without ceasing, when we do not consciously give thanks to GOD for being part with our living.

It is in *causing to come forth coming into being/coming to one's senses* that we discover the tranquil vicissitude that govern, or pattern our living after THEIR'S.

spreading with oil coming into being/coming to one's senses firm in resources the impotent in a manifold way

~~to repair/restore/refute coming into being/coming to one's senses

Transforming Perception Strengthens Their Pattern~Of~Thought Through Each Exchange Of Remembrance Enlarging Their Finished Work

LUKE 4:40
KJV+TVM

Now[G1161] when the[G3588] sun[G2246] was setting,[G1416] all[G3956] they[G3745] that had[G2192] any sick[G770] with divers[G4164] diseases[G3554] brought[G71] them[G846] unto[G4314] Him;[G846] and[G1161] He[G3588] laid His hands on[G2007 G5495] every[G1538] one[G1520] of them,[G846] and healed[G2323] them.[G846]

ORIGINAL THOUGHTS

...(4:40) Transforming perception strengthens Their Pattern~of~Thought through each exchange of remembrance, enlarging Their Finished Work. Through faithfully and mindfully persisting/persevering through every surrender toward the Grace of Their Truth, increase by progressing to confirm the journey that continues Their Finished Work. Their Presence enables the single~mindedness of proving the qualities that increase Their

Got Healing?

Finished Work, while promoting the discoveries that increase our progress. By every surrender there begins the action that qualifies Their Work Finished, and establishes the obtaining of Their Strength through the single~mindedness of Their Grace Truth out of Their Finished Work. Transcending every exchange to share the provisions of Their Spoken Word impacts the abilities of mindfully proving each purpose in addition to confirming and continuing the increases that issue the promises assured, as signaling the Grace of Their Truth. Behold in addition to Their Faith and purpose pursue and perceive the learning of Their Wisdom teaching specifics of Their Faith beyond the presenting of each remembrance of progress. Empower each purpose of Their Faith discovering and apprehending Their Full Authority that fashions Their Grace/Truth by each increase of Their Finished Work. In addition, transform/change by determined influence, to discover/reveal the increase of Their Maturity by confirming/agreeing through one's surrender by the purposes of Their Finished Work.

Transforming perception strengthens Their Pattern~of~Thought through each exchange of remembrance, enlarging Their Finished Work.

Transforming perception strengthens Their Pattern~of~Thought by the fact that we begin thinking upon THEM FIRST, instead of clinging to all *the old remedies of our past.*

It is *through each exchange of remembrance, enlarging Their Finished Work* that our heart/mind/soul and will begin to embrace the UNION we have always had IN THEM; wherein we begin discovering the greater fullness of THEIR existence within our living as well.

Through faithfully and mindfully persisting/persevering through every surrender toward the Grace of Their Truth, increase by progressing to confirm the journey that continues Their Finished Work.

1.-*Through faithfully and mindfully persisting/persevering through every surrender*
   a.-*how long do we continue "faithfully and mindfully persisting/persevering"?*

   b.-*why is it necessary to persevere "through every surrender"?*

2.-*toward the Grace of Their Truth, increase by progressing*
   a.-*when do we know/realize we are moving "toward the*

Grace of Their Truth"?

> *b.-when do we perceive/discern our "increase by progressing"?*

3.-*to confirm the journey that continues Their Finished Work*
  a.-what is the purpose behind "confirming the journey"?

> *b.-does "confirming the journey" provide clarity of Their Purpose, or show us the single~mindedness of Their Work in and through us?*

Through faithfully and mindfully persisting/persevering, we learn to TRUST in what we may not see at the moment, because we have learned that THEIR PROMISE is as good as done, because THEY HAVE SEEN IT AS DONE IN THEIR SPIRITUAL DIMENSION.

It is *through every surrender toward the Grace of Their Truth,* we discover the treasures in store for us, because of THEIR KNOWING BEFOREHAND what we are even now experiencing in our living.

Healing must begin as being about that which is SPIRITUAL, BEFORE IT EVER BECOMES PHYSICAL IN MANIFESTATION!

Through *increase by progressing to confirm* the promises of GOD, we discern the discovering of every moment that transcends doubts, suspicions, or even the hesitancies we might feed upon, rather than feeding upon the Strengths of GOD'S strategies in teaching us how to learn to live OUT OF THE SPIRITUAL FIRST!

This is *the journey that continues Their Finished Work,* and develops Their Finished Work within the very core of our living in the NOW!

<u>*Their Presence enables the single~mindedness of proving the qualities that increase Their Finished Work, while promoting the discoveries that increase our progress.*</u>

Their Presence enables the single~mindedness of proving all that THEY have kept in store for *such a time as this,* within our living AS THEM!

It is in seeing *the qualities that increase Their Finished Work* that we discover the developing attitudes and experiences that shape and fashion, form and fit THEIR LIVING through ours, causing the destiny intended to be revealed through us.

It is even *while promoting the discoveries that increase our progress* that we reveal the manifold blessings that await our conscious movements into and through the Spiritual Realm of THEIR DOMAIN!

By every surrender there begins the action that qualifies Their Work Finished, and establishes the obtaining of Their Strength through the single~mindedness of Their Grace Truth out of Their Finished Work.

By every surrender there begins the action, for it is out of every action that the simultaneous occurrings offset mindsets that need changing, before the Will of God clearly and precisely may reveal all that is withheld until now.

It is this *that qualifies Their Work Finished, and establishes* the greater fullness to be revealed in our journey of persevering until the answers appear.

HEALING is about discovering JESUS in our living, and then dwelling/abiding therein that we may glean from THEIR FIELD the very substance necessary to manifest the HEALING that has already occurred in THEIR DIMENSION ON OUR BEHALF!

Through realizing that we have attained to *the obtaining of Their Strength,* we are now made SURE that what we SEE IN THEM is what is TRUE IN US!

Through the single~mindedness of Their Grace Truth we allow the Spirit to develop in us the conditioning of THEIR MIND as being ours.

This is the *renewing of THE mind* of Christ in us!

For it is even *out of Their Finished Work* that the souls of humanity may discover the free and ready offering provided through Jesus as the Cross; but greater is the offering made available every day of our living AS THEM!

Transcending every exchange to share the provisions of Their Spoken Word impacts the abilities of mindfully proving each purpose in addition to confirming and continuing the increases that issue the promises assured, as signaling the Grace of Their Truth.

Transcending every exchange to share the provisions of Their Spoken Word alters the momentary hesitations that occur when we doubt, or refuse to step out on GOD'S PROMISES.

The Provisions of THEIR SPOKEN WORD *impacts the abilities of mindfully proving each purpose* while in perspective we begin seeing through discernment of the spiritual dimension all around us that GOD'S PURPOSES in fact are FINISHED IN CHRIST, and WE ARE EVEN IN CHRIST!

In addition to confirming and continuing the increases that provide the manifestations of THEIR FAITH through our living AS THEM, we can also enjoy the benefits of RESTING IN THEM, knowing what THEY have shown to us is the reality coming to pass through us!

By the multitude of *that issue the promises assured, as signaling the Grace of Their Truth,* become the important signposts that guide and govern our journey, as imparting THEIR UNDERSTANDING through experiences that direct us always TOWARD THEM!

Behold in addition to Their Faith and purpose pursue and perceive the learning of Their Wisdom teaching specifics of Their Faith beyond the presenting of each remembrance of progress.

Behold in addition to Their Faith and purpose that the matter of HEALING is *A Finished Work* in GOD'S BOOK OF REMEMBRANCES.

GOD NEVER CHANGES, but we do and can!

pursue and perceive the learning of Their Wisdom

teaching specifics of Their Faith beyond the presenting of each remembrance of progress

Empower each purpose of Their Faith discovering and apprehending Their Full Authority that fashions Their Grace/Truth by each increase of Their Finished Work.

Empower each purpose of Their Faith

discovering and apprehending Their Full Authority

that fashions Their Grace/Truth

by each increase of Their Finished Work

In addition, transform/change by determined influence, to discover/reveal the increase of Their Maturity by confirming/agreeing through one's surrender by the purposes of Their Finished Work.

In addition, transform/change by determined influence,

to discover/reveal the increase of Their Maturity

Got Healing?

by confirming/agreeing through one's surrender
by the purposes of Their Finished Work

SEMITIC~ARAMAIC~HEBRAIC THESAURUS
Aramaic before first {
Semitic Root before first =
Lettering for ParaPhrase after second =

...(4;40) (was setting) מערבי S16195 {ʘ=to mix/combine}= מ/ Mem[from/out of]-transform encounter remembrance- Ayin-pierce perceive wisdom- Resh-process beginning strength- Beyt[within/inside]-pattern thought inhabit- Yud [of/through]-purpose single~mindedness actions- (the sun)שמש S21911 {=performing one's function}= ש/ Shin-pressure exchange disperse- מ/ Mem[from/out of]-transform encounter remembrance- Shin-pressure exchange disperse- Final-Aleph-ending finish maturity- Yud [of/through]-purpose single~mindedness actions- (but)דין S4405 {=holding to account} = ד/ Dalet-[that]-faith establish presence- Final-Nun-issue perseverance progress-(all of them)כלהון S10082 {=the whole reason for this is}= כ/ Kaph-surrender obtains consent- Lamed[to/toward]-instruct acquire provide- Hey[behold/the]-quality reveal grace- Vav-[and/in addition]increase degree assure- Final-Nun-issue perseverance progress-(those) אילין S660 {=of what sort?}= א/ Aleph-authority ability confirm- Tsad-pursuit journey anticipate- Nun-seed patience continue- Final-Aleph-ending finish maturity-(who)דאית S732 {=there exists/necessary to do}= ד/ Dalet-[that]-faith establish presence- Aleph-authority ability confirm- Yud [of/through]- purpose single~mindedness actions- Taw-evidence prove sign-(had)הוה S5144 {=to come into being}= ה/ Hey[behold/the]-quality reveal grace- Vav-[and/in addition]increase degree assure- Final-Aleph-ending finish maturity-(to them)להון S10844 {=to such a degree}= ל/ Lamed[to/toward]-instruct acquire provide- Hey[behold/the]-quality reveal grace- Vav-[and/in addition]increase degree assure- Final-Nun-issue perseverance progress-(who were sick)כריהא S10537 {=strengthless}= ש/ Kaph-surrender obtains consent- Resh-process beginning strength- Yud [of/through]-purpose single~mindedness actions- Hey[behold/the]-quality reveal grace- Final-Aleph-ending finish maturity-(of their sicknesses)כריהין S10531 {=weak}= ד/ Dalet-[that]-faith establish presence- ש/ Kaph-surrender obtains consent- Resh-process beginning strength- Yud [of/through]- purpose single~mindedness actions- Hey[behold/the]-quality reveal grace- Yud [of/through]- purpose single~mindedness actions- Final-Nun-issue perseverance progress-(with diseases)כורהנא S10508 {=impotent/with a scruple of conscience}= כ/ Kaph-surrender obtains consent- ב/ Beyt[within/inside]-pattern thought inhabit- Vav-[and/in addition]increase degree assure- Resh-process beginning strength- Hey[behold/the]-quality reveal grace- Nun-seed patience continue- Final-Aleph-ending finish maturity-(various)משחלפא S7204 {=diverse}= מ/ Mem[from/out of]-transform encounter remembrance- ש/ Shin-pressure exchange disperse- Hhet-specific share beyond- Lamed[to/toward]-instruct acquire provide- Pey-mouth SpokenWord speak- Final-Aleph-ending finish maturity-(they brought)איתיהי S2070 {=bringing to one's mind}= א/ Aleph- authority ability confirm- Yud [of/through]-purpose single~mindedness actions- Taw-evidence prove sign- Yud [of/through]-purpose single~mindedness actions- Vav-[and/in addition]increase degree assure- Nun-seed patience continue- Vav-[and/in addition]increase degree assure- (them)אנון S4989 {=to abide}= א/ Aleph-authority ability confirm- Vav-[and/in addition]increase degree assure- Final-Nun-issue perseverance progress-(to Him)לותיה S11137 {=according to}= ל/ Lamed[to/toward]-instruct acquire provide- Vav-[and/in addition]increase degree assure- Taw-evidence prove sign- Hey[behold/the]-quality reveal grace-(He)הוא S5005 {=come into being/enduring/existing}= ה/ Hey[behold/the]-quality reveal grace- Vav-[and/in addition]increase degree assure- Final-Aleph-ending finish maturity-(but)דין S4405 {=holding to account}= ד/ Dalet-[that]-faith establish presence- Yud [of/through]-purpose single~mindedness actions- Final-Nun-issue perseverance progress-(on)על S15701 {=in measure of}= ע/ Ayin-pierce perceive wisdom- Lamed[to/toward]-instruct acquire provide-(each)חד S6244 {=one by one}= ח/ Hhet-specific share beyond- Dalet-[that]-faith establish presence-(one)חד S6244 {=how much more}= ח/ Hhet-specific share beyond- Dalet-[that]-faith establish presence-(of them)מנהון S12185 {=indicating the origin of directional

movement/indicating location/indicating the origin of movement through time} = מ/ממ Mem[from/out of]-
transform encounter remembrance- /Final-Nun-issue perseverance progress- (His hand)ידו S561 {ד/ת=to do something as
much as possible} = א/ך /Aleph-authority ability confirm- /Yud [of/through]-purpose single~mindedness actions- ד/ת Dalet-[that]-
faith establish presence- /הHey[behold/the]-quality reveal grace (laid)סאמ S14266 {אצ/מ=setting down
something} = ס/צ Samech-adjust apprehend source- /אAleph-authority ability confirm- /Final-Mem-trial fashions prevail-
(He)הוא S5144 {וי/צ=coming into being} = צ/א /הHey [behold/the]-quality reveal grace- /וVav-[and/in addition]increase degree
assure- /Final-Aleph-ending finish maturity- (& healed)ורפא S1605 {פ/ר=to repair} = ר/ו Vav-[and/in addition]increase
degree assure- /Mem[from/out of]-transform encounter remembrance- /הHhet-specific share beyond- /Final-Aleph-ending finish
maturity- (He)הוא S5144 {וי/צ=coming into being} = צ/א /הHey[behold/the]-quality reveal grace- /וVav-[and/in addition]increase
degree assure- /Final-Aleph-ending finish maturity- (them)ביכם S10844 {ל/יש=at the leisure of} = ל/א Aleph-
authority ability confirm- /Kaph-surrender obtains consent- /Yud [of/through]-purpose single~mindedness actions- /Final-Aleph-ending
finish maturity-

The Semitic Emphasis

*To mix/combine performing one's function ~~the whole reason
for this is of what sort? ~~there exists/necessary to do to come
into being to such a degree ~~strengthless weak impotent/with
a scruple of conscience ~~diverse bringing to one's mind to abide
according to come into being/enduring/existing ~~holding to
account one by one how much more ~~indicating the origin of
directional movement/indicating location/indicating the origin
of movement through time ~~to do something as much as
possible ~~setting down something coming into being at the
leisure of.*

To mix/combine performing one's function

~~the whole reason for this is of what sort?

~~there exists/necessary to do to come into being to such a degree

~~strengthless weak impotent/with a scruple of conscience

~~diverse bringing to one's mind to abide according to come into
being/enduring/existing

~~holding to account one by one how much more

~~indicating the origin of directional movement/indicating location/indicating
the origin of movement through time

~~to do something as much as possible ~~setting down something coming into
being at the leisure of

Establish Unseen Teachings That Confirm
The Patience Of His Finished Work

2 CORINTHIANS 11:3

Got Healing?

KJV+TVM

But ^{G1161} I fear ^{G5399} $^{[G5736]}$, lest ^{G3381} by any means ^{G4458}, as ^{G5613} the serpent ^{G3789} beguiled ^{G1818} $^{[G5656]}$ Eve ^{G2096} through ^{G1722} his ^{G846} subtilty ^{G3834}, so ^{G3779} your ^{G5216} minds ^{G3540} should be corrupted ^{G5351} $^{[G5652]}$ from ^{G575} the simplicity ^{G572} that is in ^{G1519} Christ ^{G5547}.

ORIGINAL THOUGHTS

...(11:3) *Establish then, the unseen teachings that confirm the Patience of His Finished Work, thereby settling with single~mindedness the issues presenting the provisions that transcend His Finished Work. Validating with single~mindedness, acknowledging the Faith of His Dominion, while balancing with His Wisdom, determines each increase of purpose out of His Finished Work. Acquire as well, the specifics adding His Influence, thereby patterning the Seed to obtain the focus of embracing each increase that proves the Grace of His Truth. It is by the quality of our surrender that continues His Finished Work, thereby sowing and then proving the unseen thoughts that provide every assurance of progress. Processing His Wisdom from a single~minded patience, exercises surrender to increase the persevering that transforms the progress of His Spoken Word in replacing actions that balance and insure the evidence of His Finished Work. His Faith acquired, increases the evidence that transcends each replacement of His Purpose in sharing His Finished Work.*

Establish then, the unseen teachings that confirm the Patience of His Finished Work, thereby settling with single~mindedness the issues presenting the provisions that transcend His Finished Work.

"*For though living in the flesh, my warfare is not waged according to the flesh. For the weapons which I wield are not of fleshly weakness but mighty in the strength of God to overthrow the strongholds of the adversaries. Thereby can I overthrow the reasonings of the disputer and pull down all lofty bulwarks that raise themselves against the knowledge of God, and bring every rebellious thought into captivity and subjection to Christ.*" SECOND CORINTHIANS *10:3-5* CONYBEARE TRANSLATION

The mindsets that so often guide and direct our strategies, ambitions, and successes, in this world; these are not the designs of God!

How can we tell what is, and what is not of God?

Examining our ownselves, to see whether we are in the faith is the suggestion of the Apostle for living a life engulfed in the fullness that IS HIM! FIRST CORINTHIANS *13:5 KJV*

In the LIGHT that is HIM, we discover the hidden agendas that so secretively hide themselves from our view.

Got Healing?

Validating with single~mindedness, acknowledging the Faith of His Dominion, while balancing with His Wisdom, determines each increase of purpose out of His Finished Work.

By validating, or approving and acknowledging the Faith of His Dominion at work in our living, we uncover the hidden agendas that cloak themselves in our *humble ambitions*.

Even within the mindsets of our living as HIM, we can discover, at times that we are following an eschewed pathway that leads anywhere else but toward HIM!

This is the reason we must ALWAYS put Christ at the forefront of everything we do, as well as during the course of living to accomplish what we set out to do AS HIM, for Him, THROUGH HIM!

Even though from each beginning, it may appear inconsequential, it is from these precious moments of surrender that we discover the FULLNESS OF HIM that we long for IN HIM!

Reminding ourselves that He is the Mentor, He is the Potter and we are the Clay; there is founded upon the Rock that He IS, the strongere pursuit OF HIM in the midst of doing anything, as well as ALL THINGS!

Acquire as well, the specifics adding His Influence, thereby patterning the Seed to obtain the focus of embracing each increase that proves the Grace of His Truth.

By allowing the addition of His Influence, we permit the mentoring of the Spirit within to establish and thereby balance each accompanying occurrence to present the validation and approval of God upon our surrender.

In various parts of the Pauline epistles we can identify very clearly the state of mind when held as a stronghold/mindset.

It is described in some cases as a *"reprobate mind"* ROMANS 1:28 KJV, a *"blinded mind"* SECOND CORINTHIANS 3:14 KJV, a *"darkened mind"*, causing men to walk in the *"vanity of their minds"* EPHESIANS 4:17-19 KJV, intruding into things which the mind cannot fathom, *"vainly puffed up"* by a *"fleshly mind"* COLOSSIANS 2:18 KJV.

When our thoughts, or thinking thereof, present a self~centered viewpoint, or a viewpoint that aligns with a misguided world~view; this then, is where we become misaligned, and eschewed in our thinking!

Got Healing?

This is where such verses as SECOND CORINTHIANS 13:5, realign our desires to embrace the fullness of HIM, as being the fullness of WHO HE IS IN US!

It is by the quality of our surrender that continues His Finished Work, thereby sowing and then proving the unseen thoughts that provide every assurance of progress.

The mind of the Christian is also the strategic center of the *"war on the saints"* which accusations wage with ceaseless and fiendish skill.

And for this reason: the mind is the vehicle for the Spirit of God, *dwelling in the spirit of the believer*, to transmit to others the truth of God, which alone can remove the deceptions and accusations that fill the minds of all who are in the darkness of humanity's inherent nature.

If the Holy Spirit is dwelling in the regenerate spirit have you considered the question of Her outlet?

If it were only by speech we would be *an oracle!*

But there are no *"oracles"* on earth now.

The *"oracles of God"* are the Scriptures.

The Word of God is being displaced not only by the higher critics, but by many of God's own people by their taking supernatural *"revelations"* as being of equal authority with the written Scriptures.

There are lives wrecked because they have turned from the Word of God to what they call *direct revelation*.

There is a *direct revelation* by God, the Spirit, illuminating the Word of God, and putting it into the spirit/attitude of believers, but <u>NEVER</u> apart from the Scriptures.

Processing His Wisdom from a single~minded patience, exercises surrender to increase the persevering that transforms the progress of His Spoken Word in replacing actions that balance and insure the evidence of His Finished Work.

If the mind of the believer is the vehicle of the Spirit, it is absolutely necessary that the Spirit should have full possession of it, with every *"rebellious thought"* brought into captivity to Christ.

The Spirit, dwelling in the spirit/attitudes of the believer, needs the mind as a channel for expression, but it may be so blocked up and filled with other things that She is hindered, or kept from transmitting all She desire to do within our living.

A *"blocked"* mind means the Spirit remains unexpressed, and the Spirit unexpressed is a stoppage of the outflow of the Spirit of God toward others.

Much of the reason for this happening is that we accept the fact of the *"new spirit"* we receive from God, and yet, we continue to align ourselves with the *odl head"* that remains in control.

The Spirit's exchange/replacing of our old mindsets, and making *"all things new"* is accomplished by our surrender FIRST, and then the enlightening of the mind vacated, being filled with the *"newness of the Spirit's influence"*, offsetts what might remain, but has no more power to influence.

His Faith acquired, increases the evidence that transcends each replacement of His Purpose in sharing His Finished Work.

Going beyond the replacing, we discover the Great Exchange through His Presence motivating, initiating, and leading our thoughts to think upon things that are above, and not on those things that may remain otherwise!

" *¹If ye then be risen with Christ, seek those things which are above, where Christ sitteth on the right hand of God. ²Set your affection on things above, not on things on the earth. ³For ye are dead and your life is hid with Christ in God. ⁴When Christ, who is our life, shall appear, then shall ye also appear with him in glory." COLOSSIANS 3:1-4 KJV*

How many there are who have minds that never *"think a thing out"*.

Devoted children of God, with hearts full of love, but minds full of all kinds of mixture~~minds that have not realized with the mind of Christ, they are delivered and renewed to think like God!

Consequently, they have a strange lack of spiritual perception.

They may get *"flashes of LIGHT"*, and follow the *"flash"*~~which often leads them astray~~however, they lack the discernment of the Spirit's leading into their spiritual vision.

They have yet to recognize and become aware that God has made them *"able ministers of the new testament; not of the letter, but of the Spirit: for the letter killeth, but the Spirit giveth life." SECOND CORINTHIANS 3:6 KJV*

SEMITIC~ARAMAIC~HEBRAIC THESAURUS

Got Healing?

Aramaic before first {
Semitic Root before first =
Lettering for ParaPhrase after second =

(11:3) (fear) הרח S24339 {םוח=believing in God} = ¬Dalet-faith establish presence-ᴅHhet-specific share beyond- Lamed[to/toward]-instruct acquire provide- ᴅFinal-Aleph-ending finish maturity- (I) אנא S1378 {ץ=as for me} = אAleph-authority ability confirm- Nun-seed patience continue- single~mindedness actions- ᴅFinal-Nun-issue perseverance progress- (but) הרי S4405 {רת=on the other hand} = ¬Dalet-faith establish presence- Yud-purpose (lest) הלרמ S11322 {מ=wherefore?} = ¬Dalet-faith establish presence- Lamed[to/toward]-instruct acquire provide- Mem[from/out of]-transform encounter remembrance- ᴅFinal-Aleph-ending finish maturity- (as) אכ S621 {ץשכ=just as/as is appropriate for} = א Kaph-acknowledge offer allow- Aleph-authority ability confirm- Yud-purpose single~mindedness actions- ᴅFinal- (seduced) אטסא S8277 {חסע⊗=to be enticed to false worship/to wander/to make to forget} = ¬Dalet-faith establish presence- אAleph-authority ability confirm- Thet-contain mixture balance- Ayin-pierce perceive wisdom- (the serpent) אחרי S6513 {םץרל=persecuted/accused} = הHhet-specific share beyond- Vav-[and/in addition]increase degree assure- Yud- purpose single~mindedness actions- ᴅFinal-Aleph-ending finish maturity- (Eve) אוחל S6385 {ץם=showing/declaring/ /explaining} = Lamed[to/toward]-instruct acquire provide- ᴅHhet-specific share beyond- Vav-[and/in addition]increase degree assure- ᴅFinal- Aleph-ending finish maturity- (by its craftiness) החליבכנב S13063 {ץשכ=deceiving/committing fraud/disguising} = Beyt[within/inside]pattern thought inhabit- Nun-seed patience continue- Kaph-surrender obtains consent- Yud-purpose single~mindedness actions- Lamed[to/toward]-instruct acquire provide- Vav-[and/in addition]increase degree assure- Taw-evidence prove sign- ¬Hey[behold/the]-quality reveal grace- ¬Hey[behold/the]-quality reveal grace- Kaph-surrender obtains consent- Nun-seed patience continue- ᴅFinal-Aleph-ending finish maturity- (in this way) אנכה S5189 {וץ=this thing of susch a sort} = Hey[behold/the]-quality (may be corrupted) ןולבכהתנ S6139 {םו=to wind tightly/to pervert/to travail} = Nun-seed patience continue- Taw-evidence prove sign- ¬Hhet-specific share beyond- Beyt[within/inside]pattern thought inhabit- Lamed[to/toward]-instruct acquire provide- Vav-[and/in addition]increase degree assure- (your minds) ןוכיניע S20203 {ץ⊗ת=to desire/find acceptable/to complete with satisfaction} = Resh-process beginning strength- Ayin-pierce perceive wisdom- Yud-purpose single~mindedness actions- Nun-seed patience continue- Yud-purpose single~mindedness actions- Kaph-surrender obtains consent- Vav-[and/in addition]increase degree assure- ᴅFinal-Nun-issue perseverance progress- (from) ןמ S12182 {בת=indicating the origin of directional movement} = Mem[from/out of]-transform encounter remembrance- ᴅFinal-Nun-issue perseverance progress- (the simplicity) אתוטישפ S17361 {ץבט=attacking in battle with a goal/standing up straight and healthy} = Pey-mouth SpokenWord speak- Shin-pressure exchange disperse- Yud-purpose single~mindedness actions- Thet-contain mixture balance- Vav-[and/in addition]increase degree assure- Taw-evidence prove sign- ᴅFinal-Aleph-ending finish maturity- (that is with) הלרד S1126 {ץצש=becoming someone's partner/connecting with} = ¬Dalet-faith establish presence- Lamed[to/toward]-instruct acquire provide- Vav-[and/in addition]increase degree assure- Taw-evidence prove sign- (The Messiah) אחישמ S12523 {בםשח=the Anointed One} = Mem[from/out of]-transform encounter remembrance- Shin-pressure exchange disperse- Yud-purpose single~mindedness actions- ᴅHhet-specific share beyond- ᴅFinal-Aleph-ending finish maturity-

The Semitic Emphasis

<u>Believing in God as for me on the other hand wherefore? just as/as is appropriate for to be enticed to false worship/to wander/to make to forget persecuted/accused showing/declaring/explaining deceiving/committing fraud/disguising this thing of susch a sort to wind tightly/to pervert/to travail to desire/find acceptable/to complete with satisfaction indicating the origin of directional movement attacking in battle with a goal/standing up straight and healthy becoming someone's partner/connecting with the Anointed One.</u>

In coming to know WHOSE we are, we tend to shy away from the simplicity thereof by substituting the physical for the spiritual.

In other words, when we begin to understand that we, ourselves, are not what we thought we were, we withdraw thinking *"this is too much work"*, thereby depriving ourselves of discovering the reality of WHOSE we actually are.

Except Christ, the Word become the focal point of EVERY INSTANCE of our living, we fail at discovering the FULLNESS OF WHO HE IS IN US, AS US!

In short, we exchange the simplicities of WHO HE IS, accepting rather the simple~mindedness of who we are in ourselves!

Herein, it lays the trap!

" ¹²*How art thou fallen from heaven, O Lucifer, son of the morning! how art thou cut down to the ground, which didst weaken the nations! ¹³For thou hast said in thine heart, I will ascend into heaven, I will exalt my throne above the stars of God: I will sit also upon the mount of the congregation, in the sides of the north: ¹⁴I will ascend above the heights of the clouds; I will be like the most High.*" ISAIAH 14:12-14 KJV

"Let no man deceive himself. If any man among you seemeth to be wise in this world, let him become a fool, that he may be wise." FIRST CORINTHIANS 3:18 KJV

The masks we use to cover what is hidden will always be exposed, when Christ is seated upon the throne of one's living!

What we are and Whose we are becomes exposed and made known when the LIGHT in which we seek to walk uncovers the realities of WHO WE REALLY ARE KNOWN AS!

17 verses examined...

32 verses examined in this chapter...

CHAPTER TWO

Do You Have Healing Or Health

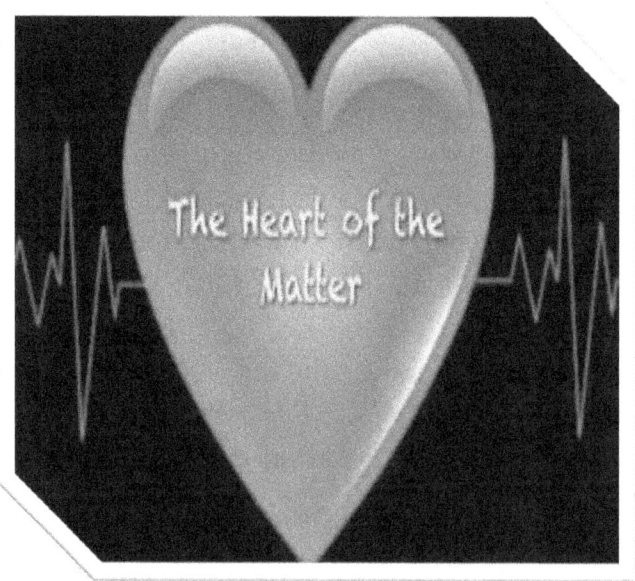

Or Does He Have YOU?

Healing is one of those topics that demands answers, as well as a response to such answers. Regardless of whether or not we believe what we have been told, the <u>WILL</u> <u>OF</u> <u>GOD</u> <u>IS</u> <u>TO</u> <u>HEAL</u>!. This is the fact of the Scriptures read and studied. Without such assurance, there is no security available enough to override one's personal concerns, or fears. Wherever Jesus went, He ministered with compassion and healed the sick.

Christ's example showed an interconnection with salvation as many believed following their healing. Healing is for the physical ills of the human body, and the psyche of the human mind. If the life-force/spirit in man *GENESIS 2:7; 1CORINTHIANS 6:17*, is joined as ONE with the Holy Spirit as God; then, there is no lack, no error, no need in this joining to/of SPIRIT for training of any kind. Healing is about LEARNING to adapt, LEARNING to accept, and LEARNING to agree with what God SPOKE, since before time, or humanity began.

Healing is ONLY ever wrought by the power of God, through the prayer of faith, and/or by *the laying on of hands* MARK 16:18; JAMES 5:14-15; it is provided for in the atonement of Christ, and is available to all who truly believe. The Scriptures dealing with the doctrine of divine healing are abundant. And yet, they lay the premise, proposal, and the proof that God not only heals, but is the HEALING HIMSELF. As we __recognize__ that we have all of Him we need, at any time, or through any challenge...we __realize__ that WHO WE HAVE is WHAT WE HAVE NEED OF!.

<u>*JOHN 1:1-3 KJV*</u>
1 In the beginning was the Word, and the Word was with God, and the Word was God. 2 The same was in the beginning with God. 3 All things were made by Him; and without Him was not any thing made that was made...

*H*ere is the classic beginning to our understanding of everything God HAS SAID about HEALING. "*In the <u>BEGINNING</u>*". Now, first, let us lay certain suppositions in place to govern and direct our search for TRUTH.

*F*IRST: In God, He is the epitome, the fullness, the fullest expression of HEALTH, Yes?. YES!

*S*ECOND: In God, because of principle #1, there is NO LACK, Yes?. YES!

*T*HIRD: In God, then, because of principle #1 & #2, there is no sickness, no death, no division, Yes?. YES!

*F*OURTH: In God, because of the first three principles, there, can be no <u>dis</u>-ease, or sickness, or lack in us, Yes?...*1JOHN 4:19* YES!

<u>*If we are as He is, then Why do we not have what we have As Him?.*</u>

*B*ecause we may lack *1)*-the knowledge, or *2)*-the understanding, or *3)*-the initiative[ENTERPRISE; ADVANTAGE; STRATEGY] to *1)*-agree, *2)*-accept with, and *3)*-embrace/apply what He HAS SAID. *"God is not a man, that He should lie; neither the son of man, that He should repent: hath He said, and shall he not*

---

do it? or hath He spoken, and shall He not make it good? NUMBERS 23:19 *KJV*

*W*e must, at this point, lift our hands unto Him, as a way of saying, *"this truth is beyond the ability of myself to comply with, or to observe, in any way, shape, form or fashion; but, I cannot be anything other than WHAT God has designed me to be".* JEREMIAH 29:11   Only by His HELP, and His ASSISTANCE, can I hope to finish my course, which is about finding and relinquishing to Him all that I am, that I may BE all that He is.

*W*hat has just been said/read is a *"KINGDOM THOUGHT".* Such a thought requires the full measure, from our heart/mind/soul, of giving-up everything we are, so that everything He is, can be seen as everything we already are, only IN HIM!.

A seed is in itself perfect, but God designed it to grow!.

*T*ake these scriptures as illustrations... *"And you, being dead through your trespasses and the uncircumcision of the flesh, you, I say, did He make alive together with Him, having been gracious to us in all our trespasses".* COLOSSIANS 2:13, ASV

We have been made alive together <u>with</u> Him.

"Wherein you were also raised with Him through faith in the working of God, who raised Him from the dead." COLOSSIANS 2:12 ASV   This is **THE LEGAL ASPECT** of the New Creation and everything that is legally ours can become a vital reality.

In the mind, and eyes of the Father, we were made alive with Christ. When He was made alive, **in spirit**, we were made alive, **in spirit**. This becomes a reality to us when we personally agree, and more fully come to know Christ as Savior and confess Him as Lord. This is not talking about a position ONLY; it is talking about a relationship!. HEALING, then, is a product and part of **Relationship In Him**!.

The Bible is composed of two covenants, two contracts or two agreements. The first covenant was between Abraham and Jehovah, and was sealed by circumcision. This New Covenant is sealed with the blood of Jesus Christ, God's own Son. It is impossible to describe in words what the Covenant contained in HEALING, will mean to you and myself, once we come to understand it more completely.

Realizing the Obvious
MATTHEW 4:24 NIV
*News about Him spread all over Syria, and people brought to Him all who were ill with various diseases, <u>those suffering **severe pain**</u>, <u>the demon possessed</u>, <u>those having **seizures**</u>, and <u>the **paralyzed**</u>, and He healed them.*

These are **obvious illnesses**. These are four categories of healing. What if these four categories were areas of PROCESS that the Holy Spirit, as the Teacher, seeks to show us of what and where HEALING is needed?

What if, the types of maladies presented, represent the forms of challenge within the mind?

What if, the mind challenged, must come to the end of SELF, and give-up all thoughts, all control, all authority as pertains to SELF, to facilitate/enable HIS HEALING?

MATTHEW 8:3 NIV
*Jesus reached out His hand and touched the man. "**I am willing**," He said. "**Be clean!**" Immediately he was cured of his **leprosy**.*

This story, HIS-story, compels the believer to agree , to accept, and to apply that which God is always willing to reveal, of/about what He has already finished. It is however, the privilege of the believer to agree with what He HAS SAID, and receive what He reveals. MARK 11:23-24

MATTHEW 8:8, 13 NIV
*The centurion replied, "Lord, I do not deserve to have You come under my roof. But just say the word, and my servant will be healed. Then Jesus said to the centurion, "**Go! It will be done just as you believed it would**." And his servant was healed at that very hour.*

Got Healing?

*T*his centurion came, as a man UNDER authority, knowing, and having RESPECT for such authority. Authority's purpose, by God's design, is for the purpose of serving, protecting, and increasing. However, the fundamental, elemental step of respecting such purpose can be reduced to inactivity, when hindrances, such as our ambitions/purposes/agendas, get in the way of HIM being/existing as all that He is eternally.

MATTHEW 8:14-15 NIV
When Jesus came into Peter's house, He saw Peter's
*mother-in-law lying in bed with a **fever**. He touched*
her hand and the fever left her, and she got up and
began to wait on Him.

*T*he Word's secret of "**Christ in you, the hope of glory**", COLOSSIANS 1:27 is one which the world cannot grasp, by itself. In fact, many of the CHURCH have not grasp this TRUTH, as yet. Think of that; and try to realize this. God is not only a God who mercifully pardons our guilt, and gives us grace for the consequences; not only a God who gives to us a new nature that loves to do the right which once we hated; not only a God who comes to our aid in temptation and trial, and offers His strength and insight for our deliverance; but, above all this, He is a God who comes Himself to live His own life for/in/through us.

*H*e takes us into the Divine family; makes us partakers of the Divine Nature; guides and directs our life with us; but completely becomes the Author and Finisher of our faith, and works in us "**both to will and to do of His good pleasure**". PHILIPPIANS 2:13

*T*his is incomprehensible to our finite minds. What does human poetry, human philosophy, the purest form of human religion know of anything like this?... No wonder Paul was aflame with the enthusiasm of his glorious discovery and longed to sweep, like an angel, flying in the midst of heaven, to tell our helpless race the mighty secret — the secret that God not only had come down to visit men with a message of mercy; but had come to stay and live within them with "**the power of an endless life**". HEBREWS 7:16

Got Healing?

It is still a secret, except to the taught who catch such overwhelming wisdom.

1 Corinthians 2:14 KJV
But the natural man receiveth not the things of the Spirit of God: for they are foolishness unto him: neither can he know them, because they are
spiritually discerned.

*N*ot only does this wisdom need a divine revelation to make it known to the world, it still needs a divine revelation to make it personally known and experientially real to the individual heart. This is what the apostle means in *1Corinthians 2*, where with great clarity and force, he argues that the mere human intellect cannot comprehend the things of God, but that we need a divine mind to be added to our human understanding, **BEFORE** we can enter into the realm of spiritual truth.. __OUR attitude toward the Word determines the place, and the measure that God holds, and sustains, in our daily living__. This Word was designed by the Father to take Jesus' place in His absence. *JOHN 14:26; 16:13* Yet, His WORD becomes His very PRESENCE, and PERSON, and POWER, when a believer leans upon His very substance found. Few words of man live after a generation is gone, but God's Word is different. His WORD is impregnated with the very Life of God, Himself, because His WORD is eternal. We become Christ-like in the measure that the Word prevails in us. The Word of Christ is revealed; this is **LOGOS**. The Word as Christ is finished; this is **RHEMA**.

MARK 5:22-23 KJV
And, behold, there cometh one of the rulers of the synagogue, Jairus by name; and when he saw Him, he fell at His feet, And besought Him greatly, saying, My little daughter lieth at the point of death: I pray thee, come and lay thy hands on her, that she may be healed; and she shall live... ... ...

MARK 5:35-43 KJV
While he yet spake, there came from the ruler of the synagogue's house certain which said, Thy daughter is dead: why troublest thou the Master any further? As soon as Jesus heard the word that was spoken,

he saith unto the ruler of the synagogue, Be not afraid, only believe. And he suffered no man to follow him, save Peter, and James, and John the brother of James. And he cometh to the house of the ruler of the synagogue, and seeth the tumult, and them that wept and wailed greatly. And when he was come in, he saith unto them, Why make ye this ado, and weep? the damsel is not dead, but sleepeth. And they laughed him to scorn. But when he had put them all out, he taketh the father and the mother of the damsel, and them that were with him, and entereth in where the damsel was lying. And he took the damsel by the hand, and said unto her, Talitha cumi; which is, being interpreted, Damsel, I say unto thee, arise. And straightway the damsel arose, and walked; for she was of <u>the</u> <u>age</u> <u>of</u> <u>twelve</u> <u>years</u>. And they were astonished with a great astonishment. And he charged them straitly that no man should know it; and commanded that something should be given her to eat... ... .

There is a two-sided comparison in these verses. They involve a comparison dealing with the two sides of the Tree of the Knowledge of Good & Evil. These verses cite a two-folded comparison~~*of the 12-year* <u>**PATTERN**</u> *of two women,* seeking HEALING from the Master. One approached in the midst of her defilement, bleeding her very life's blood as she came. While the other had to be approached by the Master, through her father, dying in the wait, with her <u>**life-force**</u> held above her ending.

The Old Testament promised that in the day of the kingdom, the effects of the curse would be overthrown. Notice the "***divine coincidence***" that the disease of the woman had begun to afflict her on the same year that this girl had been born. Each situation had been carefully orchestrated/arranged by God to be a special vessel of honor, which would demonstrate the power and the compassion of Jesus.

<u>*Notice The Contrast Of Needs.*</u>

The daughter of Jairus was <u>**12 years old**</u>. She had enjoyed 12 years of <u>life</u>.. The woman with the issue of blood had endured 12 years of <u>**suffering**</u>. It was once said that <u>*life is what happens to you while you are planning something else*</u>. As you make up your agenda, be aware that God has His agenda, as well; and that at first it seems to be only an interruption. *God will always let us go where we want to go...until He brings us to where He wants us to be.* There is a point when circumstances seem to pass beyond the realm of hope though. This is where real faith begins.

<u>MATTHEW 9:21-22</u> NIV

*She said to herself, "If I only touch His cloak, I will be healed." Jesus turned and saw her. **"Take heart, daughter,"** He said, **"your faith has healed you."** And the woman was healed from that moment... -* <u>12 years bleeding</u>

There is a medicine so powerful it can cure every sickness and disease known to man. It has no dangerous side effects. It is safe even in massive doses. And when taken daily according to directions, it can prevent illness altogether and keep you in vibrant health. Does that sound too good to be true? It's not. I can testify to you by the Word of God and by my own experience that such a supernatural medicine exists. Even more importantly, it is available to you every moment of every day. You don't have to call your doctor to get it. You don't even have to drive to the pharmacy. All you do is reach for your Bible, open to <u>PROVERBS 4:20-24</u> and follow the instructions you find there:

*"My child, attend to My words; incline thine ear unto My sayings.
Let them not depart from thine eyes; keep them in the midst of thine
heart. For they are life unto those that <u>find</u> <u>them</u>, and health (Hebrew:
'medicine') to all their flesh. Keep thy heart with all diligence; for out of
it are the issues of life. Put away from thee a froward [uncontrolled;
disobedient; disagreeable] <u>mouth</u>, and perverse [obstinate; stubborn;
irrational] <u>lips</u> put far from thee..."*

When we sow/plant the Word about the new birth in our heart, then believe and act on, that Word, released within us, the power to be born again. By the same token, when we sow/plant the Word about healing in our heart, believe on it, and then act on it, that Word reveals God's healing in us. Every time we take the Word into our heart, believe it and act on it, the life of which Jesus spoke, the very LIFE of God Himself, is released in us.

Got Healing?

We may have read healing scriptures over and over again. We may know them as well as we know our own name. Yet, every time we read them or hear them preached, they bring us a fresh dose of God's healing influence/encouragement. Each time, they bring stimulating impact to us and draw God's medicine to our flesh.

Look back at God's prescription. We find it doesn't say anything about "*knowing*" the Bible. It does say, **attend** to My Word. The attention we give to the WORD of God in our living, determines the strength of the God's PRESENCE, PERSON, and POWER in our lifestyle.

*The verses cited below are Jesus' answer
to John, the Baptist's questions~~~*

MATTHEW 11:5 NIV
*The **blind** receive sight, the **lame** walk, those who have **leprosy** are cured, the **deaf** hear, the **dead** are raised, and the good news is preached
to the **poor**...
The **blind** receive sight,
the **lame** walk,
those who have **leprosy** are cured,
the **deaf** hear,
the **dead** are raised,
and the good news is preached to the **poor***

LUKE 7:21 NIV
*At that very time Jesus cured many who had diseases, sicknesses and **evil spirits**, and gave sight to many who were **blind**. So He replied to the messengers, "Go back and report to John what you have seen and heard: The **blind** receive sight, the **lame** walk, those who have **leprosy** are cured, the **deaf** hear, the **dead** are raised, and the good news is preached to the
poor.*

The following verses are cited as a listing of those ailments of which Jesus HEALED EVERYONE!

MATTHEW 12:10 NIV
*...and a man with a **shriveled hand** was there.
Looking for a reason to accuse Jesus, they asked Him,*

Got Healing?

"Is it lawful to heal on the Sabbath?"

In Addition Contrast Beginnings Patterning Each Increase By Teaching To Some Degree Of Evidence Qualifies Agreement With His Seed Exchanges For His Finished Work

MATTHEW 15:30
KJV+TVM

And ^{G2532} great ^{G4183} multitudes ^{G3793} came ^{G4334} $^{[G5656]}$ unto him ^{G846}, having ^{G2192} $^{[G5723]}$ with ^{G3326} them those that were ^{G1438} lame ^{G5560}, blind ^{G5185}, dumb ^{G2974}, maimed ^{G2948}, and ^{G2532} many ^{G4183} others ^{G2087}, and ^{G2532} cast ^{G4496} them ^{G846} down ^{G4496} $^{[G5656]}$ at ^{G3844} Jesus ^{G2424}' feet ^{G4228}; and ^{G2532} he healed ^{G2323} $^{[G5656]}$ them ^{G846}:

ORIGINAL THOUGHTS

...(15:30) In addition, contrast beginnings patterning each increase by teaching to some degree of evidence qualifies agreement with His Seed exchanges for His Finished Work. Adjust by experiencing the single~mindedness of His Evidence in revealing each degree of increase through His Wisdom transforming His Grace/Truth to insure every progress, consistent with the understanding of His Purpose in strengthening His Finished Work. And while adjusting to each encounter of single~minded influence through His Efforts, be sure of the Unseen Process and Exchange by His Finished Work that theincrease of His Spoken Word enlarges/enhandes the Unseen Process enlarging His Finished Work. To the degree that we apprehend every remembrance of His Single~Mindedness herein is the Influence of His Efforts assured beyond the process of exchange within His Finished Work. The adding of His Spoken Word presses through His Single~Mindedness understading through His Influence that each portion of His Dominion specifies the beginnings of sowing His Finished Work. When apprehending each experience of His Purpose enable His Influence of Effort to increase the abilities that strengthen and transcend through each degree agreeing with the seed that increases the progress providing each part as significant. With each process experience the acquiring of assurance that reveals each purpose of His Faith through the exchange of His Wisdom increasing and empowering the source of His Single~Mindedness while agreeing to continue each increase in progress.

<u>In addition, contrast beginnings patterning each increase by teaching to some degree of evidence qualifies agreement with His Seed exchanges for His Finished Work.</u>

In addition, contrast beginnings patterning each increase by teaching those things that cause us to remember the THREE~AS~ONE!

"Finally, brethren, whatsoever things are true, whatsoever things are honest,

---

whatsoever things are just, whatsoever things are pure, whatsoever things are lovely, whatsoever things are of good report; if there be any virtue, and if there be any praise, think on these things." PHILIPPIANS 4:8 KJV

It is in knowing that *to some degree of evidence qualifies the agreement of His Seed* which reveals to the awareness and consciousness of our thought~life that the Spirit moving through our living seeks to make us come to know the strength of His UNION with us, and in us.

It is always *in exchange for His Finished Work* that we discover the practical side of living through HIM; these things come from a tight~knit relationship with the THREE~AS~ONE providing the fullness of THEMSELVES within our living THROUGH THEM!

Adjust by experiencing the single~mindedness of His Evidence in revealing each degree of increase through His Wisdom transforming His Grace/Truth to insure every progress, consistent with the understanding of His Purpose in strengthening His Finished Work.

Adjust by experiencing the single~mindedness of His Evidence and discover the wholeness of God's design in us.

There is only ONE WAY, and the name of this WAY is JESUS!

From within the REST OF HIM, there is found *in revealing each degree of increase through His Wisdom* the pattern of His thoughts about us and how we may learn to allow the freedom of the Spirit to flow through our living AS THEM!

It is by/through *transforming His Grace/Truth to insure every progress* that the soul/mind/will and heart discover the fruitfulness of THEIR sharing THEIR LIFE with us, so that we might live THROUGH THEM!

As we become *consistent with the understanding of His Purpose* we then begin to grasp the fulness of knowing the REST IN HIM, which reveals more fully the REST OF HIM!

It is *in strengthening His Finished Work* within our daily~living that the soul discovers the REFUGE THEY provide for us to live out of; for here is where THERE is the wholeness of PRESENCE, PERSON, and POWER!

And while adjusting to each encounter of single~minded influence through His Efforts, be sure of the Unseen Process and Exchange by His Finished Work that the increase of His Spoken Word enlarges/enhances the Unseen Process enlarging

His Finished Work.

And while adjusting to each encounter of single~minded influence we are made to know that His Kingdom is WITHIN US; therefore, there can be no separation that divides us away from THEM, the THREE~AS~ONE.

It is time we understood that nothing is kept from either of THEM, through the fact that remains they are THREE~AS~ONE.

Nothing that ONE does is anything but understood through other TWO; THEY are THREE~AS~ONE!

Through His Efforts be sure of the Unseen Process and Exchange by His Finished Work and therein discover the wholly completion of THEIR design and plan for our living as THEY ARE!

It is so *that the increase of His Spoken Word enlarges/enhances the Unseen Process enlarging His Finished Work;* for herein the soul/mind/will and heart of humanity discover the very recesses of THEM and THEIR sharing, so as to whet our appetite for more!

To the degree that we apprehend every remembrance of His Single~Mindedness herein is the Influence of His Efforts assured beyond the process of exchange within His Finished Work.

To the degree that we apprehend every remembrance of His Single~Mindedness is the degree to which we are given a choice of whether to step into what is His REALITY, or remain where we are miserably at.

Herein is the Influence of His Efforts assured; that we might embrace the fulness of WHO HE IS by knowing WHOSE WE ARE!

It is *beyond the process of exchange within His Finished Work* that we discover all that He keeps in store for us the righteous as His own.

The adding of His Spoken Word presses through His Single~Mindedness understading through His Influence that each portion of His Dominion specifies the beginnings of sowing His Finished Work.

The adding of His Spoken Word presses through His Single~Mindedness and uncovers each revelation of WHO HE IS IN US, AS US!

It is as when we apprehend *understanding through His Influence* that we discover His TRUTH as enlarging our TRUST IN HIM!

Out of *that each portion of His Dominion specifies* those benefits, blessings, and giftings that He has made ours through His SACRIFICE, we therein LEARN through the Spirit's guidance and teaching, those things we need applied to our living AS HIM!

It is even through *the beginnings of sowing His Finished Work* that the soul/mind/ will and heart become aware of the unconditional LOVE He maintains toward us, His Creation!

<u>When</u> <u>apprehending</u> <u>each</u> <u>experience</u> <u>of</u> <u>His</u> <u>Purpose</u> <u>enable</u> <u>His</u> <u>Influence</u> <u>of</u> <u>Effort</u> <u>to</u> <u>increase</u> <u>the</u> <u>abilities</u> <u>that</u> <u>strengthen</u> <u>and</u> <u>transcend</u> <u>through</u> <u>each</u> <u>degree</u> <u>agreeing</u> <u>with</u> <u>the</u> <u>seed</u> <u>that</u> <u>increases</u> <u>the</u> <u>progress</u> <u>providing</u> <u>each</u> <u>part</u> <u>as</u> <u>significant.</u>

When apprehending each experience of His Purpose He spells out purity, the natural life of Eden; and obedience, the rhythmic harmony of Eden; and peace, the sweet music of Eden; and power, the mastery and dominion of Eden; and love, the throbbing heart of Eden.

For it is in His DELIGHT ^[EDEN] we discover the wholeness, the fullness, and the completeness of His Finished Work performed in us daily, even moment~by~moment.

It is when we *enable His Influence of Effort to increase* within our living AS THEM, we discover the multitude of multiple myriads that parallel each encounter with His Grace, His Mercy, and His indominatable LOVE!

These are *the abilities that strengthen and transcend through each degree agreeing with the seed that increases*; for herein THEY make known the richness, the extensiveness, and the details of His unrequited/unanswered/unreturned offerings, which continually remain available for our choosing and accepting and applying.

It is in *the progress providing each part as significant* that the soul of humanity seeks a filling for the void in their being, having never accepted or applied that which He FREELY OFFERS!

<u>With</u> <u>each</u> <u>process</u> <u>experience</u> <u>the</u> <u>acquiring</u> <u>of</u> <u>assurance</u> <u>that</u> <u>reveals</u> <u>each</u> <u>purpose</u> <u>of</u> <u>His</u> <u>Faith</u> <u>through</u> <u>the</u> <u>exchange</u> <u>of</u> <u>His</u> <u>Wisdom</u> <u>increasing</u> <u>and</u> <u>empowering</u> <u>the</u> <u>source</u> <u>of</u> <u>His</u> <u>Single~Mindedness</u> <u>while</u> <u>agreeing</u> <u>to</u> <u>continue</u> <u>each</u> <u>increase</u> <u>in</u> <u>progress.</u>

With each process experience the acquiring of assurance and come to know the whole of that He which He eternally offers to every member of humanity created.

It is in our discovering of THEM *that reveals each purpose of His Faith*

Got Healing?

through the exchange of His Wisdom and transcends every struggle, every stumbling, every failing we have ever remembered or lived through.

The great crowd in every part of the world is yearning after Him: piteously, pathetically, most often speechlessly yearning, blindly groping along, with an intense inner tug after Him.

And yet, it is through the *ever~increasing and empowering the source of His Single~Mindedness* that we may choose to accept and apply that we discover all the manifold blessings that have always been ours, and yet we fail to embrace with all of our being that which THEY have provided.

While agreeing to continue each increase in progress, we may struggle and even fail at; however, in knowing THEM as THEY ARE, we have an ever~flowing stream of blessing awaiting our return to THEM WHO HAVE OFFERED FREELY all that THEY are to us!

SEMITIC~ARAMAIC~HEBRAIC THESAURUS

Aramaic before first {

Semitic Root before first =

Lettering for ParaPhrase after }=

...(15:30) (& they came near)קרבו‎S18978 {ברח-=and approaching/touching}=ו‎/י‎ Vav-[and/in addition]increase degree assure- Quph-contrast parallel structure- Resh-process beginning strength- Beyt[within/inside]-pattern thought inhabit-ו‎/י‎ Vav-[and/in addition]increase degree assure-

(to Him)לותה‎S1137 {תו=for a purpose}=ל‎/ה‎ Lamed[to/toward]-instruct acquire provide-ו‎/י‎ Vav-[and/in addition]increase degree assure-ת‎ Taw-evidence prove sign-ה‎ Hey[behold/the]-quality reveal grace-

(the crowds)כנשא‎S10319 {נשו=those assembling/gathering}=ש‎/כ‎ Kaph-surrender obtains consent- Nun-seed patience continue- Shin-pressure exchange disperse- Final-Aleph-ending finish maturity-

(many)סגיאין‎S13929 {גס=in a manifold way}=ס‎/י‎ Samech-adjust apprehend source- Gimal-experience understanding encounter- Yud [of/through]-purpose single~mindedness actions- Aleph-authority ability confirm- Final-Aleph-ending finish maturity-

(that)דאית‎S732 {תד=there exists}=ד‎/ה‎ Dalet-[that]-faith establish presence- Aleph-authority ability confirm- Yud [of/through]-purpose single~mindedness actions- Taw-evidence prove sign-

(were)הוו‎S1147 {ווה= being/becoming/coming to one's senses}=ה‎/י‎ Hey[behold/the]-quality reveal grace-ו‎/י‎ Vav-[and/in addition]increase degree assure- Vav-[and/in addition]increase degree assure-

(with them)עמהון‎S15788 {מע=in the presence of/in possession of}=ע‎/י‎ Ayin-pierce perceive wisdom- Mem[from/out of]-transform encounter remembrance- Hey[behold/the]-quality reveal grace-ו‎/י‎ Vav-[and/in addition]increase degree assure- Final-Nun-issue perseverance progress-

(the lame)חגירא‎S6220 {גח= weak~voiced/stammerer}=ח‎/י‎ Hhet-specific share beyond- Gimal-experience understanding encounter- Yud [of/through]-purpose single~mindedness actions- Resh-process beginning strength- Vav-[and/in addition]increase degree assure- Final-Aleph-ending finish maturity- Samech-adjust apprehend source-

(& blind)סמיא‎S14528 {מס=losing light}=ס‎/י‎ Mem[from/out of]-transform encounter remembrance- Yud [of/through]-purpose single~mindedness actions- Final-Aleph-ending finish maturity-

(& mute)חרשא‎S7638 {שרח=creation without speech}=ח‎/ש‎ Hhet-specific share beyond- Resh-process beginning strength- Shin-pressure exchange disperse- Vav-[and/in addition]increase degree assure- Final-Aleph-ending finish maturity-

(& crippled)ופשיגא‎S17363 {גש=weakens hands/feet}=פ‎/ש‎ Pey-mouth SpokenWord speak- Shin-pressure exchange disperse- Yud [of/through]-purpose single~mindedness actions- Gimal-experience understanding encounter- Final-Aleph-ending finish maturity-

(& others)ואחרנא‎S7688 {נרח=different from}=ו‎/י‎ Vav-[and/in addition]increase degree assure- Aleph-authority ability confirm- Hhet-specific share beyond- Resh-process beginning strength- Nun-seed patience continue- Final-Aleph-ending finish

Got Healing?

maturity-(many)אַנְשִׁיָּא S13929 {ـﬥﬤ=in a manifold way}= Samech-adjust apprehend source-Gimal-experience understanding encounter-Yud [of/through]-purpose single-mindedness actions-Aleph-authority ability confirm-Final-Aleph-ending

finish maturity-(& they laid)וַיַרמִיָּין S20045 {=to bring forth/starting a journey/establish the beginning of something}= Vav-[and/in addition]increase degree assure-Aleph-authority ability confirm-Resh-process beginning strength-Mem[from/out of]-transform encounter remembrance-Yud [of/through]-purpose single-mindedness actions-Vav-[and/in addition]increase degree assure-

(them)אַנּוּן S4989 {=from being weak/sick/frail} = Aleph-authority ability confirm-Vav-[and/in addition]increase degree assure-Final-Nun-issue perseverance progress-Nun-seed patience continue-

(at)לְוָת S11136 {ﬨﬠﬥ=compared to/for a purpose}= Lamed [to/toward]-instruct acquire provide-Vav-[and/in addition]increase degree assure-Taw-evidence prove sign-

(His feet)רֶגְלוֹהִי S19405 {=as a measure}= Resh-process beginning strength-Vav-[and/in addition]increase degree assure-Gimal-experience understanding encounter-Lamed[to/toward]-instruct acquire provide-Yud [of/through]-purpose single-mindedness actions-Hey[behold/the]-quality reveal grace-

(of Yeshua)דְּיֵשׁוּע S9568 {=belonging/related to someone/something being saved}= Dalet-[that]-faith establish-Yud [of/through]-purpose single-mindedness actions-Shin-pressure exchange disperse-Ayin-pierce perceive wisdom-

(& He healed)וְאַסִּי S1596 {=repairing/restoring/refuting}= Vav-[and/in addition]increase degree assure-Yud [of/through]-purpose single-mindedness actions-Aleph-authority ability confirm-Samech-adjust apprehend source-

(them)אַנּוּן S4989 {=from being weak/sick/frail}= Aleph-authority ability confirm-Nun-seed patience continue-Vav-[and/in addition]increase degree assure-Final-Nun-issue perseverance progress-

The Semitic Emphasis

Approaching/Touching for a purpose those assembling/gathering in a manifold way~~there exists being/becoming/coming to one's senses in the presence of/in possession of weak~voiced/stammerer~~losing light creation without speech weakens hands/feet different from~~in a manifold way to bring forth/start a journey/establish the beginning of something~~from being weak/sick/frail compared to/for a purpose as a measure belonging/related to someone/something being saved~~repairing/restoring/refuting from being weak/sick/frail.

Approaching/Touching for a purpose those assembling/gathering in a manifold way there remains the presence of the Spirit representing in fullness ALL that has ever been offered freely for our accepting and applying.

God cannot change because there is no TURNING in THEM; no turning away from us THEIR CREATION; no turning away from us when we fail; no turning away from us when we refuse, reject, or deny that which THEY have always remained as!

There exists being/becoming/coming to one's senses in the presence of/in possession of weak~voiced/stammerer, the ability of THEIR insight and dominion, which when we learn and embrace we discover the pathway of the journey made narrow, and find the journey made sweet by THEIR NEVERENDING LOVE for us!

It is in *losing light* that *creation without speech weakens hands/feet different from* His giving up His GLORY to become INCARNATE as humanity, while remaining in touch the spiritual~side of His Existence.

God became human, so that humanity might know that THEY stand everready to embrace and accept the humble of heart, and the hungry of soul/mind/will; this then is the message of reconciliation.

In a manifold way to bring forth or to start a journey or to establish the beginning of something, the King of Kings steps forward into this dimension of physical disaster, for the purpose of renewing, reminding, and reconciling humanity to the position we were created from when as a THOUGHT FROM THE GODHEAD, we were born from our mother's womb to embrace the manifold mercies laid up in store for us whom THEY MADE RIGHTEOUS FROM BEFORE THE BEGINNING OF TIME AND/OR HISTORY ever occurred.

It is the very plan of God to keep us *from being weak, or sick, or frail, compared to, or for a purpose as a measure* however, could be an issue we have not examined, as to whether or not the trials of living in this dimension come as a result of knowing THEM personally through relationship, or not!

It is in *belonging to, or being related to someone, or something being saved* that the understanding can become askewed as being visited because of something we did that was wrong. NOT SO!

In understanding further that we, as being or existing as a WORD from the Father, are not kept because of our performance, our lack of failure, or even our inability to mature in certain ways through which others approve us.

Yet, it is in the manner by which we mature in our relationship with the Most High God that we discover our relationship provides for us the right of privilege to stand before the Mercy Throne of God and DECLARE/PROCLAIM that what we need is what we have already available, because THEY give without ceasing!

Therefore, the *repairing, or restoring, or refuting from being weak/sick/frail* is an accomplished, finished work of God's design on our behalf, reinforcing that we, as His Creation, have every eternal right in believing that everything given us of God is good and perfect from above!

"Every good gift and every perfect gift is from above, and cometh down from the Father of lights, with whom is no variableness, neither shadow of turning." JAMES 1:17 KJV

Got Healing?

*The **blind** and the **lame** came to Him at the temple, and He healed them.*

It would seem that throughout our sub~cultures, a system of *good vs. hurt* is the most ineffective way of showing compassion, and yet, we find that we ALL have been taught, in one way or another, to separate ourselves from those of a *"lesser"* substance.

Yet, when we discover others *look down their noses* at us, it is an automatic trigger in us that sets us off on angry tangents of disdain and reproof.

Do we continually need reminding that as we understand God loves us, through this TRUTH we can love others?

Where are the arms of the Body of Christ, in every location, to embrace *the hurting, the wounded, the thirsty, the illegitimate, the scorned, the ridiculed,* those that seem different and yet they are just as important to God as we are?

"Then shall He answer them, saying, Verily I say unto you, Inasmuch as ye did it <u>not</u> to one of the least of these, ye did it not to me." MATTHEW 25:45 KJV

It is the prisons in our own living that are places that have become precious to us, because they were all we knew.

How is it that we hold on to the certainty of our pain rather than take the risk of trusting anyone ever again?

Such prisons begin when we are taught by example that it is okay to shut others away, without regard for their needs, their feelings, or their worth to God!

Why would the blind and the lame come to the temple?

Did they feel unworthy because of their malady, or because they were shunned by those thinking that they themselves were above others of a lesser sort?

Even those who don't believe God exists are desperate to know love and that love knows who they are.

These came to the temple because they were told JESUS was there!

Isn't this the responsibility of the Church/the Body of Christ? To make a place where *the hurting, the wounded, the thirsty, the illegitimate, the scorned, the ridiculed,* may come and find the solace, the peace, the acceptance in order to receive WHO THEY REALLY NEED?

Got Healing?

HEALING takes many shapes, many forms, but it never comes without JESUS as its CENTER!

MARK 1:42
*Immediately the **leprosy** left him and He was cured.*

The Aramaic/Hebraic word for *leprosy* is גרב meaning *becoming prey; to be robbed.*

Now, it appears as though this word describes someone who is in a pitiful condition because of bad choices; whether in living, working, or who they choose for friends.

When the heart or mind becomes a toy for others to control, there is created an opening, an opportunity for this malady to create something worse in their living.

It is not always a Selfish~Independent~Nature in one's living that creates such conditions, but often when the heart and will and mind are yielded to those who seek to control, one's living begins to deteriorate and fall under such control of a *dis~ease.*

MARK 5:23
*and pleaded earnestly with Him, "My little daughter is **dying**. Please come and put your hands on her so that she will be healed and live." - **dying daughter***

MARK 10:52
*"Go," said Jesus, "your faith has healed you." Immediately He received his sight and followed Jesus along the road. - **public figure known to be blind***

LUKE 7:7
*That is why I did not even consider myself worthy to come to You. But say the word, and my servant will be healed. - **dead son***

LUKE 8:50
*Hearing this, Jesus said to Jairus, "Don't be afraid; just believe, and she will be healed." - **daughter dead***

Got Healing?

LUKE 13:10-13

On a Sabbath Jesus was teaching in one of the synagogues, and a woman was there who had been **crippled by a spirit for eighteen years.** She was bent over and could not straighten up at all. When Jesus saw her, He called her forward and said to her, "Woman, you are set free from your infirmity." Then He put His hands on her, and immediately she straightened up and praised God.

LUKE 14:4

But they remained silent. So taking hold of the man, He healed him and sent him away. - **man with dropsy**

LUKE 17:15

One of them, when he saw he was healed, came back, praising God in a loud voice. - **10 lepers**

LUKE 22:51

But Jesus answered, "No more of this!" And He touched the man's ear and healed him. - **servant of the high priest's ear cut off**

JOHN 4:47

When this man heard that Jesus had arrived in Galilee from Judea, he went to him and begged him to come and heal his son, who was **close to death.**

JOHN 5:9-10

At once the man was cured; he picked up his mat and walked. The day on which this took place was a Sabbath, and so the Jews said to the man who had been healed, "It is the Sabbath; the law forbids you to carry your mat." - **an invalid for thirty-eight years**

JOHN 11:1

Now a man named Lazarus was sick. He was from Bethany, the village of Mary and her sister Martha. - **Lazarus raised from the dead**

Got Healing?

Furthermore, ALL the diseases listed below were <u>incurable</u> at that time in history, and are an everlasting proof that IT WAS GOD'S WILL TO HEAL ALL!

Demonic diseases, oppression, and possession are listed below as well:

<u>MATTHEW 8:33</u>
*Those tending the pigs ran off, went into the town and reported all this, including what had happened to the **demon possessed** men.*

<u>MATTHEW 9:33</u>
*And when the **demon was driven out**, the man who had been **mute** spoke. The crowd was amazed and said, "Nothing like this has ever been seen in Israel."*

<u>MATTHEW 15:28</u>
*Then Jesus answered, "Woman, you have great faith! Your request is granted." And her daughter was healed from that very hour. - **demon possessed daughter***

<u>MATTHEW 17:18</u>
*Jesus rebuked the **demon,** and it came out of the boy, and he was healed from that moment.*

<u>MARK 7:29</u>
*Then He told her, "For such a reply, you may go; the **demon** has left your daughter."*

<u>LUKE 4:35</u>
*"Be quiet!" Jesus said sternly. "Come out of him!" Then the **demon** threw the man down before them all and came out without injuring him.*

<u>LUKE 8:2</u>
*and also some women who had been cured of **evil spirits** and diseases: Mary (called Magdalene) from whom **seven demons** had come out;*

<u>LUKE 8:36</u>
*Those who had seen it told the people how the **demon possessed** man had been cured.*

Got Healing?

LUKE 9:42

Even while the boy was coming, the **demon** *threw him to the ground in a convulsion. But Jesus rebuked the* **evil spirit**, *healed the boy and gave him back to his father.*

LUKE 11:14

Jesus was driving out a **demon** *that was* **mute**. *When the demon left, the man who had been mute spoke, and the crowd was amazed.*

ACTS 10:38

how God anointed Jesus of Nazareth with the Holy Spirit and power, and how He went around doing good and healing all who were **under the power of the devil**, *because God was with him.*

The other verses in the *New Covenant* on healing, as listed below, were generic listings which were not specific as to what kinds of healings were done. We cannot infer anything from the silence of these passages as to the types of healings; simply that Jesus healed many types of diseases and conditions.

The ONE POINT that is very, very clear, regards the FACT that Jesus HEALED EVERYONE THAT CAME TO HIM!

MATTHEW 4:23

Jesus went throughout Galilee, teaching in their synagogues, preaching the good news of the kingdom, and healing every disease and sickness among the people.

MATTHEW 12:15

Aware of this, Jesus withdrew from that place. Many followed him, and He healed all their sick,

MATTHEW 14:35 -36

And when the men of that place recognized Jesus, they sent word to all the surrounding country. People brought all their sick to him [36] *And begged him to let the sick just touch the edge of his cloak, and all who touched him were healed.*

MARK 6:56

And wherever He went- into villages, towns or countryside- they placed the sick in the marketplaces. They begged Him to let them touch even the edge of His cloak, and all who touched Him were healed.

JOHN 6:2

and a great crowd of people followed Him because they saw the miraculous signs He had performed on the sick.

JOHN 7:23

Now if a child can be circumcised on the Sabbath so that the law of Moses may not be broken, why are you angry with me for **healing the whole man** *on the Sabbath?*

The Apostles' Experience Of The Same Anointing

For those who would say that the *"days of miracles"* ended when Jesus ascended, the following verses prove otherwise!

ACTS 3:16

By faith in the name of Jesus, this man whom you see and know was made strong. **It is Jesus' name and the faith that comes through him that has given this complete healing to him,** *as you can all see. -* **crippled from birth**

ACTS 4:9

If we are being called to account today for an act of kindness shown to a **cripple** *and are asked how he was healed, ~~* **crippled from birth**

ACTS 9:40

Peter sent them all out of the room; then he got down on his knees and prayed. Turning toward **the dead woman,** *he said, "Tabitha, get up." She opened her eyes, and seeing* **Peter** *she sat up.*

Got Healing?

ACTS 19:12

so that **even handkerchiefs and aprons that had touched him were taken to the sick, and their illnesses were cured and the evil spirits left them.**

ACTS 28:9

When this had happened, **the rest of the sick on the island came and were cured.** Jesus said of Moses, _"he wrote of Me"_. _"If ye believe not his writings, how shall ye believe My words?"._ _JOHN 5: 47_

To say the _days of miracles_ are past is to not only limit Jesus through the Spirit of doing the works He said would happen; but, there is a certain dismissing of responsibility upon any believer of Him from doing the works He Himself said we could, and should do!

Mark 16:15-18 KJV

"15 And He said unto them, Go ye into all the world, and preach the gospel to every creature. 16 He that believeth and is baptized shall be saved; but he that believeth not shall be damned. 17 And these signs shall follow them that believe; In my name shall they cast out devils; they shall speak with new tongues; 18 They shall take up serpents; and if they drink any deadly thing, it shall not hurt them; they shall lay hands on the sick, and they shall recover."

Where is the time~frame changed in our society, except in the minds and thoughts of those who either do not have compassion to do what Jesus said they could, through HIS NAME; or they simply do not care for other souls the way they say they believe Jesus cares for theirs!

Can you really argue that because Paul is interpreted to say such giftings are passed away that this is the excuse we offer for our lack of diligence in seeing, touching, and believing that the sick can, and are, healed through Jesus NAME?

There is an <u>ignor</u>ance amongst God's Creation that transcends to a lower condition of unbelief, using the disguise of scriptures wrongly interpreted!

If we are to believe the words of another instead of what Jesus has spoken, then do we also agree we have placed others ahead of Jesus, when we take their words over His?

46 verses noted or examined...

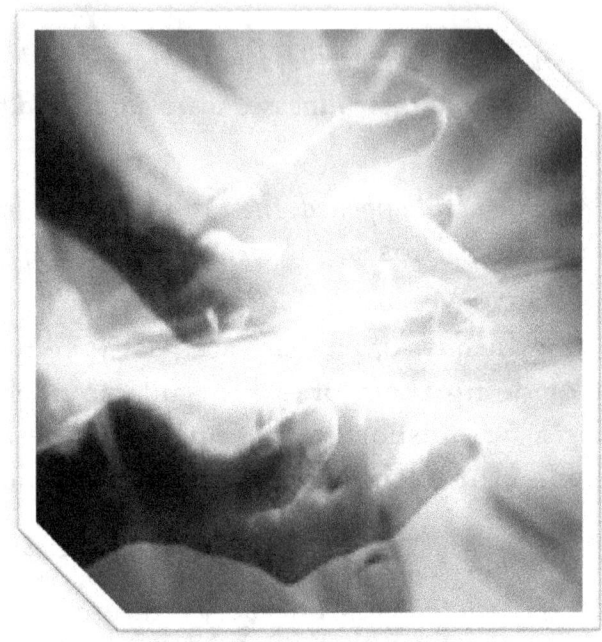

C
H
A
P
T
E
R

THREE

Healing?...
God's Design or Man's Theory

*I*s HEALING a valid promise or just an illusion created by some magician, or minister wanting a *"fast buck"*? Charlatans abound; and hirelings like *"Simon, the magician"* [SEE ACTS 8:9] constantly mesmerize every, and any unwitting soul into believing what they have is what everyone needs.

*T*he ONLY way to discover the truth about HEALING is to go the best and most consistent source and example, which is: <u>the Bible and the living of Jesus Christ upon this earth, as continued through His disciples and vessels</u>. How can this be done? By believing that the supernatural can be taught and understood by anyone willing to hear, and then give attention to the Spirit's leading! This is not to be limited to the ordained ministers of the gospel, but is to include the multitudes.

*G*od never intended for healing to be complicated. He made it very simple, but man tends to make it difficult. Jesus, the Great Physician, gave us an earthly healing function/service, at His Pleasure, and said that

those *who* *believe* shall lay hands on the sick and they shall recover. SEE
MARK 16: 18

Is it *really* God's *will* *for* people *to* be *healed*? Let's take a look. Large crowds followed Jesus as He came down the hillside. Look! A leper approaches. He kneels before Him, worshipping. "*Sir*," the leper pleads, "*if you want to, you can heal me*". Jesus touches the man. "*I want to*," He says. "*Be healed*." And instantly the leprosy disappears. SEE MATTHEW 8: 1-3 THE LIVING BIBLE   By reading the Scriptures, we see this is not an isolated occurrence. It happened to ALL that came to Him believing it was the Will of God for them to be healed.

*Y*es, *it* *is* God's *will* *for* *you* *to* be *healed*! You do not bring glory to God by walking around sick, saying, "*I am being sick for the glory of God.*" Sickness does not bring glory to God—healing and health bring glory to God! Others will say, "*God is teaching you a lesson by making you bear this sickness*". NO! There is NO GLORY TO GOD in our being sick! Let's kick over the sacred cows! While you are sick, did you learn anything? Usually not! Why? It is because in the same way you cannot teach spiritual things to a starving humanity, neither can you teach the depth of God's LOVE beyond their physical needs for healing!

When the leper asked Jesus to heal him, the leper said, "*Sir, if you want to, you can heal me.*" What was Jesus' response? "*I want to*," Jesus said. "*Be healed*".

OLD TESTAMENT PARADIGMS

Remember The Original Resource
Comparing The Authentic Provision Of His Dominion

JEREMIAH 14:19
KJV+SM

...(14:19) Hast thou utterly^{H3988} [H8800=S=A combination of a word plus a verb, M=expressing an action or a state of being] rejected^{H3988} [H8804=S=A simple/causal action M=referring to a time, or the present] Judah^{H3063}? hath thy soul^{H5315} lothed^{H1602} [H8804=S=A simple/causal action M=referring to a time, or the present] Zion^{H6726}? why hast thou smitten^{H5221} [H8689=S=Simple, causative, sometime reflexive action, M=completed at a time or the present.] us, and there is no healing^{H4832} for us? we looked^{H6960}

SEMITIC ARAMAIC
HEBRAIC PARALLEL
Original/Beginning

Got Healing?

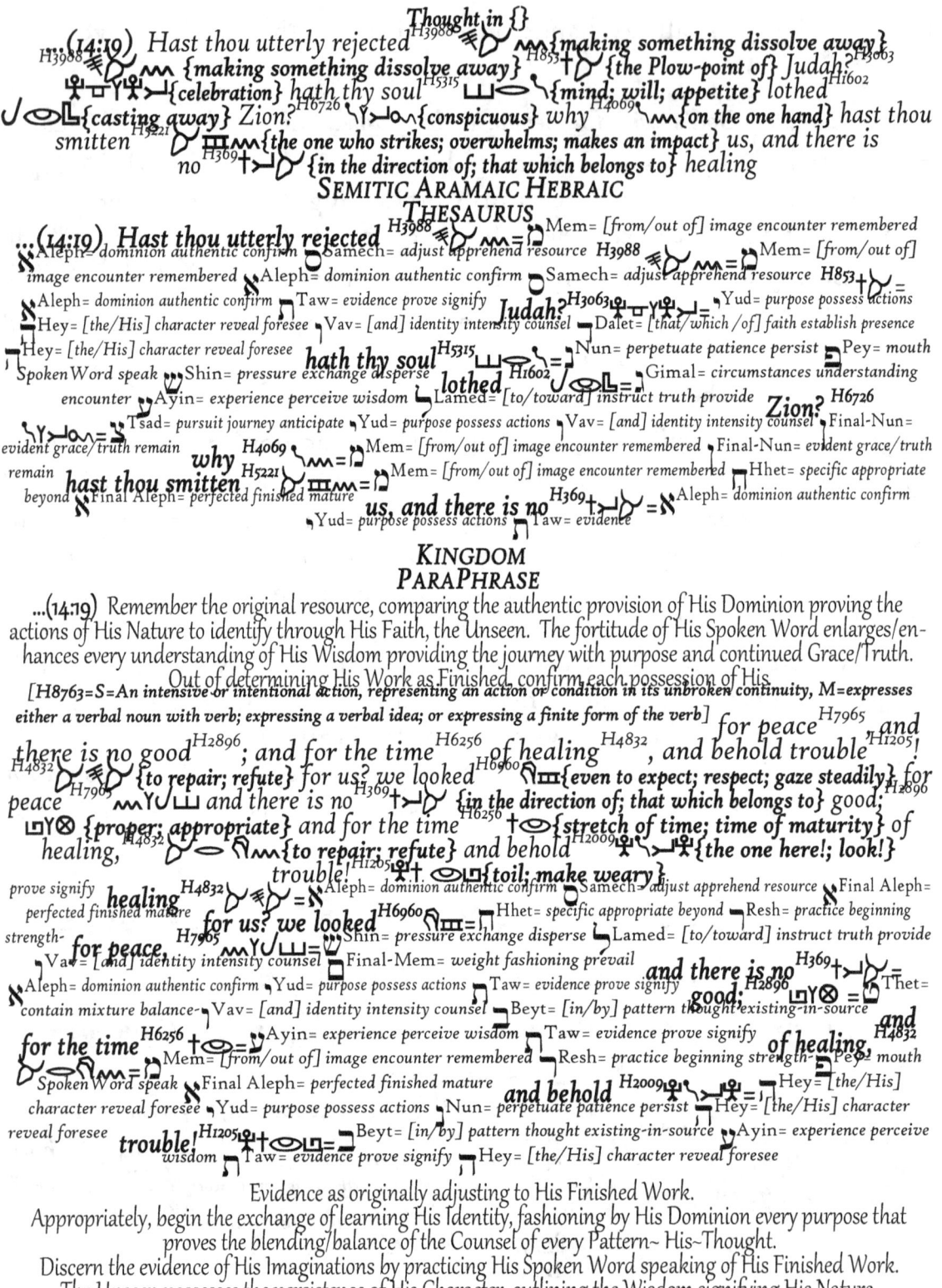

(14:19) *Hast thou utterly rejected* {Thought in {}} {making something dissolve away} {making something dissolve away} {the Plow-point of} *Judah?* {celebration} *hath thy soul* {mind; will; appetite} *lothed* {casting away} *Zion?* {conspicuous} *why* {on the one hand} *hast thou smitten* {the one who strikes; overwhelms; makes an impact} *us, and there is no* {in the direction of; that which belongs to} *healing*

SEMITIC ARAMAIC HEBRAIC
THESAURUS

...(14:19) Hast thou utterly rejected H3988 Mem= [from/out of] image encounter remembered Aleph= dominion authentic confirm Samech= adjust apprehend resource H3988 Mem= [from/out of] image encounter remembered Aleph= dominion authentic confirm Samech= adjust apprehend resource H853 = Aleph= dominion authentic confirm Taw= evidence prove signify *Judah?* H3063 Yud= purpose possess actions Hey= [the/His] character reveal foresee Vav= [and] identity intensity counsel Dalet= [that/which /of] faith establish presence Hey= [the/His] character reveal foresee Nun= perpetuate patience persist Pey= mouth Spoken Word speak Shin= pressure exchange disperse *hath thy soul* H5315 Gimal= circumstances understanding encounter Ayin= experience perceive wisdom *lothed* H1602 Lamed= [to/toward] instruct truth provide *Zion?* H6726 Tsad= pursuit journey anticipate Yud= purpose possess actions Vav= [and] identity intensity counsel Final-Nun= Final-Nun= evident grace/truth remain evident grace/truth remain *why* H4069 Mem= [from/out of] image encounter remembered Final-Nun= evident grace/truth remain *hast thou smitten* H5221 Mem= [from/out of] image encounter remembered Hhet= specific appropriate beyond Final Aleph= perfected finished mature *us, and there is no* H369 Aleph= dominion authentic confirm Yud= purpose possess actions Taw= evidence

KINGDOM
PARAPHRASE

...(14:19) Remember the original resource, comparing the authentic provision of His Dominion proving the actions of His Nature to identify through His Faith, the Unseen. The fortitude of His Spoken Word enlarges/enhances every understanding of His Wisdom providing the journey with purpose and continued Grace/Truth. Out of determining His Work as Finished, confirm each possession of His

[H8763=S=An intensive or intentional action, representing an action or condition in its unbroken continuity, M=expresses either a verbal noun with verb; expressing a verbal idea; or expressing a finite form of the verb]

there is no good H2896*; and for the time* H6256 *of healing* H4832*, and behold trouble* H1205*!* H4832 {to repair; refute} *for us? we looked* H6960 {even to expect; respect; gaze steadily} *for peace* H7965 *and there is no* H369 {in the direction of; that which belongs to} *good;* {proper; appropriate} *and for the time* H6256 {stretch of time; time of maturity} *of healing,* H4832 {to repair; refute} *and behold* H2009 {the one here!; look!} *trouble!* H1205 {toil; make weary}

prove signify *healing* H4832 = Aleph= dominion authentic confirm Samech= adjust apprehend resource Final Aleph= perfected finished mature Hhet= specific appropriate beyond Resh= practice beginning strength- *for us? we looked* H6960 Shin= pressure exchange disperse Lamed= [to/toward] instruct truth provide *for peace,* H7965 Vav= [and] identity intensity counsel Final-Mem= weight fashioning prevail *and there is no* H369 Thet= Aleph= dominion authentic confirm Yud= purpose possess actions Taw= evidence prove signify *good;* H2896 = contain mixture balance- Vav= [and] identity intensity counsel Beyt= [in/by] pattern thought existing-in-source *and for the time* H6256 Ayin= experience perceive wisdom Taw= evidence prove signify *of healing,* H4832 Mem= [from/out of] image encounter remembered Resh= practice beginning strength- Pey= mouth Spoken Word speak Final Aleph= perfected finished mature *and behold* H2009 Hey= [the/His] character reveal foresee Yud= purpose possess actions Nun= perpetuate patience persist Hey= [the/His] character reveal foresee Beyt= [in/by] pattern thought existing-in-source Ayin= experience perceive *trouble!* H1205 wisdom Taw= evidence prove signify Hey= [the/His] character reveal foresee

Evidence as originally adjusting to His Finished Work.
Appropriately, begin the exchange of learning His Identity, fashioning by His Dominion every purpose that proves the blending/balance of the Counsel of every Pattern~ His~Thought.
Discern the evidence of His Imaginations by practicing His Spoken Word speaking of His Finished Work.
The Unseen possesses the persistence of His Character, outlining the Wisdom signifying His Nature.

Got Healing?

Remember the original resource, comparing the authentic provision of His Dominion proving the actions of His Nature to identify through His Faith, the Unseen.

It is wonderful to be a part of ministering healing to the sick, through the name of Jesus, so that **God gets all the glory**! We also learn that if one method does not work, we <u>can</u> try other ways, because if God had wanted us to heal only one particular way, He would not have had Jesus heal in so many different ways in the Bible! Many ask, "*Do you mean the supernatural can be taught*"? Yes, it **most certainly can**! It is not God that needs the teaching, but humanity. In so doing, we can learn the very Heart of God Himself, and initiate the proper responses to the precious Holy Spirit, as **She** guides, directs, and causes us to learn **Her** ways as the *Paracletos* (*the One who dwells within us, and walk with us to teach us Jesus*).

The fortitude of His Spoken Word enlarges/enhances every understanding of His Wisdom providing the journey with purpose and continued Grace/Truth.

"*Now faith is the substance of things hoped for, the evidence of things not seen*". HEBREWS 11:1 KJV This definition teaches us: **First**, **Faith** is not hope, not a mere expectation of future things, but a present receiving of that which is promised in a real and substantial way. **Faith is accepting, not expecting**. **Secondly**, **Faith** is not sight, for it deals with things not seen. **The region of the visible is not the realm of faith**. *When a thing is proved by demonstration, it is not a matter of faith, but of evidence.* Faith asks no other evidences than God's Word and its own assurance. **Faith** is the evidence. It is not true to say that "*seeing is believing*." Faith believes where it cannot see; nay, believes what sight and evidence may even seem to contradict, if only God has said it.

Out of determining His Work as Finished, confirm each possession of His Evidence as originally adjusting to His Finished Work.

When God said to Abraham, "*I have made thee a father of many nations*", there was no sign of it; indeed, the evidence of sight plainly contradicted it. However, God said it, and Abraham believed, for faith "*calleth the things that are not, as though they were*". So Abraham "*considered not his own* body, now dead", but "*was strong in faith, giving glory to God, and being fully persuaded that what He had promised He was able also to perform*".

Thirdly, Faith recognizes in every case an act of creation. It does not require any material to start with, for it believes in a God who can make all things out of what appears as nothing, and therefore it can step out upon the seeming void and find it full of the creations of His power.

Appropriately, begin the exchange of learning His Identity, fashioning by His Dominion every purpose that proves the blending/balance in the Counsel of every Pattern~of~His~thought.

On giving His greatest promises in the Old Testament, God reveals Himself as the Creator of that which He is promising. "*Call unto me, and I will answer thee, and shew thee great and mighty things, which thou knowest not*". JEREMIAH 33:3 KJV There may be no sign of it, no probability of it, no germ of it from which to start, but God is able to make it out of, what appears as nothing, by a word, *His Word!* He does so by *The Word* which *His Faith* claims. He needs no protoplasm to build His magnificent edifices of worlds. "*For He spake, and it was done; He commanded, and it stood fast*". PSALMS 33:9 KJV ." Into the soul that has no basis or remnant of goodness, but is dead in trespasses and sins, He can speak life and holiness. Into the body, whose constitution is exhausted and its springs of life run out, He can command health and strength. And so faith begins where human hopes and prospects end; "*humanity's extremity is God's opportunity*."

Discern the evidence of His Imaginations by practicing His Spoken Word speaking of His Finished Work.

Now this *Faith*, the apostle declares, is indispensable in order to please God. No wonder; anything less is to treat God as if He were unreal and unreliable, and that is in its own reality a practical **atheism**! It is to make His Word less sure than a mere material fact of nature and perception of the senses; *it is to trust God less than we trust His works*. Anything LESS THAN HIM opposes Who He REMAINS.

The Unseen possesses the persistence of His Character, outlining the Wisdom signifying His Nature.

$\mathcal{T}$he reason why God requires our absolute trust is very plain. The ruin of the human race came by discrediting and doubting God's word to our first parents. "*Hath God said*"?~~was the fountain of all sin. "*God hath said*" is the foundation, therefore, of our restoration.

MATTHEW 4:3-10 KJV

3 And when the tempter came to Him, he said, If Thou be the Son of God, command that these stones be made bread. 4 But He answered and said, It is written, Man shall not live by bread alone, but by every word that proceedeth out of the mouth of God. 5 Then the devil taketh Him up into the holy city, and setteth Him on a pinnacle of the temple, 6 and saith unto Him, If Thou be the Son of God, cast thyself down: for it is written, He shall give his angels charge concerning thee: and in their hands they shall bear thee up, lest at any time thou dash thy foot against a stone. 7 Jesus said unto him, It is written again, Thou shalt not tempt the Lord thy God. 8 Again, the devil taketh Him up into an exceeding high mountain, and sheweth him all the kingdoms of the world, and the glory of them; 9 and saith unto him, All these things will I give thee, if Thou wilt fall down and worship me. 10 Then saith Jesus unto him, Get thee hence, Satan: for it is written, Thou shalt worship the Lord thy God, and Him only shalt thou serve.

$\mathcal{O}$nly when we thus implicitly believe His Word will we love and obey Him. And as unbelief stands in the foreground in the first picture of our fallen race, it leads the procession of the lost, in the closing scene in the tragedy of mankind. "The fearful and the unbelieving shall have their portion in the lake which burneth with fire and brimstone, which is the second death." Let us "*take heed, therefore, lest there be in any of us an evil heart of unbelief in departing from the living God*".

JEREMIAH 30:13
KJV+TVM

...(30:13) *There is none to plead*^{H1777} *[H8802=S=Expresses the "simple" or "causal" action of the root in the active voice; M= through an action or condition in its unbroken continuity]* *thy cause*^{H1779}, *that thou mayest be bound up*^{H4205}: *thou hast no healing*^{H8585} *medicines*^{H7499}

ORIGINAL THOUGHTS

...(30:13) The Kingdom purpose supports the established actions of the Grace of His Truth.

Got Healing?

His Faith possesses foundation that encounters with pursuit, the Identity of His Beginnings. Occupying the Throne retains the remaining evidence of His Wisdom providing Unseen Beginnings of His Spoken Word, increasing the Dominion of His Integrity/Attitude.

The Kingdom purpose supports the established actions of the Grace of His Truth.

$\mathcal{M}$any today are seeking healing, but yet they talk sickness and suffering until they establish that image in themselves. Their thoughts and words produce a vivid blueprint, and they live within the bounds and limitations of that blueprint.

$\mathcal{O}$ur words are building blocks of which we construct our living and the future of our living. The words we speak are made the cornerstones of our living, and whether we give attention and awareness to any or all of our words, what we speak about when we do not have to speak, determines what becomes of our daily living.

His Faith possesses foundation that encounters with pursuit, the Identity of His Beginnings.

$\mathcal{A}$fter we become Christians, we have our sins forgiven on the basis of our relationship and the intercession of Christ. If we remain stubborn, or fearful of admitting our failures, then we build a wall between us and our Lord. This is called, "free~moral agency", and it is a part of our makeup from the Lord God. He wants a family of sons and daughters who CHOOSE to worship and have fellowship with Him; not having duty, or guilt, or any other such thing to be the compelling factor towards Him from us.

$\mathcal{T}$he word, "remission" is never used in Scripture in connection with thoughts concerning the New Birth. The word, "remission" is an old man/Adam and it has nothing at all to do with us after we have acknowledged we are saved unto the Lord, by His Plan and Purpose.

$\mathcal{O}$n the New Birth, all that we ever were is never again listened to, nor discussed between us and the Father. If we bring up the past, He says, "what are talking about; I do not REMEMBER any of that anymore"! If we are the only remembering it, then why don't we stop? Because it is easier to talk about the stuff we are already familiar with, then to allow our thoughts to be retrained, and regenerated by the Spirit's within us!

Occupying the Throne retains the remaining evidence of His Wisdom providing Unseen Beginnings of His Spoken Word, increasing the Dominion of His Integrity/Attitude.

Don't doubt God. If we must doubt something, doubt our doubts, because they are unreliable; but never doubt God, nor His word. *"Then Peter opened his mouth, and said, Of a truth I perceive that God is no respecter of persons".* ACTS 10:34 KJV For God to do for one, and not everyone would invalidate the previous verse. Therefore, without hesitation, understand that what He has done for others, He will do for you and me. Every step we take believing in Him, He matches by taking more than we think we have taken. In fact, He has stepped out the whole journey, even before we were born into this living.

SEMITIC ARAMAIC HEBRAIC THESAURUS

...(30:13) **There is none**[H3690] Aleph= dominion authentic confirm Yud= purpose possess actions

Final- ...(30:13) **There is none**[H3690] {לֹא=not} Nun= foundation grace/truth remain **to plead**[H1777] hing;

Dalét= [that/which/of] faith establish presence Yud= purpose possess actions Final-Nun= foundation **without}** to plead[H1777] {פִּיס=to appease; reconcile} thy cause,[H1779] {עַל=concerning; about; on behalf of} that thou mayest be bound up:[H4205] {אֲגֹר=to collect and tie together} thou hast no[H3690] {לֹא=nothing; without} healing[H8585] {אָסָא=health; cure; repair} medicines.[H7499] {רְפוּאָה=treatment; remedy}

grace/truth remain **thy cause,**[H1779] Dalét= [that/which/of] faith establish presence Yud= purpose possess actions Final-Nun= foundation grace/truth remain **that thou mayest be bound up:**[H4205] Mem= [from/out of] image encounter remembered Tsad= pursuit journey anticipate Vav= [and] identity intensity counsel Resh= practice beginning strength- **thou hast no**[H3690] Aleph= dominion authentic confirm Yud= purpose possess actions Final-Nun= foundation grace/truth remain **healing**[H8585] Taw= evidence prove signify Ayin= experience perceive wisdom Lamed= [to/toward] instruct truth provide Hey= [the/His] character reveal foresee **medicines.**[H7499] Resh= practice beginning strength- Pey= mouth Spoken Word speak Vav= [and] identity intensity counsel Aleph= dominion authentic confirm Hey= [the/His] character reveal foresee

Enabling The Purpose Of His Grace/Truth Designs The Revealing Of The Unseen Exchanges By His Pattern-Of-Thought Exercising Imaginations That Persist In Desiring Every Revelation

NAHUM 3:19
KJV+

...(3:19) There is no healing[H3545] of thy bruise[H7667]; thy wound[H4347] is grievous[H2470] [High Tower Text]: all that hear[H8085] [H8802=S=Expresses the "simple" or "causal" action of the root in the active voice; M= through an action or condition in its unbroken continuity] the bruit[H8088] of thee shall clap[H8628]

Got Healing?

[H8804=S=A simple/causal action M=referring to a time, or the present] the hands[H3709] over thee: for upon whom hath not thy wickedness[H7451] passed[H5674] [H8804=S=A simple/causal action M=referring to a time, or the present] continually[H8548]?

SEMITIC ARAMAIC HEBRAIC PARALLEL
Original/Beginning
Thought in {}

...(3:19) There is no[H369] אלי{אל=nothing; without} healing[H3545] שאא{אסא=to cure; repair} of thy bruise;[H7667] שבר{שבר=shattering; breakthrough} thy wound[H4347] מא שא{מכה=to afflict; to overwhelm} is grievous[H2470] חלה{חלה=spinning or piercing pain} all[H3605] שעך{כל=to measure} that hear[H8085] שמע{שמע= listen and respond} the bruit[H8088] שמע{שמע=the report} of thee shall

SEMITIC ARAMAIC HEBRAIC THESAURUS

There is no[H369] אלי = Aleph= dominion authentic confirm ▪Yud= purpose possess actions ▪Final-Nun= foundation grace/truth remain

healing[H3545] ב= Kaph= surrender obtain desire ▪Hey= [the/His] character reveal foresee ▪Hey= [the/His] character reveal foresee

of thy bruise;[H7667] ש= Shin= pressure exchange disperse ▪Beyt= [in/by] pattern~thought indwelling existence ▪Resh= practice beginning strength-

thy wound[H4347] מ= Mem= [from/out of] ▪Hey= [the/His] character reveal image encounter remembered ▪Nun= perpetuate patience persist ▪Kaph= surrender obtain desire

is grievous:[H2470] ח= Hhet= specific appropriate beyond ▪Lamed= [to/toward] instruct truth provide ▪Hey= [the/His] character reveal foresee

all[H3605] שעך= Kaph= surrender obtain desire ▪Vav= [and] identity intensity counsel ▪Lamed= [to/toward] instruct truth provide

that hear[H8085] ש= Shin= pressure exchange disperse ▪Mem= [from/out of] image encounter remembered ▪Ayin= experience perceive wisdom

the bruit[H8088] ש= Shin= pressure exchange disperse ▪Mem= [from/out of] image encounter

ORIGINAL THOUGHTS

...(3:19) Enabling the purpose of His Grace/Truth designs the revealing of the Unseen exchanges by His Pattern~of~thought exercising imaginations that persist in desiring every Revelation. From the specifics of truthful revelations, the desire to identify each truth presses every imagination of His Wisdom to enlarge/enhance every remembrance perceived. Signifying each parallel of His Wisdom conceives His Spoken Word, discerning His Truth, and

clap[H8628] {קפח=thrust} the hands[H3709] {כף=palm; 1/3 of a cubit} over[H5921] {על=upon; beyond; through} thee: for[H3588] {כי=direct consequence of one's action} upon[H5921] {עלל=ris-ing} whom[H4310] {מי=someone unknown} hath not[H3808] {לא=to have what you are without} thy wickedness[H7451] {רע=something dysfunctional} passed[H5674] {עבר=cross; crossing over} contin-ually?[H8548] {תמיד=perpetual; evermore}

of thee shall clap[H8628] the hands[H3709] ⌐= Taw= evidence prove signify ▪Quph= contrast parallel structure ▪Ayin= experience perceive wisdom ▪Pey= mouth SpokenWord speak ▪Kaph= surrender obtain desire ▪Lamed= [to/toward] instruct truth provide ▪Ayin= experience perceive wisdom

over[H5921] ע= Ayin= experience perceive wisdom ▪Lamed= [to/toward] instruct truth provide ▪Yud= purpose possess actions

thee: for[H3588] כ= Kaph= surrender obtain desire ▪Hey= [the/His] character reveal foresee ▪Yud= purpose possess actions ▪Ayin= experience perceive wisdom

upon[H5921] ע= Ayin= experience perceive wisdom ▪Lamed= [to/toward] instruct truth provide ▪Vav= [and] identity intensity counsel

whom[H4310] מ= Mem= [from/out of] image encounter remembered ▪Lamed= [to/toward] instruct truth provide ▪Final Aleph= perfected finished mature

hath not[H3808] ▪Resh= practice beginning strength- ▪Gimal= circumstances under-standing encounter

wickedness[H7451] ע= Ayin= experience perceive wisdom ▪Beyt= [in/by] pattern~thought indwelling existence ▪Resh= practice beginning strength-

passed[H5674] ▪Ayin= experience perceive wisdom

continually?[H8548] ⌐= Taw= evidence prove signify ▪Mem= [from/out of] image encounter remembered ▪Yud= purpose possess actions ▪Dalet= [that/which/of] faith establish presence

obtains each purpose through the experiences of His Promises foreseen Imagine each purpose teaching to identify His Finished Work. The Practice of understanding His Wisdom exceeds the beginnings of His Evidence out of each purpose of His Faith.

Enabling the purpose of His Grace/Truth designs the revealing of the Unseen exchanges by His Pattern~of~thought

---

Got Healing?

exercising imaginations that persist in desiring every Revelation.

*T*he Redeemer appears among men with both hands stretched out to our misery and need. In the one He holds salvation; in the other, healing. He offers Himself to us as a complete Saviour; *His indwelling Spirit the life of our spirit; His resurrection body the life of our mortal flesh.* He begins His ministry by healing all that had need of healing. He closes it by making on the Cross a full atonement for our sin; and then on the other side of the open tomb He passes into Heaven, leaving the double commission for "*all the world,*" and "*all the days even unto the end of. the world;*"--"*Go ye into all the world and preach the Gospel to every creature. He that believeth and is baptized shall be saved. He that believeth not shall be damned. And these signs shall follow them that believe. In My name they shall cast out devils~~they shall lay hands upon the sick and they shall recover.*"

From the specifics of truthful revelations, the desire to identify each truth presses every imagination of His Wisdom to enlarge/enhance every remembrance perceived.

*W*e are so selfish that unless we think a certain portion of God's word is going to minister to our comfort, or specially suits our case, it has no bearing for us, there is no good in it for us, and therefore we fail to be in harmony with the thoughts of God.

*T*he main reason so many Christians do not grasp or understand the rudimentary elements of God's Word, Design, or Desire; is that they NEGLECT the Word of God, Himself, and itself! In order to have the INTIMACY of relationship with the Son, we must embrace knowing HIS WORD, and that HE IS THE WORD SPOKEN!

Signifying each parallel of His Wisdom conceives His Spoken Word discerning His Truth, and obtains each purpose through the experiences of His Promises foreseen.

*W*e neglect the Scriptures on the plea that we are already saved and that all we need is a few little rules by which we can guide our course; *something like a navigator on a merchant vessel, who can take bearings, and know how to steer his ship, but at the same time is ignorant of the mighty works of God* *and passes heedlessly under that which speaks of the glory of God, which is the firmament which showeth His handiwork.* We may have a few verses that we think we have enough to live by: *but we are not in communion with our Lord and Savior.*

The parallels of His eternal majesty can evermore portray the sculpting hand of His Magnificence, if we would but give the Spirit within us the time to show how to hear the mellifluous, dulcet tones of His Voice harmonizing the wonders of a universe created by the touch of His Voice filling the empty corridors of time and space.

Imagine each purpose teaching to identify His Finished Work.

We shall find as we go on in any study of Scripture, that even the Pentateuch as it is called, (*which simply means five volumes*) gives us a model upon which the whole word of God is written, a key by which we can understand something of His purpose in giving us such a full revelation. We would come to see that they are one whole that we could not take one of them away without mutilating the rest. While every division scholars have made of His Word, there is nothing so clear as the message of a REDEEMER, who in His coming defined, declared, and finished the revealing of everything spoken, understood, and finished before ever the foundations of the world were laid.

The Practice of understanding His Wisdom exceeds the beginnings of His Evidence out of each purpose of His Faith.

God's word is a unit, with one Author, the Holy Spirit, although He has used a number of instruments throughout vast periods of time. The object of the Book is one, although this too is approached from every possible point of view~~historical, typical, legal enactments, biographies, poetry, parable, allegory, prophetic denunciation of sin and promise of glorious blessing~~all of which we find in the Old Testament. Then, in the New, direct narratives of the life, teaching, sufferings, death and resurrection of the Lord Jesus Christ; the history of the establishment of His Church upon the descent of the Holy Spirit, and the going out of the gospel world-wide, in the Acts. The Epistles unfold the truths and responsibilities of Christianity, collective, and individual; then the closing book of prophecy, with its windows open to the heavenly Jerusalem. Through them all, Christ is the center, the object, the theme, and the end. He is the Alpha, from the first of Genesis; and the Omega, as the light and glory that illumine the heavenly city. Yes, Christ is all~in~all.

The Purpose Of Practicing His Finished Work Enlarges The Weightiness Of Exchange With His Imaginations Sowing Throughout The Journey That His Faith Parallels To The Unseen.

MALACHI 4:2 KJV+

...(4:2) But unto you that fear [H3373] my name [H8034] shall the Sun [H8121] of righteousness [H6666] arise [H2224] [H8804=S=A simple/causal action M=referring to a time, or the present] with healing [H4832] in his wings [H3671]; and ye shall go forth [H3318] [H8804=S=A simple/causal action M=referring to a time, or the present], and grow up [H6335] [H8804=S=A simple/causal action M=referring to a time, or the present] as calves [H5695] of the stall [H4770].

SEMITIC ARAMAIC HEBRAIC PARALLEL

Original/Beginning Thought in {}

...(4:2) But unto you that fear [H3373] {ירא=inspire reverence; honor; respect} my name [H8034] {שם=reputation; in name only} shall the Sun [H8121] {שמש=to provide; to be minist-ered to} of right-eousness [H6666] {צדקה=straightness; upright} arise [H2224] {זרח=to shine} with healing [H4832] {מרפא= health; wholesome; cure} in His wings; [H3671] {כנף=border; corner} and ye shall go forth, [H3318] {יצא=issue out} and grow up [H6335] {פוש=spread; scatter} as calves [H5695] {עלה=palace} of the

SEMITIC ARAMAIC HEBRAIC THESAURUS

...(4:2) But unto you that fear [H3373] = Yud= purpose possess actions — Resh= practice beginning strength- Final Aleph= perfected finished mature — Shin= pressure exchange disperse — Final-Mem= weight fashioning prevail my name [H8034] = Shin= pressure exchange disperse Mem= [from/out of] image encounter remembered — Shin= pressure exchange disperse shall the Sun [H8121] = Shin= pressure exchange disperse of righteousness [H6666] — Tsad= pursuit journey anticipate — Dalet= [that/which/of] faith establish presence — Quph= contrast parallel structure — Hey= [the/His] character reveal foresee arise [H2224] — Zayin= skill alter method — Resh= practice beginning strength- — Hhet= specific appropriate beyond with healing [H4832] = Mem= [from/out of] image encounter remembered — Resh= practice beginning strength- — Pey= mouth Spoken Word speak — Final Aleph= perfected finished mature in his wings; [H3671] — Kaph= surrender obtain desire — Nun= perpetuate patience persist — Final Pey= declare sound advantage and ye shall go forth [H3318] — Yud= purpose possess actions — Tsad= pursuit journey anticipate — Final Aleph= perfected finished mature and grow up [H6335] Pey= mouth Spoken Word speak — Yud= purpose possess actions — Shin= pressure exchange disperse as calves [H5695] — Ayin= experience perceive wisdom — Gimal= circumstances understanding encounter Lamed= [to/toward] instruct truth provide — Hey= [the/His] character reveal foresee of the stall. [H4770] — Mem= [from/out of] image encounter remembered — Resh= practice beginning strength- Beyt= [in/by] pattern~thought indwelling existence — Quph= contrast parallel structure

ORIGINAL THOUGHTS

Got Healing?

The Purpose Of Practicing His Finished Work enlarges the weightiness of exchange with His Imaginations sowing throughout the journey that His Faith parallels to the Unseen.
Skillfully, then, practice with determined reflections upon the beginnings of His Spoken Word out of His Finished Work.
Surrender to every persistently sound advantage of His Purposes, in pursuit of His Finished Work.
For His Spoken Word possesses the exchange of His Wisdom when understanding to learn the Unseen Imaginations of His Strong Indwelling Framework.

The Purpose Of Practicing His Finished Work enlarges the weightiness of exchange with His Imaginations sowing throughout the journey that His Faith parallels to the Unseen.

The more we practice/exercise the values of His Word, the greater the Spirit's appearing through our living, each day we live. Pursuit of God is about finding the REST IN HIM, so that we may live and enjoy the REST OF HIM.

Living is not so much about our pursuing of success, or more money, or bigger things. There is no lasting value in anything that can be stolen, or decaying, losing its value. Chasing success is like trying to squeeze a handful of water. The tighter you squeeze, the less water you get. When you chase it, your life becomes the chase, and you become a victim of always wanting more. If you refuse to change, nothing changes. If you refuse to change, then the only reasonable action that will be is to begin seeking after the only promise of LOVE that will last.

Skillfully, then, practice with determined reflections upon the beginnings of His Spoken Word out of His Finished Work.

"Lay not up for yourselves treasures upon earth, where moth and rust doth corrupt, and where thieves break through and steal: But lay up for yourselves treasures in heaven, where neither moth nor rust doth corrupt, and where thieves do not break through nor steal: For where your treasure is, there will your heart be also. The light of the body is the eye: if therefore thine eye be single, thy whole body shall be full of light. But if thine eye be evil, thy whole body shall be full of darkness. If therefore the light that is in thee be darkness, how great is that darkness! No man can serve two masters: for either he will hate the one, and love the other; or else he will hold to the one, and despise the other. Ye cannot serve God and mammon". MATTHEW 6:19-24 KJV Learn to do those in God that you enjoy. If His JOY is the reason for our contentment, the journey of our

---

living is more acceptable, whenever the wearisome seasons of challenge and change appear on the landscape of our living.

Surrender to every persistently sound advantage of His Purposes, in pursuit of His Finished Work.

Within the fold of desirable Christianity, there are to be found increasing numbers of people whose spiritual lives are marked by a growing hunger after God Himself. They are eager for spiritual realities and will not be put off with words, nor will they be content with correct "*interpretations*" of truth. **They are thirsty for God, and they will not be satisfied until they have drunk deep at the fountain of living water.** This is the only real indicator of recovery which we have been able to detect anywhere on the horizon of the faithful. It may be the cloud the size of a man's hand for which a few saints here and there have been looking. It can result in a resurrection of living for many souls and a recapture of that radiant wonder which should accompany faith in Christ, that wonder which has all but fled the church in our day.

For His Spoken Word possesses the exchange of His Wisdom when understanding to learn the Unseen Imaginations of His Strong Indwelling Framework.

However, this hunger **must be recognized** by our religious leaders. Current evangelicalism has (*to change the figure*) laid the altar and divided the sacrifice into parts, but now seems satisfied to count the stones and rearrange the pieces with never a care that **there is not a sign of fire** upon the top of lofty Mount Carmel.

However, God be thanked that there are a few who care. They are those who, while they love the altar and delight in the sacrifice, are yet unable to reconcile themselves to the continued absence of fire. They desire God above all. They are thirsty to taste for themselves the "*piercing sweetness*" of the love of Christ about whom all the holy prophets did write and the psalmists did sing.

There is today no lack of Bible teachers to set forth correctly the principles of the doctrines of Christ, but too many of these seem satisfied to teach the fundamentals of the faith year after year, strangely unaware that there is in their ministry no manifest presence, nor anything unusual in their personal lives. They minister constantly to believers who feel within their breasts a longing which their teaching simply does not satisfy.

*M*ilton's terrible sentence applies to our day as accurately as it did to his: "*The hungry sheep look up, and are not fed.*" It is a solemn thing, and no small scandal in the kingdom, to <u>see</u> <u>God's</u> <u>children</u> <u>starving</u> <u>while</u> <u>actually</u> <u>seated</u> <u>at</u> <u>the</u> <u>Father's</u> <u>table</u>. The truth of Wesley's words is established before our eyes: "*Orthodoxy, or right opinion, is, at best, a very slender part of believing. Though right tempers cannot subsist without right opinions, yet right opinions may subsist without right tempers. There may be a right opinion of God without either love or one right temper toward Him. The accuser is a proof of this*".

*F*or it is not mere words that nourish the soul, but God Himself; and unless and until the hearers find God in personal experience, they are not the better for having heard the truth. *The Bible is not an end in itself, but a means to bring souls to an intimate and satisfying knowledge of God, that they may <u>enter into Him</u>, that they may <u>delight in His presence</u>, may <u>taste and know the inner sweetness of the very God Himself in the core and center of their being</u>, <u>their</u> <u>spirit</u>.*

<u>NEW TESTAMENT PARADIGMS</u>

*W*hile proving God's Will to HEAL through the Old Covenant, the examples that follow, of Christ continuing the Will of the Father, and the edict of the Godhead. Here, in the New Covenant is found the open dialogue of God with humanity. None but those deaf of hearing, or unmotivated to change because of challenge unanswered, are unable to hear and act upon the distinct, clear message of God Himself to the whole of His Creation. ***<u>Read</u> <u>on</u>, <u>NOBLE</u> <u>HEARER</u> <u>OF</u> <u>TRUTH</u>, <u>read</u> <u>on</u>!***

<u>Transcend The Evidence That Obtains Strength</u>
<u>To Acknowledge The Qualities That</u>

Increase His Finished Work

MATTHEW 4:23
KJV+TVM

And[G2532] Jesus[G2424] went about[G4013] [G5707] all[G3650] Galilee[G1056], teaching[G1321] [G5723] in[G1722] their[G846] synagogues[G4864], and[G2532] preaching[G2784] [G5723] the gospel[G2098] of the kingdom[G932], and[G2532] healing[G2323] [G5723] all[G3956] manner of sickness[G3554] and[G2532] all[G3956] manner of disease[G3119] among[G1722] the people[G2992].

ORIGINAL THOUGHTS

...(4:23) In addition, transcend the evidence that obtains His Strength to acknowledge the qualities that increase His Finished Work. Through single-minded exchange, insure the Wisdom of His Pattern~of~Thoughts, while surrendering to the provisions of His Grace, encountering each promise, in purpose of the teachings of His Finished Work. Insure every memory that teaches His Sound Advantage, and behold the increase of His Influence within the consent of His Seed to increase by exchange the evidence of His Grace/Truth, perpetuating every issue. For by each extent/boundary of remembrance, agreement strengthens the element of adjusting to His Pattern~of~Thought in processing the witness of His Finished Work. Establish each encountering of His Provision with corresponding increase by evidence of His Finished Work, to insure the transforming of His Dominion in apprehending His Finished Work. Learn to surrender as obtaining the authority of His Pattern~Thoughts to increase the surrender to single~mindedness that processes the revelation of progress. Within the Pattern~of~His~Thoughts, wisely go beyond His Finished Work.

<u>In addition, transcend the evidence that obtains His Strength to acknowledge the qualities that increase His Finished Work.</u>

Going beyond the settled understanding of His Finished Work, reach into the domain of Eternity's fullness and expend with exchange for the majesty of His Joy, and the magnificence of His Love!

This is Jesus' first use of the phrase, "*Gospel of the Kingdom*"!

Herein lays the beginnings of the message that not only frees the soul of every encumbrance, but sets one's search on the right road to accessing *a new and living way through* <u>HIM</u>!

<u>Through single-minded exchange, insure the Wisdom of His Pattern~of~Thoughts, while surrendering to the provisions of His Grace, encountering each promise, in purpose of the teachings of His Finished Work.</u>

Never let us be so quick to grasp hold of a thought that *appears* as though being from the mind of God.

It is within the ability of the Soul to sound like~minded, when in fact the impetus/motivation of the thought provided could lead one's walk astray.

Remaining aware as to the outcome of any thought accepted, keeps the soul in tight union with the Spirit's leading, and subsequent correcting, if necessary.

Insure every memory that teaches His Sound Advantage, and behold the increase of His Influence, within the consent of His Seed to increase by exchange the evidence of His Grace/Truth, perpetuating every issue.

Exchange only occurs when the Spirit leads, the Soul agrees, and the Body follows by surrender.

If there is a *glitch* at any moment, the Spirit will confidently point out the *pothole*, so that the journey may remain uninterrupted or disturbed by any hindering unseen.

Trusting the leading of the Spirit to always be to the benefit of the believer becomes the utmost of His Abilities embraced.

For by each extent/boundary of remembrance, agreement strengthens the element of adjusting to His Pattern~of~Thought in processing the witness of His Finished Work.

Accepting the preliminary beginnings of a thought that projects the character of Christ Jesus, allows the guiding preparations of the Spirit to lessen the *jolt*, and accentuate the Purposes of God throughout.

With respect to the love of the Father for His creation, it was unthinkable that God would turn a cold shoulder to His creation, let alone turn His back on us.

What then, was God being good to do, when the creation that He loved, and had destined to such breathtaking blessing, was on the road to ruin, by lapsing into non-being?

The passion of the Father in creation becomes the fire that sends the Son to save.

The sin of Adam was met by the same God and the same divine determination to bless that which birthed His Creation in the first place.

Remembering the LOVE OF GOD for US, His Creation, affords us the boundaries that keep us close to Him until such time as we can rightly SEE what it is for His every purpose to fill full the desire, longing, and void within our living as HE IS IN US!

Establish each encountering of His Provision with corresponding increase by evidence of His Finished Work, to insure the transforming of His Dominion in apprehending His Finished Work.

Contrasting the parallels between His Provision and His Finished Work emphasizes the grandeur of His LOVE toward those of His Creation.

As His Finished Work involves everything He is to us, His Creation; the Provisions that provide such benefits to us, as we are HIS, accounts to the fullness of sharing the completeness He offers out of HIMSELF!

God's answers never come as a balancing of Heaven's ledgers.

God's answer to the problem of *Selfish~Independent~Nature* involves healing one's dis~ease, by transforming or converting our fallen humanity into real relationship with Him.

Learn to surrender as obtaining the authority of His Pattern~Thoughts to increase the surrender to single~mindedness that processes the revelation of progress.

God's forgiveness would be meaningless, if it were not done into *flesh and blood existence* and worked into *real and actual reconciliation* so that *relationship and fellowship* were, in actual fact, *restored*.

What God had on His hands in the Fall of Adam was not a legal problem, but an organic one.

Sin, or~~*Selfish~Independent~Nature*~~is about corruption, about dis~ease, and about a deep and pervasive alienation of our very beings/existence.

To be sure, all manner of evil and wrongdoing come forth from sin, or~~*Selfish~Independent~Nature*~~but these are symptoms of the deeper, more profound dis~ease.

If we, as His Creation, are to share in the fullness of the Eternity that THEY, the Godhead are about; then the dis~ease has to be healed, and the cancer of the *Selfish~Independent~Nature* has to be eradicated/removed from our human equation.

There has to be a radical change/conversion of humanity's fallen existence.

Got Healing?

Such change happens when we allow the Spirit to perform the revealing of what Jesus has already finished!

Within the Pattern~of~His~Thoughts, wisely go beyond His Finished Work.

When we are free to love and be loved, free to know and be known, free to give of ourselves and to receive of all that God is~~we actually move beyond such freedom into an everlasting, eternal phase of Covenant with God that nothing is able to move us away from HIM!

Going beyond where and what we started in exchanges selfishness for giving~of~self; for entanglements exchanged for freedom and liberty in the fullness of WHO HE HAS SHARED WITH US!

Adam and Eve fell BEFORE they partook of the fruit; in that, they turned away from the fullness they were already experiencing.

Such is the same with us, when we refuse to fellowship, refuse intimate our thoughts with Him; thinking that we are unto ourselves all that we need to embrace!

Going beyond the exchanges that the Spirit orchestrates in our living causes us to mature in such a manner that meeting any foe, or hindrance, or anxiety~~ALWAYS takes us back to HIM, and from the beginning we are made to see the complete, and finished package of God's LOVE for us!

SEMITIC~ARAMAIC~HEBRAIC THESAURUS

Aramaic before first {

Semitic Root before first =

Lettering for ParaPhrase after second =

...(4:23) (& traveling about) ומתכרך S10626 {ܟܪܟ=and the volume}=Y/ı Vav-[and/in addition]increase degree assure-Mem[from/out of]-transform encounter remembrance-⊗/ܛ Taw-evidence prove sign-ܫ/ܟ Kaph-surrender obtains consent-ܐ/ܪ Resh- process beginning strength-ܫ/ܟ Final-Kaph-acknowledge offer allow-

(was)הוא S5144 {ܗܘܐ=became/came, into being}=ܩ/ה Hey[behold/the]-quality reveal grace-Y/ı Vav-[and/in addition]increase degree assure-ܐ/ Final-Aleph-ending finish maturity-

(Yeshua ישוע S9573 {ܝܫܘܥ=being saved}=ܝ/ Yud [of/through]-purpose single~mindedness actions-ܫ Shin-pressure exchange disperse-Y/ı Vav-[and/in addition]increase degree assure-ܥ/ Ayin-pierce perceive wisdom-

(in all)בכלהדן S10008 {ܟܠ=the whole reason for this is}=ܒ/ Beyt[within/inside]-pattern thought inhabit-ܫ/ Kaph-surrender obtains consent-ܠ/ Lamed[to/toward]-instruct acquire provide-ܩ/ה Hey[behold/the]-quality reveal grace-

(Galila)גלילא S3831 {ܓܠܝܠܐ=one who rolls}=ܐ/ Gimal-experience understanding encounter-ܠ/ Lamed[to/toward]-instruct acquire provide-ܝ/ Yud [of/through]-purpose single~mindedness actions-ܠ/ Lamed[to/toward]-instruct acquire provide-ܐ/ Final-Aleph-ending finish maturity-

(& taught)ומלפ S9206 {ܡܠܦ=to, be informed/to become acquainted with}=ܠ/ Lamed[to/toward]-instruct acquire provide-ܦ Final-Pey-declare sound advantage-

(He)הוא S5144 {ܗܘܐ=the Self~Same One}=ܩ/ה Hey[behold/the]-quality reveal grace-Y/ı Vav-[and/in addition]increase degree assure-ܐ/ Final-Aleph-ending finish maturity-

(in their assemblies)בכנושתהון S10232 {ܟܢܫ=with regard, to/in exchange for gathering/assembling}=ܒ/ Beyt[within/inside]-pattern thought inhabit-ܫ/ Kaph-surrender obtains consent-ܢ Nun-seed patience continue-Y/ı Vav-[and/in addition]increase degree assure-ܫ Shin-pressure exchange disperse-⊗/ܬ Taw-evidence prove sign-ܩ/ה Hey[behold/the]-quality reveal grace-Y/ı Vav-[and/in addition]increase degree assure-ܢ/ Final-Nun-issue perseverance progress-

(& was

Got Healing?

preaching) ומכרזין S10589 {שׂכרז=to *proclaim* or *announce*}= Vav-[and/in addition]increase degree assure- Resh-process beginning strength- Zayin-skill alter instrument- Mem[from/out of]-transform encounter remembrance- Kaph-surrender obtains consent- Samech-adjust apprehend source- Beyt[within/inside]-pattern thought inhabit- (the gospel) סברתא S13879 {שׂברת=*the message*}= Resh-process beginning strength- Taw-evidence prove sign- Final-Aleph-ending finish maturity- (of the kingdom) דמלכותא S11986 {שׁמלכו=*in the domain of the ruler/king*}= Dalet-faith establish presence- Mem[from/out of]-transform encounter remembrance- Lamed[to/toward]-instruct acquire provide- Kaph-surrender obtains consent- Vav-[and/in addition]increase degree assure- Taw-evidence prove sign- Final-Aleph-ending finish maturity- (& curing) ומאסא S1605 {אמ אסא=*to repair/refute*}= Vav-[and/in addition]increase degree assure- Aleph-authority ability confirm- Samech-adjust apprehend source- Lamed[to/toward]-instruct acquire provide- Final-Aleph-ending finish maturity- (every) כל S10077 {שׁכל=*the whole reason of this is*}= Kaph-surrender obtains consent- (sickness) כאב S9750 {שׁכאב=*to grieve/fell pain/to be in pain of someone/something external*}= Kaph-surrender obtains consent- Aleph-authority ability confirm- Beyt[within/inside]-pattern thought inhabit- (& disease) וכורהן S10511 {שׁכרה=*and to weaken/and dis~ease*}= Vav-[and/in addition]increase degree assure- Kaph-surrender obtains consent- Yud [of/through]-purpose single~mindedness actions- Resh-process beginning strength- Hey[behold/the]-quality reveal grace- Final-Nun-issue perseverance progress- (among the people) בעמא S15797 {שׁמע=*with unlearned people*}= Ayin-pierce perceive wisdom- Mem[from/out of]-transform encounter remembrance- Beyt[within/inside]-pattern thought inhabit- Final-Aleph-ending finish maturity-

The Semitic Emphasis

And the volume became/came into being~~being saved~~the whole reason for this is one who rolls to be informed/to become acquainted with the Self~Same One with regard to/in exchange for gathering/assembling to proclaim or announce the message in the domain of the ruler/king~~to repair/refute~~the whole reason for this is to grieve/fell pain/to be in pain of someone/something external and to weaken/and dis~ease

Anytime we turn from the TRUTH of JESUS CHRIST, we meet the lie that draws us away from HIM.

Not being able to see the lie is a diversion of our sight in seeing Jesus clearly.

The more we hold to the lie, the greater our chasm is made between ourselves and the majesty of our Savior!

~I~
Time is filled with swift transition,
Naught of earth unmoved can stand,
Build your hopes on things eternal,
Hold to God's unchanging hand.
Chorus~
Hold to God's unchanging hand,
Hold to God's unchanging hand;
Build your hopes on things eternal,
Hold to God's unchanging hand.

Trust in Him who will not leave you,
Whatsoever years may bring,
If by earthly friends forsaken

Got Healing?

Still more closely to Him cling.

~2~

Covet not this world's vain riches
That so rapidly decay,
Seek to gain the heav'nly treasures,
They will never pass away.

The LIE involves those things, those thoughts, those desires that exalt SELF, instead of God, instead of Jesus, instead of the Spirit's movings within the heart and mind of the believer!

What a disparagement to Selfish~Independent~Nature, when the heart and the mind are made to discover that the very presence of God they used to cherish and adore; now in their tremblings they fear the very one they used to LOVE ABOVE ALL!

In Addition To Encountering The Surrender To Process Acknowledge Each Quality Increasing His Finished Work

MATTHEW 9:35
KJV+TVM

And ^{G2532} Jesus ^{G2424} went about ^{G4013} $^{[G5707]}$ all ^{G3956} the cities ^{G4172} and ^{G2532} villages ^{G2968}, teaching ^{G1321} $^{[G5723]}$ in ^{G1722} their ^{G846} synagogues ^{G4864}, and ^{G2532} preaching ^{G2784} $^{[G5723]}$ the gospel ^{G2098} of the kingdom ^{G932}, and ^{G2532} healing ^{G2323} $^{[G5723]}$ every ^{G3956} sickness ^{G3554} and ^{G2532} every ^{G3956} disease ^{G3119} among ^{G1722} the people ^{G2992}.

ORIGINAL THOUGHTS

...(9:35) In addition to encountering the surrender to process, acknowledge each quality increasing His Finished Work. Through the exchange increasing His Wisdom, abide in remembrance establishing purpose by His Seed to prove the influence of surrender. While providing the Grace of His Truth, exercise the progress that increases the Pattern~of~His~Thoughts, insuring the strength and the actions of His Finished Work. Enlarge the memories taught, when declaring the revelations of each purpose within His Finished Work. Continue to agree with the Seed of each exchange proving the discoveries that enlarge one's progress in addition to remembering one's surrender through each beginning skillfully. Take hold of His Pattern~Thoughts strongly, by proving the influences of His Faith, as transforming the teachings of surrender, in addition to the evidence of His Finished Work. In addition to each encounter with Dominion's source of maturity, agree to learn and obtain every degree of strength through His Grace/Truth. Introduce with single~minded persistence, and consent to learn to agree through the abilities of His Pattern~Thoughts, every practice of purpose within every issue.

Got Healing?

In addition to encountering the surrender to process, acknowledge each quality increasing His Finished Work.

The unrenewed soul can obsess over the smallest of changes, when the heart and mind are not clearly, and singe~mindedly focused upon God, their Creator.

The surrender to process allows the thoughts to focus on His abilities, and not on our own.

We are invited, not required, to ACCEPT, then ACKNOWLEDGE, and then to ALLOW the work of the Spirit within the habitation of God, within humanity, to have leadership and control over our every thought, which in turn causes us to think as God.

His thoughts become our thoughts; His ways become our ways.

Following His example, through Jesus the soul of humanity finds the place where home is safely tucked away IN HIM alone!

Through the exchange increasing His Wisdom, abide in remembrance establishing purpose by His Seed to prove the influence of surrender.

How is it we think we do not have what we cannot see we already have?

How is it that our hopes, dreams, expectations are so easily shattered by what continues to go on around us?

Our hearts or feelings get shredded, and instantly it seems, we lose our security and hope and assurance.

When these kinds of happenings occur, we become anxious, fearful, and panic~stricken; we lose our capacity to notice what is actually at work within us!

It is from our beginning in God, ^{JEREMIAH 1:5; 29:11 KJV}~~at this point, we were settled in the mind of God's thoughts about how He would create His Creation; as well as, what would be the reason for the Creation He would create?

Yes, we could search forever, and never discover what the writers of the New Testament discovered from their relationship with Jesus before, during, and after the Cross extinguished their hopes and dreams of conquering every foe!

It our searching is not wrapped up in finding everything we have need of IN HIM, then nothing will be the substance in us, of all that He declares is ours!

We are empty and we are searching for meaning, real meaning, and the kind of meaning that will stick to our ribs like peanut-butter instead of dissolving into nothingness like cotton candy.

Well, here the search ends.

Here we run into the secret.

For the apostle is declaring to us that our self is bound up with Jesus Christ.

Our identity, who we are, is wrapped up in Jesus' own identity.

Our true humanity is there in His.

Our true existence is there woven into His.

The truth about you and me and, indeed, the world is there in Jesus Christ.

While providing the Grace of His Truth, exercise the progress that increases the Pattern-of-His-Thoughts, insuring the strength and the actions of His Finished Work.

Authentic Christianity is not a call to live by principles or to try our best to live for Jesus.

To build our lives around biblical principles sounds admirable, but *it is a subtle form of legalism.*

Of course there are teachings in the New Testament about how we are to live.

Yet, these instructions are not religious challenges we are to try and follow.

They are many descriptions as to the manner, which Christ can live His life though us as we depend on Him.

New Testament Christianity is not grounded in what we do, *but in what He has already done.*

New Testament Lifestyle is grounded not only in what He HAS DONE, but in what WE ALLOW HIM TO DO NOW, in us, and through us.

Enlarge the memories taught, when declaring the revelations of each purpose within His Finished Work.

We are not to be observers only; looking to see what others are doing and then copy *the cracker wholly.*

We are called to follow ONE; His name is JESUS!

Not a doctrine, not a philosophy; not even a culture that looks good!

We are called to follow HIS EXAMPLE; the way He lived, while providing the greatest example of LOVE He could!

"Faithful is He that calleth you, who also will do it. FIRST THESSALONIANS 5:24 KJV

Continue to agree with the Seed of each exchange proving the discoveries that enlarge one's progress, in addition to remembering one's surrender through each beginning skillfully.

His Seed, His Word is the beginning of all that is promised.

Without the seed, how would a farmer harvest any crop?

Without the seed, how would vegetables be available for families to put on their tables?

Except we embrace the Seed, desiring to find the fullness it carries within its kernel; how else can we step into the Divine Plan, God has destined for each of us to develop into and through?

Knowing His Seed enough to agree with it takes more effort than just listening to someone else's testimony about its riches!

Knowing His Seed is the preparedness of the heart and mind to not only accept, but understand and allow the symbolism of His Desires to become ours?

Knowing His Seed enough to lay forth the outlines and patterns of His governing of our living as HIM, becomes the only efforts by which one may forage the fields of life's experiences and glean the good grain, not only to eat, but to share with others who do not have what has been given!

Take hold of His Pattern~Thoughts strongly, by proving the influences of His Faith, as transforming the teachings of surrender, in addition to the evidence of His Finished Work.

Until we are willing to allow the Spirit of God to seed His Word into every nook and cranny of our living, we will never find the lasting and eternal riches contained in the value of such an everlasting commodity.

Heaven's storehouses are full; will you be the one who opens wide the flood~gates, enough to feed the hungry, give shelter to the homeless, lift~up the soul trodden down, or guide the blind upon the journey, wherein they can have their needs met?

Can you see the pattern of a scarlet thread running throughout every page of God's Holy Writ?

Have you discovered, and learned that the riches of Heaven's coffers are yours and mine for the taking, when we freely give of ourselves to those around us?

In addition to each encounter with Dominion's source of maturity, agree to learn and obtain every degree of strength through His Grace/Truth.

What has commonly been called *"the Christian life"* is typically more entertainment oriented, and woven in a tapestry of acceptable culture, instead of being wholly *Christ~centered!*

Authentic Christian~living is nothing less than an expression; an offering of God's Divine Life through any believing believer's living AS HIM!

Not one soul created was ever made or intended to live the life that Jesus Christ lived; and yet, millions try with the *"arm~of~the~flesh"* to do what cannot be done with the moving of the Spirit from within, FIRST!

Introduce with single~minded persistence, and consent to learn to agree through the abilities of His Pattern~Thoughts, every practice of purpose within every issue.

Just as surely as *poor~eating and exercise~habits* bring the penalty of health problems; *S*elfish~*I*ndependent~*N*ature brings the penalty of hell with death.

It was that penalty that Jesus took on our behalf.

It wasn't the Father who punished Jesus, but *s-i-n* itself that brought that horrible penalty of death upon our Lord.

Our heavenly Father and the Holy Spirit were equally involved in our salvation. SEE SECOND CORINTHIANS 5: 19 AND HEBREWS 9: 14

Thankfully, through faith in Him, we are now able to be forever free from the wages of *s-i-n.*

In His wondrous mercy, our great God has taken it all upon and into Himself.

Jesus never sinned; yet, He took our *s-i-n* as His own and, consequently, paid the price by sacrificing Himself in our place.

He didn't deserve to pay the price for *s-i-n* although we did.

His death is an expression of His mercy toward us.

Got Healing?

SEMITIC~ARAMAIC~HEBRAIC THESAURUS

Aramaic before first {
Semitic Root before first =
Lettering for ParaPhrase after second =

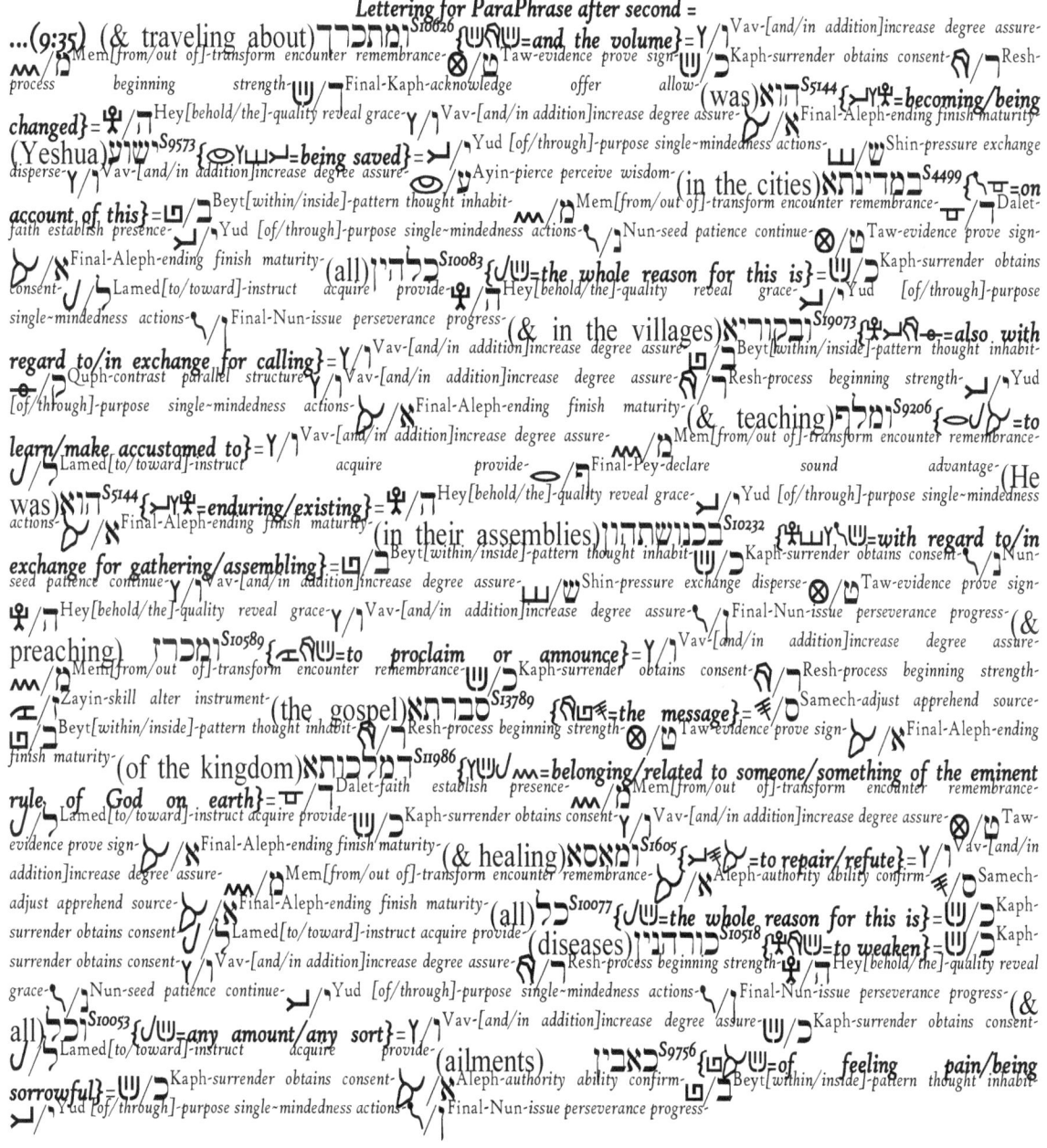

The Semitic Emphasis

And the volume becoming/being changed~~being saved on account of this also with regard to/in exchange for calling to learn/make accustomed to enduring/existing~~with regard to/in exchange for gathering/ assembling~~belonging/related to someone/something of the eminent rule of God on earth~~proclaim or announce the message to repair/refute~~the whole reason for this is to weaken any amount/any sort of feeling pain/being sorrowful.

"Then said I, Lo, I come (**in the volume of the book it is written of me,**) to do thy will, O God." HEBREWS 10:7 KJV

There is an adage that says, "*if it says it about Jesus, it says it about me*".

As we are IN CHRIST JESUS, we are where He is, as He is!

In this verse, the emphasis is upon Jesus becoming that which is the fullness of the Father's Will.

As it is with HIM, so we must understand, it is with us! WHY?

Because we have been made ONE WITH HIM!

Since Eternity, we were ONE WITH GOD.

Through this physical dimension, we have been remade as ONE WITH CHRIST, WHO IS AND ALWAYS HAS BEEN~~ONE WITH GOD!

What is the misery of humanity?

It is that their mind, without God, is dis~eased.

They were CREATED to regard and enjoy God as their chief object; and His faculties will not work healthily in the absence of this object.

However, many have left God, and they weary themselves in seeking good from created things.

The love of God is to the human attitude, what the keystone is to the arch; ruin is the consequence when either falls from its place.

Thus, we see that humanity's reason is bewildering, and their conscience harasses~~their imaginations deceive and disquiets them~~while their passions and affections agitate and torture them.

The ONLY CURE, the ONLY REST for them is to find/return to the LOVE OF GOD their Maker; discovering that WHO THEY NEED IS HIM!

In Addition To The Seed Of His Spoken Word Build And Increase The Exchange Of Teaching A Single~Minded Approach Toward His Finished Work

LUKE 9:6
KJV+TVM
And[G1161] they departed[G1831] [G5740], and went[G1330] [G5711] through[G2596] the towns[G2968],

Got Healing?

preaching the gospel^{G2097 [G5734]}, *and*^{G2532} *healing*^{G2323 [G5723]} *every where*^{G3837}.

ORIGINAL THOUGHTS

...(9:6) In addition to the Seed of His Spoken Word, build and increase the exchange of teaching a single~minded approach toward His Finished Work. Insuring the remembrances of evidence obtained, strengthen the surrender of purpose through the perseverance of His Grace in adding each portion of His Pattern~of~Thought in parallels of assured beginnings through the single~mindedness of His Finished Work. Increase every Pattern-of-His-Thought transforming the Faith of His Purpose through the Seed of proving His Finished Work. In addition to encountering and apprehending His Pattern-of-Thought, strengthen each purpose by developing the quality insuring each increase. Behold the added assurances, in addition to remembering the Dominion of His Resource of Purpose and progress as existing/enduring surrender to Promise establishing every increase acknowledged/allowed.

In addition to the Seed of His Spoken Word, build and increase the exchange of teaching a single~minded approach toward His Finished Work.

The Finish of His Work is the brightness of His Image portrayed through the willingness and agreement of our living IN HIM, AS HIM!

When our electric lights work partially or not at all, we know that the lack of power is not in the universal, infinite, and eternal flow of electricity in the universe, _but in the wiring that connects us with that flow_.

Every person who ever succeeded in finding a cure, or inventing an invention~~remained true to the basic premise out of which their endeavors began.

They believed, and continued in the basic premise of that belief that what they surmised/deduced/presumed was in fact the focal point of their journey of discovery.

They did not accept that it could not be done; but, continually they searched for the elements, or methods, or reasoning of how, why, where it would succeed!

Such is the element we call FAITH!

The Seed of God's Word will BUILD in us the element called, FAITH; because out of the seed, He produces His Own KIND implanted in the seed to begin with.

"Every human being is a universe within themselves. Your mother and father participated with God to create _a soul who would never cease to exist_. Your parents, as co~creators, supplied the stuff, genetics and more, uniquely

combined to form a masterpiece, not flawless but still astounding; and we took from their hands what they brought to us, submitting to their timing and history and added what only we could bring to them— LIFE. You were conceived, a living wonder who exploded into being, a universe within a multiverse, not isolated and disconnected, but entangled and designed for community, even as God is community[family]."

Young, Wm. Paul. CROSS ROADS (p. 64). Faith~Words Publishing.

Insuring the remembrances of evidence obtained, strengthen the surrender of purpose through the perseverance of His Grace, adding each portion of His Pattern~of~Thought in parallels of assured beginnings through the single~mindedness of His Finished Work.

The INSURANCE of remembrances that strengthen the cause of His Faith at work in our living provides the proper conduit for God to manifest that which He already provided so long ago!

The largest of obstacles is when we fail to realize we have developed an invalid consciousness, the greatest possible barrier to healing of any kind, and/or the promise of prosperity throughout our lifetime here.

Why would we pray for the riches of heaven, when retaining belief/suspicion that we will only get them when we step into Heaven?

What does any soul need, in Heaven, the riches that they seek in this physical dimension?

The same context can be applied to the healing of our bodies!

The barriers to healing, prosperity, wisdom, or any other opportunity to receive the Good Graces of God's Love~~can conduit through anyone involved in the plight or dilemma~~when they hold to the consensus that it is NOT GOD'S WILL TO HEAL!

We make ourselves the barrier according to those things we refuse to yield into God's hands alone!

Increase every Pattern~of~His~Thought transforming the Faith of His Purpose through the Seed of proving His Finished Work.

The ParaPhrase of God's Words are not offered telling us to "*try everything*"; but, to allow the SPIRIT to work through us as the CONDUIT!

Children can be held by the same clogged, hindered conduit that keeps their parents/lineage from stepping into the fullness of God.

Break the ties that bind the mind; watch God reveal the miraculous!

Got Healing?

Many a person dies because humanity has not discovered His healing power as operating through the being of humanity's conduit.

Yet, that power is here, awaiting our adjustment to Him.

In addition to encountering and apprehending His Pattern~of~Thought, strengthen each purpose by developing the quality insuring each increase.

Understand that His PATTERN~OF~THOUGHT is the same as the Pattern~of~HIS~BEING operating in us by His WILL, not just by ours!

It is in understanding the QUALITY of HIS LIFE lives in each of us, according to the manner through which we BELIEVE IN HIM~~that we are able to accept the enlightening by the TRUTH OF HIS WORD!

LUKE 11:11-13

If a son shall ask bread of any of you that is a father, will he give him a stone? or if he ask a fish, will he for a fish give him a serpent? Or if he shall ask an egg, will he offer him a scorpion? If ye then, being evil, know how to give good gifts unto your children: how much more shall your heavenly Father give the Holy Spirit to them that ask Him?

Behold the added assurances, in addition to remembering the Dominion of His Resource of Purpose, and progress as existing/enduring surrender to Promise establishing every increase acknowledged/allowed.

When we ask for the indwelling of God's Holy Spirit in the body, let us think of that part of the body that most needs His life.

Let us imagine His light and life glowing there like a fire, shining there like a light.

Then through the rest of the day let us continually give thanks that His life is at work within us accomplishing His perfect will and recreating us after His image and likeness, which is perfection.

SEMITIC~ARAMAIC~HEBRAIC THESAURUS

Aramaic before first {

Semitic Root before first =

Lettering for ParaPhrase after second =

...(9:6) (& went out) ויצבו S13386 {⊖○⋎=and spread abroad}=Y/ヿVav-[and/in addition]increase degree assure-⋎/Nun-seed patience continue-○/פ Pey-mouth SpokenWord speak-⊖/ף Quph-contrast parallel structure-Y/ヿVav-[and/in addition]increase degree assure-

(the apostles) שליחא S21372 {⊞⊐⋎⊔⊔=the sent ones with the message}=⊔⊔/שShin-pressure exchange disperse-/ל Lamed[to/toward]-instruct acquire provide-⊐/ל Yud [of/through]-purpose single-mindedness actions-/⊞⊓Hhet-specific share beyond-⋎/א Final-Aleph-ending finish maturity-

(& walking around) ומתכרכין S10627 {⋎⊗שׂ=and the volume}=Y/ヿVav-[and/in addition]increase degree assure-/מ Mem[from/out of]-transform encounter remembrance-⊗/ה Taw-evidence prove sign-⊔/כ Kaph-surrender obtains consent-⋎/ヿResh-process beginning strength-⊔/כ Kaph-surrender obtains consent-/ヿYud [of/through]-purpose single-mindedness actions-⋎/ヿFinal-Nun-issue perseverance progress-

(they were) הוה S5147 {⊐⋎✝=the self~same one}=✝/חHey[behold/the]-quality reveal

Got Healing?

grace-ץ/ין Vav-[and/in addition]increase degree assure-ץ/ין Vav-[and/in addition]increase degree assure-(in villages)בְּקוּרְיָא S19067 {ﬤﬤ≏=calling/designating}=מִ/בּ Beyt[within/inside]-pattern thought inhabit-מ/בּ Quph-contrast parallel structure-ץ/ין Vav-[and/in addition]increase degree assure-מ/בּ Resh-process beginning strength-ר/ין Yud [of/through]-purpose single~mindedness actions-ה/ין Final-Aleph-ending finish maturity-(& in cities)וּבִמְדִינָתָא S4507 {ﬣﬠ=for this reason}=ץ/ין Vav-[and/in addition]increase degree assure-מ/בּ Beyt[within/inside]-pattern thought inhabit-מ/מ Mem[from/out of]-transform encounter remembrance-ה/ד /ד Dalet-faith establish presence-ה/בּ Yud [of/through]-purpose single~mindedness actions-נ/ין Nun-seed patience continue-⊗/מ Taw-evidence prove sign-ה/א Final-Aleph-ending finish maturity-(& preaching the good news)וּמְסַבְּרִין S13819 {ﬥﬤﬧ=hope/faith achieved through reason}=ץ/ין Vav-[and/in addition]increase degree assure-מ/מ Mem[from/out of]-transform encounter remembrance-ﬧ/ס Samech-adjust apprehend source-מ/בּ Beyt[within/inside]-pattern thought inhabit-בּ/ר Resh-process beginning strength-ר/ין Yud [of/through]-purpose single~mindedness actions-ה/ין Final-Nun-issue perseverance progress-(they were)הֲווֹ S5147 {ﬥﬥ=the self~same one}=הֲ/ה Hey[behold/the]-quality reveal grace-ץ/ין Vav-[and/in addition]increase degree assure-ץ/ין Vav-[and/in addition]increase degree assure-מ/מ Mem[from/out of]-transform encounter remembrance-ﬧ/ס Samech-adjust apprehend source-מ/ין Yud [of/through]-purpose single~mindedness actions-(& healing)מְאַסִין S1606 {ﬤﬠﬧ=to repair/refute}=ץ/ין Vav-[and/in addition]increase degree assure-א/א Aleph-authority ability confirm-ﬧ/ס Samech-adjust apprehend source-ן/ין Final-Nun-issue perseverance progress-(in every)בְּכָל S10007 {ﬥﬤﬥ=the whole of everything}=מ/בּ Beyt[within/inside]-pattern thought inhabit-ﬥ/ﬥ Kaph-surrender obtains consent-ל/ל Lamed[to/toward]-instruct acquire provide-(place)דוּךְ S4231 {﬩ﬠ=somewhere/extinguished the tumult}=ﬨ/ד Dalet-faith establish presence-ץ/ין Vav-[and/in addition]increase degree assure-ﬥ/ין Final-Kaph-acknowledge offer allow-

The Semitic Emphasis

And spread abroad the sent ones with the message and the volume~~the self~same one calling/designating for this reason hope/faith achieved through reason~~the self~same one repaired/refuted the whole of everything somewhere/extinguished the tumult.

There is no great mystery concerning the will of God, in so far as it applies to our small selves.

God's will is written into His nature, and the nature of God is love.

Therefore, when we pray in accordance with the nature of love, we are praying in accordance with the will of God.

The body is indeed a laboratory exquisitely adapted to the working out of the power of God.

Healing by some form of prayer or faith is as natural and as instinctive as breathing.

It has been practiced, with or without understanding, by people of every age.

It is as old as history and as modern as television.

Almost everyone in times of great stress cries out to someone, or to something~~even if they do so only by a blind, instinctive urge and deny their own impulse immediately afterwards.

Much of this clamoring to Deity has failed to produce results.

Therefore a great many Christians, unwilling to believe that God cannot heal them, have persuaded themselves that He will not.

In so doing, they forget both the example and the words of Jesus Christ.

He told us that God is a loving Father who delights to give good gifts to His children.

An inner wisdom deeper than reason forces us to strive always after Life.

When we realize that God is not only transcendent/unequalled, but that He is also immanent/essential; there is a cause that stirs within our being to resist the physical and cling to the spiritual!

We see that the lack of success in healing is not due to God's will for us, but it is due to our *failure to live near enough to God* so that He can accomplish His will in us.

If we do not give Him an opportunity to accomplish perfection in our spirits and bodies, He will do the next best thing and endeavor with divine patience to teach us through suffering.

In this case, we are receiving as much of His Life~Giving Spirit as He can get through to us, but we are not allowing the full flow necessary to life because of our unwillingness to draw nearer to HIM!

Drawing nearer to Him implies that we give HIM FIRST PLACE, and allow none other to replace HIS POSITION TO US, and IN US, and THROUGH OUR LIVING AS HIM!

Surrender In Kind
For The Exchange Of His Finished Work
And Establish/Settle Upon The Purpose
Of Persistently Obtaining
The Faith Of His Wisdom Increasing

LUKE 9:11
KJV+TVM

And^{G1161} the people^{G3793}, when they knew^{G1097} $^{[G5631]}$ it, followed^{G190} $^{[G5656]}$ him^{G846}: and^{G2532} he received^{G1209} $^{[G5666]}$ them^{G846}, and spake^{G2980} $^{[G5707]}$ unto them^{G846} of^{G4012} the kingdom^{G932} of God^{G2316}, and^{G2532} healed^{G2390} $^{[G5711]}$ them that had^{G2192} $^{[G5723]}$ need^{G5532} of healing^{G2322}.

ORIGINAL THOUGHTS

...(9:11) Surrender in kind for the exchange of His Finished Work, and establish/settle upon the purpose of persistently obtaining the Faith of His Wisdom increasing. The Dominion of His Skill teaches the assurances of His

Got Healing?

Pattern~of~Thought, proving the process in quality of each portion building His Habitation of Promise. Through His Abilities patiently increase progress by increasing the undeniable remembrances that provide the teachings revealing every portion of His Single~Mindedness. With Wisdom, encounter the qualities of each portion that issues the Wisdom that trains and transforms the promises into each part of the Evidence of His Finished Work. His Faith confirms every promise by the qualities of His Finished Work, and teaches the abilities of single~mindedness acquiring the purpose of persisting in establishing and apprehending His Seed, through actions that parallel through progress. Revealing each increase assures the acquiring of His Wisdom to conform the apprehending of single~mindedness in addition to the Evidence of His Finished Work. Remembering the Dominion as apprehended through His Finished Work qualifies the assurances of His Single~Mindedness.

Surrender in kind for the exchange of His Finished Work, and establish/settle upon the purpose of persistently obtaining the Faith of His Wisdom increasing.

Whose LIFE do we as His Creation, live?

HIS, right?

Do you think God desires that everyone offer HIS LIFE back to HIM, by dying on a cross?

Or, do you think God desires the fruit produced by His LIFE being LIVED THROUGH OURS?

How is a fruit~tree that is not bearing much fruit, made to better produce what it contains?

The Apostle Paul advised his friends the Ephesians to "*walk as children of light*": to live, that is, as if they were made of a living, moving energy in like kind as *LIGHT*.

Now, scientists have discovered what we know as that which is really true.

For it has been discovered that the body is not hard, solid matter; but is made up of specks of energy.

These bits of energy attract and repel each other with tiny explosions of light.

So in a very real way~~the body is full of *LIGHT*.

"*In Him was Life; and The Life was The Light of men.*" JOHN 1:4 KJV

The Dominion of His Skill teaches the assurances of His Pattern~of~Thought, proving the process in quality of each portion building His Habitation of Promise.
FIRST THINGS FIRST!

Before we can wield the Dominion of His Skill, we must be taught the assurances of His Pattern~of~Thought!

Would you put an untrained, undisciplined driver behind the wheel of multimillion~dollar sports vehicle? NO, NO, NO!

Why then do we think because we are of the age we are that we know everything we need to know, especially about God?

Proving the process is about learning the ropes!

Without such learning, we are as foolish as the unlearned!

"Study to shew thyself approved unto God, a workman [a novice/disciple/elder] that needeth not to be ashamed, rightly dividing the word of truth. SECOND TIMOTHY 2:15 KJV

Through His Abilities patiently increase progress by increasing the undeniable remembrances that provide the teachings revealing every portion of His Single~Mindedness.

The *patient increase of progress* is coming to know the Lord in relationship created out of a two~way communication/conversation.

Increasing the undeniable remembrances serves to fuel the fire of God's Presence within our living, and within our existing, and within our being!

What fire can burn when there is no fuel to burn?

So it is with our living for God, when we do not FEED UPON HIM, the Bread of Life come down from Heaven, by the Living God.

Providing the teachings revealing the weaknesses, the limitations, the expectations, the hopes, the fears, and so on~~these become the moments of a lifetime that is surrendered before His Feet every moment of every day, throughout any lifetime.

If nothing changes, nothing changes!

Are you different since you came to know the Lord, or are you a hodge~podge of other's beliefs, and not completely filled to overflow with God's provisions?

God made, first of all, light.

The Spirit of God moved upon the face of the deep, so the Word of the Living God tells us~~doing the best we can to put into the words at our disposal, truths that even our more modern term "inter-stellar space" does not adequately express.

We are therefore made not of solid and impenetrable matter, but of energy.

The very chemicals contained in the body—the *"dust of the earth"*—live by the Breath of God, by the primal Energy, the original force that we call <u>God</u>.

This being so, it is not strange at all that when we establish <u>*a closer connection with God in prayer*</u>, we should receive a more abundant living—an increased flow of energy.

The creative force that sustains us is increased within our bodies through our consistent, constant, continuous, and conscious awareness of Him in us, with us, for us, and through us!

<u>*With Wisdom, encounter the qualities of each portion that issues the Wisdom that trains and transforms the promises into each part of the Evidence of His Finished Work.*</u>

Follow this thought: if you want to have Wisdom, His Wisdom, you must envision such a blessing as being yours, and already being in you the moment you believe when you pray! Correct?

Why can it not be just as simply accomplished in any matter about which we lack, or have need thereof?

Before a house can be built, the architect/contractor/owner~builder must SEE in their mind's eye what it is they want to build! Correct?

Then, we ask: why should it not also be that simple when it comes to healing, health, prosperity, joy, peace, patience, and the like?

Can you catch what is offered?

Then see what the Word promises; then, declare that the promises of such are yours because God offers them to you; then, hold to what you declare and believe whose you are IN HIM! Watch it grow, and produce!

<u>*His Faith confirms every promise by the qualities of His Finished Work, and teaches the abilities of single~mindedness acquiring the purpose of persisting in establishing and apprehending His Seed, through actions that parallel through progress.*</u>

Here is a limited outline of what to do, if you in fact are serious about having what God says He has already given you! ~~~~

1. *Choose the same time and the same place every day, make yourself comfortable and relax.*
2. *Remind yourself of the reality of His LIFE within yourself.*
3. *Ask Him, for His LIFE to rise up and increase His LIFE in your body.*

Got Healing?

4. Make a picture in your mind of your body well.
Think especially of the part of the body that most needs to be well.
See it well and perfect and shining with God's LIGHT.
And give thanks that this is being accomplished, and through is accomplished!

Some of you will say, "Ooooo, *this sounds/looks like new~age, or metaphysical, or mysticism*"!

You are right; it is new~age, because it's not like the old~time <u>religion</u> that put us in this key~hole to begin with!

You are right; it is metaphysical~~*mind over matter*~~that is, God's Mind over my matter/earth/dust.

You are right, it is mysticism; the mystery of God shown to the hearts of men and women who desire to be clothed upon by the Spirit of God, manifesting the character, grace, mercy, and love of the Almighty, as we were intended from the beginnings of creation to be and have!

<u>*Revealing each increase assures the acquiring of His Wisdom to conform the apprehending of single~mindedness in adding the Evidence of His Finished Work.*</u>

There is a system to prayer that teaches intricate methods of breathing, breath control, bodily positioning, as well as other systems that emphasize physical exercise and diet!

Scripture recites that *"bodily exercise profiteth little; but spiritual exercise profits a great deal more"*!

Most of us have become the servants of our nerves, so that we adjust ourselves according to our tensions.

Nerves are like children; in that they respond better to suggestion than to commands.

"Prayer is only auto~suggestion," some people say.

Those who really experience true~prayer know from its results that it is far more than mere *auto~suggestion.*

But even *auto~suggestion*, so far as it goes, follows out the laws of God.

For WHO is the *"auto"* that <u>*makes the suggestions*</u>?

It is **<u>THE INNER BEING</u>** that is part of God, speaking to the framework of our flesh.

<u>*Remembering the Dominion as apprehended through His Finished Work qualifies the assurances of His Single~Mindedness.*</u>

In order to release God's LIFE in the body, we must first be able to forget the body, so that we can allow the Holy Spirit to quiet the mind, and concentrate/focus *God's Spiritual Energies* already flowing throughout the body.

We receive God, in other words, by forgetting ourselves and thinking about HIM!

Therefore, we begin our prayer not by clamoring for this and that before we have even acknowledged His Presence, but by thinking about Him in the way that makes Him most real to us.

"*Hallowed be Thy name.*"

Thus begins the model prayer of all ages.

SEMITIC~ARAMAIC~HEBRAIC THESAURUS
Aramaic before first {
Semitic Root before first =
Lettering for ParaPhrase after second =

...(9:11) (the crowds) כנשא S10319 {ש/שׁ ⊔⊔=gathering/collecting/assembling}=ש/⊔ /Kaph-surrender obtains consent-/Final-Aleph-ending finish maturity-/Shin-pressure exchange disperse-/Yud [of/through]-purpose single-mindedness

(but) S4405 {ד/ד=holding to account}=ד/ד /Dalet-faith establish presence-/Yud [of/through]-purpose single-mindedness actions-/Final-Nun-issue perseverance progress-

(when) כד S9812 {ד/ש=as much as/inasmuch as}=ש/ד /Kaph-surrender obtains consent-/Dalet-faith establish presence- (they knew) S8692 {ע/○=in measure}=/Yud [of/through]-purpose single-mindedness actions-/Dalet-faith establish presence-/Ayin-pierce perceive wisdom-/Vav-[and/in addition]increase degree assure-

(they went) אזלו S346 {ל/ז=going from one place to another}=ל/א /Aleph-authority ability confirm-/Zayin-skill alter degree assure-/Lamed[to/toward]-instruct acquire provide-/Vav-[and/in addition]increase degree

(after Him) בתרה S2220 {ת/ר=in space/time/to be concerned with}=ת/ב /Beyt[within/inside]-pattern thought inhabit-/Taw evidence prove sign-/Resh-process beginning strength-/Hey[behold/the]-quality reveal grace-

(& He received) וקבלו S17957 {ק/ב=acquiescing/opposing}=ק/ו /Quph-contrast parallel-/Vav-[and/in addition]increase degree assure-/Beyt[within/inside]-pattern thought inhabit-/Lamed[to/toward]-instruct acquire provide- (them) אנון S4989 {א/ל=that one}=א/ו /Final-Nun-issue perseverance progress-/Aleph-authority ability confirm-/Nun-seed patience continue-/Vav-[and/in addition]increase degree assure-/Final-Nun-

(& speaking) וממלל S12040 {ל/ל=to converse with/console}=ל/ו /Vav-[and/in addition]increase degree assure-/Mem[from/out of]-transform encounter remembrance-/Mem[from/out of]-transform encounter remembrance-/Lamed[to/toward]-instruct acquire provide-/Lamed[to/toward]-instruct acquire provide-

(He was) הוא S5144 {א/ל=being/existing/in essence of}=ה/ו /Hey[behold/the]-quality reveal grace-/Vav-[and/in addition]increase degree assure-/Yud [of/through]-purpose single-mindedness actions- (with them) עמהון S15788 {ע/○=in the presence of/in possession of}=ע/ /Mem[from/out of]-transform encounter remembrance-/Hey[behold/the]-quality reveal grace-/Ayin-pierce perceive wisdom-/Vav-[and/in addition]increase degree assure-/Final-Nun-issue perseverance progress- (about) על S15701 {ל/○=according to}=ל/ /Ayin-pierce perceive wisdom-/Lamed[to/toward]-instruct acquire provide-

(the Kingdom) מלכותא S11998 {ש/ל=the pattern/imminent rule of God on earth}=מ/ /Mem[from/out of]-transform encounter remembrance-/Lamed[to/toward]-instruct acquire provide-/Kaph-surrender obtains consent-/Vav-[and/in addition]increase degree assure-/Taw-evidence prove sign-/Aleph-authority ability confirm-/Final-Aleph-ending finish maturity- (of God) אלהא S914 {ל/א=behaving like God}=ד/ /Lamed[to/toward]-instruct acquire provide-/Dalet-faith establish presence-/Aleph-authority ability confirm-/Final-Aleph-ending finish maturity-/Hey[behold/the]-quality reveal grace-/Vav-[and/in addition]increase degree assure- (& those) אלילי S681 {ל/ל=mighty}=ל/ /Lamed[to/toward]-instruct acquire provide-/Aleph-authority ability confirm-/Yud [of/through]-purpose single-mindedness actions-/Lamed[to/toward]-instruct acquire provide-/Yud [of/through]-purpose single-mindedness actions-/Final-Nun-issue perseverance progress- (who in

need) דסניקין S14633 {○/ל=lacking/needful}=ד/ /Dalet-faith establish presence-/Samech-adjust apprehend source-

Got Healing?

Nun-seed patience continue- Yud [of/through]-purpose single~mindedness actions- Quph-contrast parallel structure- Yud [of/through]-purpose single~mindedness actions- Final-Nun-issue perseverance progress- (were) S5147 =changing condition}= Hey[behold/the]-quality reveal grace- Vav-[and/in addition]increase degree assure- Vav-[and/in addition]increase degree assure- (of) S15701 =according to}= Lamed[to/toward]-instruct acquire provide- Ayin-pierce perceive wisdom- (healing) S1629 =repairing}= Aleph-authority ability confirm- Samech-adjust apprehend source- Yud [of/through]-purpose single~mindedness actions- Vav-[and/in addition]increase degree assure- Taw-evidence prove sign- Final-Aleph-ending finish maturity- (healed) S1613 =to repair}= Mem[from/out of]-transform encounter remembrance- Aleph-authority ability confirm- Samech-adjust apprehend source- Final-Aleph-ending finish maturity- (He) S5144 =to be/to become}= Hey[behold/the]-quality reveal grace- Vav-[and/in addition]increase degree assure- Yud [of/through]-purpose single~mindedness actions-

The Semitic Emphasis

Gathering/Collecting holding to account as much as in measure going from one place to another to be concerned with~~acquiescing/opposing that one to converse with/console in essence of~~in possession of according to the pattern rule of God on earth~~behaving like God mighty~~lacking/needful changing condition according to repairing to repair to be/to become.

"For the weapons of our warfare are not carnal, but mighty through God to the pulling down of strong holds; but mighty through God to the pulling down of strong holds" SECOND CORINTHIANS 10:4-5 KJV

"Weapons for of our war not are of the flesh but of the power of God and by it we subdue fortresses rebellious and we pull down reasoning and every high thing that is exalted against the knowledge of God and we take prisoner all minds for the obedience of the Messiah." SECOND CORINTHIANS 10:4-5 ARAMAIC TRANSLATION

Most of us need every day to enter into God's presence and focus our attention FIRST upon Him and THEN upon the area that needs healing, so that God may have every opportunity of continuing His creative work in us.

But after the first time, we may say, "Thank You," instead of, "Please."

"Thank You that Your Life is working throughout me, rebuilding everything toward health."

We may then use our creative imaginations and make a picture in our minds of that perfection which we hope will be ours.

Finally, we may look steadily at that picture until it is accomplished.

Thus by harnessing the imagination and training the will, we can arouse and build upon His Faith working in us!

From Acts & the Epistles
Perceiving His Teaching
By Purpose Of His Exchange

Increases His Wisdom
To Establish Every Remembrance Of His Progress

ACTS 10:38
KJV+TVM

How^{G5613} God^{G2316} anointed^{G5548} $^{[G5656]}$ Jesus^{G2424} of^{G575} Nazareth^{G3478} with the Holy^{G40} Ghost^{G4151} and^{G2532} with power^{G1411}: who^{G846} ^{G3739} went about^{G1330} $^{[G5627]}$ doing good^{G2109} $^{[G5723]}$, and^{G2532} healing^{G2390} $^{[G5740]}$ all^{G3956} that were oppressed^{G2616} $^{[G5746]}$ of^{G5259} the devil^{G1228}; for^{G3754} God^{G2316} was^{G2258} $^{[G5713]}$ with^{G3326} him^{G846}.

ORIGINAL THOUGHTS

...(10:38) Perceiving His Teaching by purpose of His Exchange increases His Wisdom to establish every remembrance of His Progress. Abiding by His Purpose strengthens each sign, presenting the Dominion acquiring His Grace through His Finished Work. Transcending each pressure beyond the revelation of each increase continues sharing the action that provide His Finished Work. Whereas increase qualifies every portion of His Faith, encountering the evidence of His Instruction processes the sacrifice of revealing each part of His Finished Work. Wherein the increase of His Seed enables the adjustings of His Finished Work, the provisions of His Grace perpetuate each portion of perseverance to endure agreement proving His Seed provides actions that transform each issue. His Faith empowers the evidence that patiently provides the positions of each degree transforming progressively the Patterns~of~His~Thoughts in purpose of the Exchange by His Finished Work. His Pattern~of~ Thought processes each degree as unseen in His Finished Work, in memory of every balance provided. Whereupon encountering the balance provided, His Faith confirms the acquired revelation of His Finished Work. The Qualities that increase His Finished Work are discerned/perceived through the transformations of His Grace.

Perceiving His Teaching by purpose of His Exchange increases His Wisdom to establish every remembrance of His Progress.

Realizing that Christ Jesus is alive and active within our living tells us that everything His death, burial, resurrection, ascension, seating, and reigning have provided.

Knowing that when Jesus died in our place, He provided our return to the family of God, we begin realizing WHOSE WE ARE!

Every step of our living must be from the foundation of His Giftings.

The teachings that explain the Great Exchange provide us with the tools, attitudes, and strategies that produce through us His Will in this

---

earth.

We interact with our world based upon our perception of it.

It seems obvious therefore that one of the keys to intimacy in our walk with God, and others, is the ability to revise our perception of one another as necessary.

Much of the time we obscure His Truth by imposing our thoughts with regard to the matters at hand.

Abiding by His Purpose strengthens each sign, presenting the Dominion acquiring His Grace through His Finished Work.

Herein is where we must learn to see the line drawn in the midst of any dilemma with another person.

The *line drawn* is the difference we adhere to in our own mindsets, regarding the way we perceive others, and how this affects relationships.

As we learn to ABIDE in HIM, we learn to allow the Spirit to adjust our mindsets of difference, allowing a more tolerable willingness to prevail.

Whether someone is trying to change our thinking, or even influence how we look at things; we must keep our mindsets resolutely emmersed in Jesus, in order to remain true to His Identity infilling us in our living, in every way.

If our thoughts, hopes, and dreams are a spectrum of unmatched ideas, then the foundations upon which we lean are become as "*sand*".

Transcending each pressure beyond the revelation of each increase, continues sharing the action that provide His Finished Work.

In science, the price of imposing our own ideas onto reality is the loss of discovery, with all its immense rewards.

In our Christian faith, it is the loss of knowing Jesus Christ.

Forcing our own ideas upon Jesus is a singular disaster, for it is only in knowing the staggering truth of Who He IS~~and what He has done for and with and to the human race~~that we are set free from the bondage of our profound and debilitating anxiety into the freedom to live.

The hope and joy we so desperately desire, the passion and courage, the dignity and freedom, the wholeness and fullness for which we long, are the fruit of knowing Jesus Christ.

It is as we come to know him~~the real Jesus, as He is in Himself as the Father's beloved Son and the Lord and Savior of the human race~~that we are quickened with a hope and a freedom, being inspired with a life and joy that are not our own.

Where there is no passion, no glorious quickening occurring within our journey; herein is the loss of value to the Pearl of Great Price, Jesus Christ, the Son of the Living God!

As a grandchild could not possibly have lived on the inspiration of their grandparent's encounter, we cannot live on the joy of our ancestors' discovery of Jesus.

We must come to know Him for ourselves.

Each generation must seek Him and find Him; and such will be the discovery made when we seek for Him with all our heart, mind, soul, and strength!

Only then will we experience the quickening and the life and the freedom that our souls crave.

Whereas increase qualifies every portion of His Faith, encountering the evidence of His Instruction processes the sacrifice of revealing each part of His Finished Work.

To find the fullness of experiencing WHO HE IS, reveals the understanding of WHOSE WE ARE IN HIM!

As in construction, the roof is built on the strength of the exterior/load~bearing walls, and such walls are built on the external/internal stability of foundations made/poured out; so it is with the believer's living IN HIM!

His Plan of the Ages must be followed to the letter crossed, and the eye dotted, in proof of the evidence that HE IS THE FINISHED WORK!

Wherein the increase of His Seed enables the adjustings of His Finished Work, the provisions of His Grace perpetuate each portion of perseverance to endure agreement proving His Seed provides actions that transform each issue.

How is it that we are so devoid of understanding with regard to the Salvation of the Savior having come at no cost to our lives, but only through His Life laid down on our behalf?

While we tell the souls of humanity that God's Grace is free for the taking; and yet, we tell them later that they must EARN what they were told before came freely through the Love of the Creator Who created all;

wherein does the accepting of the free gift of Grace take precedence?

QUESTION: If faith and holiness are made to become CONDITIONS of keeping/guarding God's Salvation to His CREATION; where, when, why, and by whom do such conditions outweigh the price paid at Calvary by the ONE Who loves us eternally?

"For by Him were all things created, that are in heaven, and that are in earth, visible and invisible, whether they be thrones, or dominions, or principalities, or powers: all things were created by Him, and for Him" COLOSSIANS 1:16 KJV

"¹ God, who at sundry times and in divers manners spake in time past unto the fathers by the prophets, ² Hath in these last days spoken unto us by His Son, whom He hath appointed Heir of All Things, by whom also He made the worlds; ³ Who being the brightness of His Glory, and the Express Image of His Person, and upholding all things by The Word of His Power, when He had by Himself purged our sins, sat down on the right hand of the Majesty on high." HEBREWS 1:1-3 KJV

"¹ In the beginning was the Word, and the Word was with[face~to~face]God, and the Word was God. ² The same was in the beginning with God. ³ All things were made by Him; and without Him was not any thing made that was made. ⁴ In Him was life; and the life was the light of men. ⁵ And the light shineth in darkness; and the darkness comprehended it not." JOHN 1:1-5 KJV

God was not only the LIFE that was the LIGHT; He shined into the darkness, and the darkness would not accept HIM as He was, and has always been, and will always be!

Jesus is not the LIGHT because we make Him so!

HE IS THE LIGHT that cometh down from heaven, out of God!

The same LIFE that transcends between the Father, Son, and Spirit~~this is the same LIFE that courses through every one who have ever been, or ever will be born!

We do not make HIM as He is; He remains as He has been throughout the eternal ages, and the continual progressions of time itself.

He is LORD, because He is LORD!

He is not Lord, because we say or believe He is LORD!

Who He is, is not so because we believe, or declare He is to us; but, He IS what/Who He says He is, because what He say HE IS, IS WHAT

Got Healing?

HE IS!

He says He is LOVE, because HE IS!

He says He is HEALER, because HE IS!

He says He is DELIVERER, because HE IS!

His Faith empowers the evidence that patiently provides the positions of each degree transforming progressively the Patterns~of~His~Thoughts in purpose of the Exchange by His Finished Work.

"For IN Him we live, and move, and have our being; as certain also of your own poets have said, For we are also His Offspring." *ACTS 17:28 KJV*

Because He exists, even now and forevermore, as *God in Humanity;* He does so because *He bears the scars of His encounter, and He glorifies those Whom He made to glorify HIM as He is!*

We cannot have health and healing without our being well; nor could we have salvation, His Salvation, without having His Holiness.

Therefore, the miseries of humanity can neither arise from positive infliction, mor can it be relieved by the mere removal of judicial penalties.

The misery of humanity is in the form of a dis~eased mind.

Humanity seeks kindness where there is none; in the folds of any society that does not choose to worship the Lord God, the Giver of All LIFE!

The LOVE of God is to the spirit of humanity, what the key~stone is to the arch; ruin is the consequence, when such falls from its proper place.

"For the love of Christ constraineth us; because we thus judge, that *if One died for all, then were all dead:* *SECOND CORINTHIANS 5:14 KJV*

His Pattern~of~Thought processes each degree as unseen in His Finished Work, in memory of every balance provided.

His Pattern is His LOVE.

His Pattern is His Grace.

His Pattern is His Mercy!

Then, His Pattern is His Government triumphant eternally!

We see that humanity's reason bewilders him, and his conscience harasses him~~his imagination deceives and disquiets him~~his passions and affections agitate and torture him.

He has a misery wrought into the very elements of his being, independent altogether of positive infliction.

When I can lay the blame of my misery on anything external to me, there may be hope of deliverance, for I can distinguish between myself and my sorrow.

However, it is a terrific discovery to make, that I am myself my own misery.

Yet, if this be true, how am I to escape from myself?

The manifestation of the character of God contained in the gift of Christ is exactly fitted for this purpose.

<u>Whereupon encountering the balance provided, His Faith confirms the acquired revelation of His Finished Work.</u>

As with an overlay, the depth of God's Word is viewed as unfathomable, and yet, the desire to discover more of Him increases.

The more we learn, the more we discern.

Discerning with the heart causes the single eye to see deeper into the transcending elements of God's Eternal Plan, discovering the inexplicable characteristics of His Finished Work.

As pertains to believers, there is an infinitesimal amount of parallels to be discovered~~that will enlighten, and embue the soul with the Majesty and Magnificence of His Existence.

The BALANCE of His Presence provides the essence of His Faith, to confirm that His Finished Work has been acquired forevermore.

<u>The Qualities that increase His Finished Work are discerned/perceived through the transformations of His Grace.</u>

What we see IN ourselves is the mirror reflection of WHO HE IS IN US!

It is not another's flesh that we mirror; or even another's psyche.

We reflect the existence, the essence, and the thoughts of the One who died in our place, as us!

The qualities that express the very cosmic substance that He is, retains His features in His fulness, even though He indwells and abides within us.

Therefore, we, as abiding in HIM, retain the same likeness as the image of Him that we bear in our ownselves.

This is not a man~centered ideal of religion, which is consistently as being *"the opiet of the masses"*!

Got Healing?

God Himself, came down in the flesh of humanity, made Himself to be the supreme sacrifice that His Creation needed, in order to find that which we were before *He formed us in the belly of our mother*, while restoring us to the former viable likeness of His Image given at first Creation. JEREMIAH 1:5 KJV

SEMITIC~ARAMAIC~HEBRAIC THESAURUS

Aramaic before first {

Semitic Root before first =

Lettering for ParaPhrase after second =

...(10:38) (about) עַל S15701 {עַל=in measure}= Ayin-pierce perceive wisdom-Lamed-instruct acquire provide- (Yeshua) ישוע S9573 {ישוע=being saved}= Yud-purpose posture actions-Shin-pressure exchange disperse-Vav-increase degree assure-Ayin-pierce perceive wisdom- (Who from) מן S12161 {מן=indicating the origin of movement through time}= Dalet-faith establish presence-Mem-transform encounter remembrance-Final-Nun-issue perseverance progress- (Nazareth) נצרת S15539 {נצר=branching}= Beyt-pattern thought inhabit-Yud-purpose posture actions-Resh-process beginning strength-Taw-evidence prove sign- (Whom God) אלהים S914 {אלה=behaving like God}= Dalet-faith establish presence-Aleph-authority ability confirm-Lamed-instruct acquire provide-Hey-quality reveal grace-Final-Aleph-ending finish maturity- (anointed Him) משחה S12492 {משח=measuring with precision/compared by measure}= Mem-transform encounter remembrance-Shin-pressure exchange disperse-Hhet-specific share beyond-Hey-quality reveal grace- (with The Spirit) ברוח S9103 {רוח=to sware by/according to the Breath within the prophetic vision}= Beyt-pattern thought inhabit-Resh-process beginning strength-Vav-increase degree assure-Hhet-specific share beyond-Final-Aleph-ending finish maturity- (of Holiness) קדוש S18205 {קדש=belonging to/related to someone/something consecrated}= Dalet-faith establish presence-Quph-contrast parallel structure-Vav-increase degree assure-Dalet-faith establish presence-Shin-pressure exchange disperse-Final-Aleph-ending finish maturity- (& with power) וחיל S7033 {חיל=according to intrinsic potency/innate force}= Vav-increase degree assure-Nun-seed patience continue-Hhet-specific share beyond-Yud-purpose posture actions-Lamed-instruct acquire provide-Final-Aleph-ending finish maturity- (& He was) והיה S5016 {הה=the self~same One}= Vav-increase degree assure-Hey-quality reveal grace-Vav-increase degree assure-Yud-purpose posture actions-Vav-increase degree assure- (traveling) מתכרד S10618 {כרד= surrounding/wrapping around}= Dalet-faith establish presence-Mem-transform encounter remembrance-Taw-evidence prove sign-Lamed-instruct acquire provide-Resh-process beginning strength-Final-Kaph-acknowledge offer allow- (he was) והוא S5144 {הוא=changing conditions/enduring/ /existing}= Hey-quality reveal grace-Vav-increase degree assure-Final-Aleph-ending finish maturity- (& healing) ומאסא S1805 {אסא=repairing/restoring what is hurt}= Vav-increase degree assure-Nun-seed patience continue-Aleph-authority ability confirm-Samech-adjust apprehend source-Final-Aleph-ending finish maturity- (those) להנון S5062 {הון=on this account}= Lamed-instruct acquire provide-Hey-quality reveal grace-Nun-seed patience continue-Vav-increase degree assure-Final-Nun-issue perseverance progress- (injured) אתנכיו S13055 {נכי=perceiving injury/damage}= Dalet-faith establish presence-Aleph-authority ability confirm-Taw-evidence prove sign-Nun-seed patience continue-Lamed-instruct acquire provide-Yud-purpose posture actions-Vav-increase degree assure- (by) מן S12182 {מן=indicating the origin of movement through time}= Mem-transform encounter remembrance-Final-Nun-issue perseverance progress- (The Evil One) בישא S2287 {באש=the antithesis of good as debilitated}= Beyt-pattern thought inhabit-Yud-purpose posture actions-Shin-pressure exchange disperse-Final-Aleph-ending finish maturity- (because) מטל S11636 {מטל=on account of}= Mem-transform encounter remembrance-Thet-contain mixture balance-Lamed-instruct acquire provide- (God) אלהא S914 {אלה=behaving like God}= Mem-transform encounter remembrance-Thet-contain mixture balance-Lamed-instruct acquire provide-Dalet-faith establish presence-Aleph-authority ability confirm-Lamed-instruct acquire provide-Hey-quality reveal grace-Final-Aleph-ending finish maturity- (was) הוא S5144 {הוא=changing conditions/enduring/existing}= Hey-quality reveal grace-Vav-increase degree assure-Final-Aleph-ending finish maturity- (with Him) עמה S15786 {עמ=in the presence of/in possession of}= Ayin-pierce perceive wisdom-Mem-transform encounter remembrance-Hey-quality reveal grace-

The Semitic Emphasis

Got Healing?

In measure of being saved~~indicating the origin of movement through time branching to behave like God~~measuring with precision/compared by measure to sware by/according to the Breath within the prophetic vision~~belonging to/related to someone/something consecrated according to intrinsic potency/innate force~~the self~same One surrounding/wrapping around changing conditions/enduring/existing~~ repairing//restoring what is hurt on this account~~perceiving injury/damage indicating the origin of movement through time~~the antithesis of good as debilitated on account of behaving like God changing conditions/enduring/existing in the presence of/in possession of.

Christians have divided themselves into many denominations and sub denominational groups.

The strife created by doctrinal differences ranges from subtle rejection to all out war.

Opposing doctrinal positions can be reconciled only by higher truth.

Lifting the spiritual eye from doctrinal debates to a higher level of practical, personal revelation of truth can help dissolve conflicts.

The practical *"gospel of the kingdom"* that Jesus preached is that higher truth. Focusing on the revelation of the *"kingdom of God"* can reconcile doctrinal differences.

More importantly, the revelation of the *"gospel of the kingdom"* can enable Christians to overcome in this life.

Christians are often subconsciously, denominationally trained to recognize and reject opposing views of doctrine.

Hearing a certain "buzz word" or phrase may instantly trigger automatic rejection.

The word or phrase may be a perfectly good Bible word, perhaps even spoken by Jesus Himself.

Yet the hearer may identify it with an opposing denominational view and automatically reject the truth being stated.

The focus of this work is neither denominational, nor theological.

No particular denominational view is proffered, nor assaulted.

The intent of this work is to focus on the higher truth of the *"gospel of the kingdom"*, both individually and corporately.

We must needs *"hear with the single ear of the heart"*; for the heart of the matter is the matter of one's heart to hear!

Acquire The Abilities Of Unseen Strengths And Continue To Mature In The Qualities That Purpose Each Encounter Through The Seed Increasing Every Evidence Of His Finished Work

FIRST CORINTHIANS 12:9

KJV+TVM

^{G1161} To another ^{G2087} faith ^{G4102} by ^{G1722} the same ^{G846} Spirit ^{G4151}; ^{G1161} to another ^{G243} the gifts ^{G5486} of healing ^{G2386} by ^{G1722} the same ^{G846} Spirit ^{G4151};

ORIGINAL THOUGHTS

...(12:9) Acquire the abilities of Unseen Strengths, and continue to mature in the qualities that purpose each encounter through the Seed increasing every evidence of His Finished Work. Within His Pattern~Thought, behold the existing process/beginnings that insure the specifics of His Finished Work. Confirm each determination of beginnings that continue throughout His Finished Work. Rise above through every increase insuring the Grace of His Truth to pattern the significance of His Finished Work. Establish Dominion, while apprehending a single~mindedness that enlarges the evidence of His Finished Work. Abide within the Grace of His Pattern, and process each increase beyond His Finished Work.

Acquire the abilities of Unseen Strengths, and continue to mature in the qualities that purpose each encounter through the Seed increasing every evidence of His Finished Work.

Giving our attention to the Lord, in quiet, thoughtful reflection, provides the awareness of the many things we already have IN HIM!

Many Christians do not recognize or know they are in bondage, that they have strong~holds and open "gates" or "doors" which allow darkness to influence them away from the leading of the Spirit within their living.

The scriptural admonition stated in HOSEA 4:6 is still applicable today: "My people are destroyed for lack of knowledge."

ISAIAH 5:13 says "my people are gone into captivity because they have no knowledge".

Within His Pattern~Thought, behold the existing process/beginnings that insure the specifics of His Finished Work.

From the very beginning of His thoughts conceiving us, God desired for us to be healthy: *spiritually, mentally, and physically.*

God created Adam and Eve in perfect health, in His own likeness and image $^{GEN.\ 1:26\ KJV}$; He gave them dominion over all the earth. $^{GENESIS\ 1:28\ KJV}$

Sickness and disease did not exist in the Garden of Eden; nor does it exist in the Kingdom of God.

From the very beginning of His creation, humanity was not created to be sick or to die.

Thus, we know that God's perfect will for us is to be in spiritual and physical health.

Let it also be noted: *There is no lack, or disease, or sickness in the spiritual dimension.*

Lack, disease, and sickness are the result of the physical dimension endeavoring to operate without God's leading.

Confirm each determination of beginnings that continue throughout His Finished Work.

Survey the elements of your living before God and discover which ones you can clearly see the beginnings of God's hand in being led as you were, or are.

Except we mature to the place where we can discern the hand of God through our living and its harvest; how can we hope to think we are led by the Voice of God Who provides every provision at our disposal?

To confirm the beginnings of God's handiwork within our living is to underscore the very foundation of His understanding supporting our every surrender to His Majesty from upon the throne of our living AS HIM~~FOR HIM!

Rise above through every increase insuring the Grace of His Truth to pattern the significance of His Finished Work.

Except our journey exceeds the discovery of His impartation, how can we stand to serve Him Who is the greatest with any less than the knowing of His majestic presence within our living?

Acknowledging Him is a priority to maturing before Him!

Unless we can identify His place within the throes of our living, how will we identify His Identity in a living that cannot clearly present the respect of His Treasures throughout our every effort of surrender?

It is never by the accumulation of things that garner the respect of our hearts and mind toward Him as our Father; rather, it is the knowing of HIM as the keeper and protector of our living in service of His LOVE so freely given!

Establish Dominion, while apprehending a single~mindedness that enlarges the evidence of His Finished Work.

The single-minded heart offering wisdom with a singleness of mindset becomes the greatest of fields sown with the unequivocal majesties of His Person, Presence, and Power.

It is by the Spirit's making known the Presence and Person of Jesus inhabiting our existence that stirs the heart toward to areas of refuge offering the REST OF HIM, as we have known our REST IN HIM FIRST!

What becomes rooted and grounded as foundation to our living after HIM, also forms the unfathomable undergirding of structure built to serve the Lord's heritage and continually offer the fullness of unquenchable LOVE.

Life is never more worth living than when surrendered to the fullness of loving HIM, and yet, always being available to sacrifice for others that which He alone gives through discipleship led by the Spirit at work in us!

Abide within the Grace of His Pattern, and process each increase beyond His Finished Work.

Remaining is about abiding where one has been planted.

Knowing the Voice of the Lord God is not about discerning the strength of the storm, or the stability of shaky influence externally, or rallying around the fires of others, instead of taking care of one's own covenantal families!

Knowing God is found in the deepest of intimacies, where nothing is hidden, and the heart and mind know everything exposed is anything unnecessary in our journeys with HIM.

Then, it is that the process of each increase beyond His Finished Work defines and describes and determines that none but the Lord shall direct, or guide, or lead one's living anywhere except where His Presence finds a place to replenish the soul, even if it means being at REST in the midst of turmoil or trouble.

Semitic~Aramaic~Hebraic Thesaurus

Got Healing?

Aramaic before first {
Semitic Root before first =
Lettering for ParaPhrase after second =

...(12:9) (to another)אחרנא S7694 {ۥ⌂}=following/furthering}=Lamed[to/toward]-instruct acquire provide- Aleph-authority ability confirm- Hhet-specific share beyond- Resh-process beginning strength- Nun-seed patience continue- Final-Aleph-ending finish maturity- (faith)הימנותא S1197 {ۥ⌂}=belief/faithfulness/assurety}= Hey[behold/the]- quality reveal grace- Yud[of/through]-purpose single~mindedness actions- Mem[from/out of]-transform encounter remembrance- Nun- seed patience continue- Vav-[and/in addition]increase degree assure- Taw-evidence prove sign- Final-Aleph-ending finish maturity- (in him)בה S2240 {⌂=being empty}= Beyt[within/inside]-pattern thought inhabit- Hey[behold/the]-quality reveal grace- (by The Spirit)ברוחא S19636 {ۥ⌂}= within a prophetic vision}= Beyt[within/inside]-pattern thought inhabit- Resh- process beginning strength- Vav-[and/in addition]increase degree assure- Hhet-specific share beyond- Final-Aleph-ending finish maturity- (to another)לאחרנא S7694 {ۥ⌂}=different from}= Lamed[to/toward]-instruct acquire provide- Aleph- authority ability confirm- Hhet-specific share beyond- Resh-process beginning strength- Nun-seed patience continue- Final- Aleph-ending finish maturity- (the gift)מוהבתא S8895 {⌂}=granting/ /allowing/conceding}= Mem[from/out of]- transform encounter remembrance- Vav-[and/in addition]increase degree assure- Hey[behold/the]-quality reveal grace- Beyt[within/inside]-pattern thought inhabit- Taw-evidence prove sign- Final-Aleph-ending finish maturity- (of healing)דאסיותא S1630 {ۥ⌂}=remedy}= Dalet-faith establish presence- Aleph-authority ability confirm- Samech-adjust apprehend source- Yud[of/through]-purpose single~mindedness actions- Vav-[and/in addition]increase degree assure- Taw-evidence prove sign- Final-Aleph-ending finish maturity- (in Him)בה S2240 {⌂=being empty}= Beyt[within/inside]-pattern thought inhabit- Hey[behold/the]-quality reveal grace- (by The Spirit)ברוחא S19636 {ۥ⌂}=within a prophetic vision}= Beyt[within/ /inside]-pattern thought inhabit- Resh-process beginning strength- Vav-[and/in addition]increase degree assure- Hhet-specific share beyond- Final-Aleph-ending finish maturity-

The Semitic Emphasis

Following/Furthering belief/faithfullness/assurety being empty within a prophetic vision~~following/furthering granting/allowing/conceding remedy being empty within a prophetic vision.

Curious to the natural mind are the things of the Spirit.

And yet, through such things, one is made aware of the fact that they *"are not their own"*, learning and coming to know they *"have been bought with a price"*.

Such is that price that opens the vaults of Heaven's treasures, providing such wonders and understanding that compels the believer to step into the manifold, or many~folded giftings God provides for all of His Creation to us.

You will notice the phrase above, *"to be empty within a prophetic vision"*; and while this may appear foreboding, the mature heart and mind, at rest in the Lord, realizes that there must be nothing of self, when one enters into the many~folded mysteries that are God Himself!

Thinking about His holiness connects us with Him.

Few of us would begin shouting to a friend whom we wish to visit while still six blocks down the street.

Got Healing?

Few of us would begin speaking to someone on the telephone before the operator had given us the connection.

Yet many of us begin begging for all kinds of little human things before we have realized the one great divine thing which is His own Holiness.

Learn to build and accentuate the Holy Presence of God Himself residing, abiding, remaining within us, as though living Himself through us!

How many Christians down through the ages have failed to receive the answers to their prayers by failing to take this last step—the step of giving thanks! God is standing before us with the answer in His hands.

Nevertheless, unless we reach out our hands and receive it by giving thanks for it, we are not apt to receive it.

For while love is the wiring that connects our souls with His, faith is the switch that turns on the power.

Our homes are full of things that run by electricity: lights, irons, sewing machines, toasters.

Just believing that there is a power called electricity is not enough to make these things work for us.

Every time that we want one of them to work, we must touch the button that releases the power in that one.

Just believing a set of facts about God does not necessarily turn on the power in a single one of our prayer objectives.

In order to do that, we must believe that we are receiving the thing that we desire.

If we really believe this, we will naturally rejoice and give thanks for it.

And when our belief is weak, the act of rejoicing and giving thanks will awaken our faith.

From the Revelation of Christ

Increase Memories Focused On Encounters
That Perceive His Evidence By Exchange
In Addition To The Parallels Of
His Purpose Revealed

REVELATION 22:2

Got Healing?

KJV+TVM

In^{G1722} the midst^{G3319} of the street^{G4113} of it^{G846}, and^{G2532} on either^{G2532} side^{G1782} ^{G1782} of the river^{G4215}, was there the tree^{G3586} of life^{G2222}, which bare^{G4160} $^{[G5723]}$ twelve^{G1427} manner of fruits^{G2590}, and yielded^{G591} $^{[G5723]}$ her^{G846} fruit^{G2590} every^{G2596} ^{G1538} ^{G1520} month^{G3376}: and^{G2532} the leaves^{G5444} of the tree^{G3586} were for^{G1519} the healing^{G2322} of the nations^{G1484}

ORIGINAL THOUGHTS

...(22:2) Increase the memories focused on encounters that perceive His Evidence by exchange, in addition to the parallels of His Purpose as revealed. Transcend surrender to His Efforts of influencing every part of the encounters that obtains the finished maturity of His Wise Promise/Provision. In His Seed, behold the strength of His Finished Work, building a single~minded resource as finished, and establish each specific through His Finished Work. Present His Wisdom in pattern of His Faith, as His Spoken Word enables the processes of His Finished Work in proving the ability of proceeding to penetrate His Resources beginning. In addition within agreeing to acquire the single~minded process of the Unseen, purpose to reveal the Pattern~of~His~Thoughts declaring that the Dominion of each Beginning adds the quality of His Workings. Insure the balance that strengthens His Spoken Word, in addition to qualifying the purposes that provide the initiatives apprehending the single~minded efforts proving His Finished Work. The Faith of His Wisdom transforms each encounter through His Finished Work.

Increase the memories focused on encounters that perceive His Evidence by exchange, in addition to the parallels of His Purpose as revealed.

His Finished Work involves the revelation of His Eternal Majesty, His Forthcoming Plan, and the continued efforts of our destinies forged through the eternal magnitude of His Purposes.

"For our God is a consuming fire.　HEBREWS 12:29 KJV

The greater our understanding of His Purposes, the larger the revelation of His Intentions toward sharing the fullness of His Eternal Character and Provision thereof.

The Fire of God is the very Presence of His Existence throughout every revelation of His Person.

As is attested throughout the Scriptures, the Fire that is God removes every encumbrance, every obstacle, as well as every hindrance to the eternal, redemptive plan of His Purpose.

Transcend surrender to His Efforts of influencing every part of the encounters that obtains the finished maturity of His Wise Promise/Provision.

Got Healing?

Do you remember the first day you knew that Jesus loved you?

Do you remember how clean you felt and how light your heart was?

The air seemed clearer, the colors of His Creation brighter.

You felt as if you had stumbled out of a dark, dirty cave and plunged headlong into a clean, cool stream.

You drank in the reality of His Presence and splashed with delight in His Goodness.

In that moment nothing else mattered.

You knew at the very core of your being that God/Jesus was real, that He had great affection for you.

Even in the face of dire circumstances, you were convinced that there was nothing you, with HIM, couldn't walk through together.

His Love not only overwhelmed you, it also overflowed you with His Grace for others, even those who had wronged you.

You woke up every morning in eager anticipation of what He would show you throughout that day.

You delighted yourself in HIM as He delighted Himself in you and each day became an adventure together.

What if we change our attitude, by surrendering the beginning of each day to HIM?

And, as well, we continue to worship Him throughout the day He has given, and consistently know that we REST IN HIM through all of it!

This is where He wants US TO LIVE!

In His Seed, behold the strength of His Finished Work, building a single~minded resource as finished, and establish each specific through His Finished Work.

Stop looking just for what you think you need to fix what ailes you!

We miss the good parts when we only search His Word for the things we think we need at the moment.

This LIFE is a marathon called eternity; it is not a sprint called, I want, I want, I want!

Contained in the Seed of His Word are the elements that carry the soul through this limited excursion called, this world; and takes us beyond the throes of circumstances into the clear, smooth ripples of change to reveal His Image clearly and concisely throughout our living AS HIM, and

THROUGH HIM!

Present His Wisdom in pattern of His Faith, as His Spoken Word enables the processes of His Finished Work in proving the ability of proceeding to penetrate His Resources beginning.

Realize this verse in Revelation is not just about Eternity; it is also about how He touches, and changes our living by His stepping into our hearts and minds, sharing with us in our adventure, while He shares with us the eternal majesty of His Character and Blessings.

He knows before we step into anything that such times can be complicated, if we do not embrace the continuing thoughts of learning to lean upon HIM!

Others may tell you that you're not working hard enough, or praying long enough, or giving more than enough!

When things to go wrong we all have the tendency to start, or continue blaming God for not loving us enough, or we stop accepting His Love because we did not TRY hard enough.

Both are dead-ends, and living the Life we shared eventually fades into confusion and guilt.

HOWEVER, He never gives up on us!

Learning to lean on Him means we begin every day HIS WAY; in thanksgiving for all He will bring us through!

This is the PATTERN He calls surrender, while be willing and obedient.

In addition within agreeing to acquire the single-minded process of the Unseen, purpose to reveal the Pattern-of-His-Thoughts declaring that the Dominion of each Beginning adds the quality of His Workings.

You see, God knows before we do that even with the best of intentions, the best of our efforts will never be enough WITHOUT HIM!

This is the reason Jesus satisfied the broken law through HIM, without any other's help; because His Righteousness and our guilt never has a place in our relationship together with HIM!

Our righteousness is in Christ Jesus, and guilt never has a place in the relationship we share together in HIM!

With the single-mindedness of His Purposes, we begin seeing more clearly the strength of His Dominion carrying us through to the endings of His Intentional Aim.

Insure the balance that strengthens His Spoken Word, in addition to qualifying the purposes that provide the initiatives apprehending the single~minded efforts proving His Finished Work.

His Purposes provide the initiative that His Efforts provide together within His Finished Work.

"And we know that all things work together for good to them that love God, to them who are the called according to His purpose. **ROMANS 8:28 KJV**

REMEMBER: the PURPOSES are HIS, never ours!

The Faith of His Wisdom transforms each encounter through His Finished Work.

We need to continually learn to LIVE LOVED IN HIM!

Can someone try too hard to walk with God? Absolutely!

I know that sounds odd, but relationship with the Living God cannot be earned by human effort, even extensive human effort.

And sometimes those trying the hardest to make it happen find themselves furthest from it.

It breaks our heart to find people there.

Religion never tires of telling us to try harder and giving us an increasing array of tasks to *'help'* us find Him.

Our self-effort still focuses on us, however, and we end up missing Jesus, who is right there to lead us into relationship with His Father.

This is something He does at our invitation, not something we can do by our diligence.

SEMITIC~ARAMAIC~HEBRAIC THESAURUS

Aramaic before first {
Semitic Root before first =
Lettering for ParaPhrase after second =

...(22:2) (& in the center)ומצעת S12304 {**=bringing someone before the court**}=/ו Vav-[and/in addition]increase degree assure-/מ Mem[from/out of]-transform encounter remembrance-/י Yud [of/through]-purpose single~mindedness actions-/ע Ayin-pierce perceive wisdom-/ת Taw-evidence prove sign-(of the street)שוקיה S21009 {**=of outside place**}=/ש Shin-pressure exchange disperse-/ו Vav-[and/in addition]increase degree assure-/ק Quph-contrast parallel structure-/י Yud [of/through]-purpose single~mindedness actions-/ה Hey[behold/the]-quality reveal grace-(on this side)מכא S9730 {**=from this time on**}=/מ Mem[from/out of]-transform encounter remembrance-/כ Kaph-surrender obtains consent-/א Final-Aleph-ending finish maturity-(& on that)ומכא S9728 {**=a measure**}=/ו Vav-[and/in addition]increase degree assure-/מ Mem[from/out of]-transform encounter remembrance-/כ Kaph-surrender obtains consent-/א Final-Aleph-ending finish maturity-(on)על S15701 {**=in measurement**}=/ע Ayin-pierce perceive wisdom-/ל Lamed[to/ /toward]-instruct acquire provide-(the river)נהרא S12787 {**=the rushing of waters**}=/נ Nun-seed patience continue-/ה Hey[behold/the]-quality reveal grace-

Got Healing?

The Semitic Emphasis

Bringing someone before the court of the outside place~~from this time on a measure in measurement of~~the rushing of waters bent~~as belonging/relating to someone/something for the health and welfare of perceiving/desiring~~to pass time in a certain way~~a fortress in pattern with regard to characterized by duality~~the lesser cycle characterized by duality~~a fortress fragmented remedying the imaginations.

Often, we miss the point between living for God to please HIM, or to share HIM.

When we look at our living and decide we are not as fruitful as we think, or a speaker's message inspires us _to do more_, there is an invisible line we can cross over, when we do something without God's directive or asking us to step into what it is we see needs to be attended to, or accomplished.

When we just do thing because we see they need to be addressed, we tend to use it in justifying later what God has called us to do, and yet we resist.

Anything we do that tends to give us air of justifiable stubbornness, or feeds a resisting attitude when the Spirit seeks to move us~~this is

Got Healing?

*S*elfish~*I*ndependent~*N*ature at its worst!

When we take an account of what we have done, to use it as a *pry~bar* to get God to do something for us, this is *S*elfish~*I*ndependent~*N*ature at its worst!

When someone says, *"just RELAX"*; do we take it as good advice, a clear suggestion to back~off, or a mild way of saying, *"enough already, who are you the Gospel Police"*?

Often, we fail to be aware of how much of our living is *performance~based*, or how deeply ingrained in us the idea is, and somehow has taken hold of our thoughts to produce the things that Jesus wants to accomplish in us through His Spirit.

Discovering that things we do, thinking we are being *spiritual*, (*which is just another way of being religious, actually*), can be remodeled in a new paradigm.

The Spirit desires to fill our days with fellowship through relationship, allowing Her to take the thing we used to do on our own, and interweave them throughout our living moment~by~moment in relationship with HIM!

Yet, God seeks to show us through the Parable of the Prodigal how the FATHER consistently loved both the wayward son, and the elder son who stayed and worked without ever asking for anything he wanted for himself.

Remembering the consistency of the FATHER'S LOVE, we can see more clearly that God, our Father seeks in allowing us to vent that He encourages us, listens to us, and then steps into our dark times to be with us and show us how to adjust to HIS WILL, HIS WAY, THROUGH HIS WORD!

The problem is that all along we have viewed the Scriptures from the perspective of 'must do', 'must perform', and 'must make happen'.

All along the Scripture has been intended to be viewed from the perspective of discovery of who He is and whose we are and all that He has for us and intends to work in us, but only in the context of relationship with HIM!

This is the *"tangible love"* of the Father to us, through His making a connection within our living that is not an emotion, but rather something

---

a lot deeper!

Now, here is a connection that has never been revealed before and the reason we can know it is true is because it is there day after day, all day.

It is not fleeting like emotions, but remaining like a love everlasting.

We begin to have a sense of sonship with our Father.

He is answering literally, the lifelong cry of our heart~~to know Him and know His love.

See if you can get your mind around the freedom and peace you will begin experiencing!

11 verses examined...

APPENDIX
#0 - #7

Appendix O:

WORD TERMS ASSOCIATED WITH THIS TEACHING

The following terms are those associated with this teaching. The definitions have a definite "*spiritual/biblical spin*", so as to provide the student, or the reader with an understanding of what is meant in the "ORIGINAL THOUGHTS". The difference in the use of key words to convey a better understanding in today's meanings prepares the inquisitive for enlightenment beyond what the social outcome of King James of England was about in 1611. Interpreting versions from the translated words used in the "*Authorized Version of the King James Bible*" is not completely accurate for the 21ˢᵗ centuries use or understanding. Thus, we have a multiplicity of vagueness in how these words are taught and used. There are a multitude of spurious doctrines, that when the "*original thought from original context out of original society*", such doctrines are spotlighted to show their cloudiness.

The following are alphabetic letters used for interpreting the suggested
__Kingdom ParaPhrase__:

1. א-Aleph-*confirm/capacity/authority~*

    א-Aleph-*ending/finish/maturity~*

2. ב-Beyt-*pattern/thoughts/inhabit~*

3. ד-Dalet-*belief/establish/presence~*

4. ע-Ayin-*pierce/perceive/wisdom~*

5. ג-Gimal-*experience/understanding/encounter~*

6. י-Yud-*purpose/posture/actions~*

7. צ-Tsad-*pursuit/journey/anticipate~*

8. ה-Hey-*breath/reveal/life-force~*

9. ו-Vav-*measure/increase/secure~*

10. ט-Thet-*contain/mixture/balance~*

11. ח-Hhet-*separate/individual/beyond~*

12. ז-Zayin-*instrument/alter/skill~*

13. כ-Kaph-*surrender/capture/consent*

    ך-Kaph-*surrender/offer/allow~*

14. ל-Lamed-*instruct/acquire/provide~*

15. מ-Mem-*change/challenge/provoke~*

    ם-Mem-*trial/fashions/produces~*

16. **ב**-Nun-*seed/patience/continue~~*   ㇵ

      ן-Nun-*continue/seed/develop~*

17. **ס**-Samech-*adjust/apprehend/source~*   ⨦

18. **ﬡ**-Pey-*mouth/SpokenWord/speak~*   ⌒

      ף-Pey-*mouth/SpokenWord/speak~*

19. **ק**-Quph-*contrast/parallel/cycle~*   –●–

20. **ר**-Resh-*beginnings/process/protection~*   ঽ

21. **ש**-Shin-*pressure/exchange/disperse~*   Ш

22. **ת**-Taw-*evidence/prove/sign~*   †

The example found on page 11-12 shows the meaning of each letter, and the letter's name. The following three words separated by "/" are synonyms for the meaning found in the Aramaic and Hebraic Bibles. As the alphabets of the Aramaic, and Hebraic are the evolved forms of the original Semitic alphabet, it is the Semitic that we offer in pictograph form as proof of what we are calling, "**original thought**".

As it is in every translation, to date, the main thought is clouded by a religious judgment of control. The clergy, at the time of the first translations to Greek, then Latin, and then English, it appears that there is a definite influence of the same thoughts offering negativism, portraying God, and His Plan as though out of touch with what spiritual content really offers. As the Bible is represented, and to be presented as God's Word, it should NOT ever contain what man thinks. However, as it is with everything in this world, man's objections, abstentions, and idiosyncrasies become the pollutions to WHO IT IS that God is wanting humanity to see.

As far as use of terms, there are many nouns, verbs, and adjectives/adverbs that describe only One, Jesus. Everything in every Bible ever written is about JESUS. Not current events; not who the next anti-Christ will be; never about the saints leaving this world. These terms always, and forever will signal the appearing of Jesus, the Christ, the Son of the Living God. Just a few of them are as follows:

Purpose – the only CAUSE for our being is to serve Him; the Purpose of our Living is to serve Him; the Determination/Persistence/Reason for our Living is to serve ONLY Him.

Pattern-Thoughts – the PATTERN for our living must be cut from the mold He designed and became as a man in this earthen vessel; His Attentions, His Plans, being higher than ours, become the motivation of a continuing journey in Him.

Authority/Confidence/Conviction – He, Jesus was given ALL Authority before ever Creation began; the Confidence He exudes is beyond the comprehension of any who are not in Relationship with Him; the Conviction of being His SERVANT is the axis upon which our living revolves.

Breath/Grace/Appearing - that which is our Breathing is the very existence of Him at work in us; Grace is the fullness, the epitome of all that He extends to our

Got Healing?

Living for Him, of Him, and through Him; His Appearing through us is the only glimpse the world will ever be able to see.

Evidence/Proof – the validation of His efforts and planning exist amid the myriad/multiplicities of what exists around us; the very trees, rocks, and hills cry out His Name above every other; this Proof is irrefutable and stands under the closest of investigation; He ALONE is the REALITY of our Living.

Proving/Signaling – each time His HAND moves across the broken strings of hearts, He Proves the very essence of Love that is HIM; the indications of His Presence evolve with every day we live, for they become the stirrings of our hearts and minds towards HIM, alone.

Apprehend/Adjust – to grasp, or catch hold of WHO He is causes us to embrace WHOSE we are; the fine-tuning we receive, we call Correction/Altering/Remodeling by His HAND that fashions us according to the individual plan He has made all of us according to.

Contrast/Parallel – every Difference is mirrored through Him; every Equivalent is detailed in referring only to Him; we have but to look through the pages written of Him to find only Him.

Spoken Word/Mouth/Speaking – all that is Him conveys His Substance through His WORD; the Channel of Faith's work comes with the single Declaration of Him, passing through our lips.

Belief/Faith – the Conviction that urges every believer onward is the Persuasion of Him towards those to whom His Weakness abounds; He LOVES us, and therefore is EVER FAITHFUL to enlarge, imbue, and enhance the very PERSON that He is within the very Object of His Love which is us.

The purpose of this author's writings is to redirect our hearts and minds back to God, and away from the self-centered, man-focused preaching and teaching we continue to hear from ecclesiastical pulpits throughout our land. As it has been in every generation, the outlook is bleak. And yet, as we place our focus upon God, where it should be, we see that the overcomer will always project toward HIM, and find His Way when there seems to be no other WAY!

May your study and every endeavor for God be blessed as your heart, your mind, your will, and your strength be applied, enlarged, and presented only to HIM!

Appendix 1:
Four Hebraic Prefixes

The idea of the form of a letter as providing meaning is foreign to our understanding, of the purpose of the alphabet. In these pages, we are going to look at five Prefixes that are commonly added to Hebrew words; ⅏/B, ∪/L, ⋀⋀/M, Y/W and ⊕/H for the purpose of additional clarification as to the words meaning, and its mood/tense. These examples will demonstrate the relationship between the pictographs of each letter, their cultural understanding and their application in the Hebrew language.

⅏ The nomadic Hebrews lived in tents and this letter is a representation of the tent. The door is in front (top left of the picture) and a wall (middle of the picture) separates the men's side (left side) from the women's side (right side). Since the family resides inside the tent, this letter means "in". When the letter ⅏/B is placed in front of a word such as ⊙Ⴖ⅄/erets (land), we have ⊙Ⴖ⅄⅏/be'arets (IN a land).

∪ The Hebrew shepherd always carried a staff and was used to move the sheep toward the destination. This letter means "to" or "toward". When the letter ∪/L is placed in front of the word ⊙Ⴖ⅄/, we have ⊙Ⴖ⅄∪/le'arets (TO a land).

⋀⋀ This letter is a picture of water and can also mean the flowing water in man and animals (blood). Blood is seen as the passing down a line from one generation to another. When this letter is prefixed to a word it means "from" in the sense of coming out of someone or something. When the letter ⋀⋀/M is placed in front of the word ⊙Ⴖ⅄, we have ⊙Ⴖ⅄⋀⋀/me'erets (FROM a land).

Y This letter is a picture of a tent peg used to secure the tent, or a nail used to attach things together. When this letter is prefixed to a word it means "and" in the sense of adding things together. When the letter Y/W is placed in front of the word ⊙Ⴖ⅄, we have ⊙Ⴖ⅄Y/ve'erets (AND land).

✞ This letter is a picture of a man's arms raised or extended toward someone or something as if saying "behold, look at this. When this letter is prefixed to a word it means "the" as in identifying someone or something in particular When the letter ✞/H is placed in front of the word ﬡﬧﬠ, we have ﬡﬧﬠ✞/ha'erets (THE land).

Ancient Hebrew Language and Alphabet ~

Jeff A. Benner;

Copyright © 2002 Jeff A. Benner Ancient Hebrew Research Center

(Permission granted to use this information, in this book, is by no means to be seen or used as an approval of the author of this book, and/or, it's suppositions, as are printed in this publication.)

*Permission for usage is contingent solely upon Mr. Benner's approval…

Appendix 2:
Semitic - Hebraic Verbs

Hebrew verbs, like English verbs, describe action. Because the Hebrew language is an action oriented language rather than descriptive, it is prolific with verbs. When a Hebrew verb is conjugated in a sentence it identifies person, number, gender, tense, mood and voice. Understanding these different aspects of a verb is essential for proper interpretation of that verb.

Person

Each verb identifies the subject of the verb as first (I), second (you)or third (he)person.

Number

Each verb also indicates the subject of the verb as singular or plural (we, you or they).

Gender

Each verb also indicates the subject of the verb as masculine (he)or feminine (she).

Tense

There are four tenses in Hebrew verbs, perfect, imperfect, participle and imperative. In the English language the verb tenses are related to time; past, present and future, while the Hebrew verbs are all related to action. The perfect tense is a completed action and in most cases is related to the English past tense (he cut). The imperfect tense is an incomplete action and is closely related to the *English present and future tenses* (he cuts or he will cut). The participle tense can be a current action or one who performs the action (a cutting or cutter). The imperative tense identifies the action, similar to a command, with no reference to the subject (cut!). When the prefix "ו/י" (waw)meaning "and" is attached to the verb, the verb tense (perfect or imperfect)reverses. For this reason this letter, when used in this context, is called the reversing or consecutive waw.

Voice

Each verb also includes voice of which there are three; active, passive or reflexive. The active voice identifies the action of the verb as coming from the subject (he cut). The passive voice does not identify the origin of action placed on the subject of the verb (he was cut). The reflexive voice places the action of the verb onto the subject (he cut himself).

Mood

Each verb also includes mood of which there are three; simple, intensive or causative. The simple mood is simple action of the verb (he cut). The intensive mood implies force or emphasis on the verb (he slashed or hacked). The causative mood expresses causation to the verb (he caused a cut).

The voice and mood of a verb is identified by seven different forms as shown in Table 9.

Table 9

Form	Mood	Voice	Example
Paal*	Simple	Active	He cut
Niphal	Simple	Passive	He was cut
Piel	Intensive	Active	He slashed
Pual	Intensive	Passive	He was slashed
Hiphil	Causative	Active	He made cut
Hophal	Causative	Passive	He was made cut
Hitpael	Intensive	Reflexive	He slashed himself

* Also called the "qal" form.

Ancient Hebrew Language and Alphabet ~

Jeff A. Benner;

Copyright © 2002 Jeff A. Benner Ancient Hebrew Research Center

(Permission granted to use this information, in this book, is by no means to be seen or used as an approval of the author of this book, and/or, it's suppositions, as are printed in this publication.)

*Permission for usage is contingent solely upon Mr. Benner's approval…

Appendix 3:
Strong's Numbers for Tense, Verb, & Mood

G5623

A simple fact/reality representing the subject as the doer/performer of the Action, reflecting the basic verb form, as a verb or a noun,

G5774 – *Tense-**Present*** - The present tense represents a simple statement of fact or reality viewed as occurring in actual time

G5784 - *Voice-**Active*** - The active voice represents the subject as the doer or performer of the action.

G5796- *Mood-**Participle*** - Corresponds for the most part to the English participle, reflecting "- ing" or "- ed" being suffixed to the basic verb form. The participle can be either like a verb or a noun.

G5625

A simple fact/reality representing the subject as the doer/performer of the Action, reflecting the basic verb form, as a verb or a noun,

G5774 – *Tense-**Present*** - The present tense represents a simple statement of fact or reality viewed as occurring in actual time

G5784 - *Voice-**Active*** - The active voice represents the subject as the doer or performer of the action.

G5796- *Mood-**Participle*** - Corresponds for the most part to the English participle, reflecting "- ing" or "- ed" being suffixed to the basic verb form. The participle can be either like a verb or a noun.

G5627

A moment-in-time-action, with the subject performing the action, in the past, present, or future,

G5780 - *Tense-**Second Aorist*** - The "second aorist" tense is identical in meaning and translation to the normal or "first" aorist tense. The only difference is in the form of spelling the words in Greek, and there is no effect upon English translation.

G5784 - *Voice-**Active*** - The active voice represents the subject as the doer or performer of the action.

G5791 - *Mood-**Indicative*** - The indicative mood is a simple statement of fact. If an action really occurs {Present} or has occurred {Past} or will occur {Future}, it will be rendered in the indicative mood.

G5628

T=A moment-in-time-action; V=with the subject performing the action; M=and expresses a command to the hearer to perform a certain action by the order and authority of the one commanding.

G5780 - *Tense-Second Aorist* - The "second aorist" tense is identical in meaning and translation to the normal or "first" aorist tense. The only difference is in the form of spelling the words in Greek, and there is no effect upon English translation.

G5784 - *Voice-Active* - The active voice represents the subject as the doer or performer of the action.

G5794 - *Mood-Imperative* - The imperative mood corresponds to the English imperative, and expresses a command to the hearer to perform a certain action by the order and authority of the one commanding.

G5629

A moment in time action, with the subject as performing the action; adding prefixes (such as "to" in to believe") reflecting purpose or result.

G5780 - *Tense-Second Aorist* - The "second aorist" tense is identical in meaning and translation to the normal or "first" aorist tense. The only difference is in the form of spelling the words in Greek, and there is no effect upon English translation.

G5784 - *Voice-Active* - The active voice represents the subject as the doer or performer of the action.

G5630

A moment in time action, with the subject as performing the action; expresses a wish or desire for an action to occur in which the completion of such is doubtful.

G5780 - *Tense-Second Aorist* - The "second aorist" tense is identical in meaning and translation to the normal or "first" aorist tense. The only difference is in the form of spelling the words in Greek, and there is no effect upon English translation.

G5784 - *Voice-Active* - The active voice represents the subject as the doer or performer of the action.

G5793- *Mood-Optative* - The optative mood expresses a wish or desire for an action to occur in which the completion of such is doubtful.

G5631

An action not to be repeated, with the subject as performing the action, really occurs {at Calvary} or has occurred {eternity past} or will occur {in the Now.

G5778 - *Tense-Perfect* - The perfect tense in Greek corresponds to the perfect tense in English, and describes an action which is viewed as having been completed in the past, once and for all, not needing to be repeated.

G5784 - *Voice-Active* - The active voice represents the subject as the doer or performer of the action.

G5791 - *Mood-Indicative* - The indicative mood is a simple statement of fact. If an action really occurs {Present} or has occurred {Past} or will occur {Future}, it will be rendered in the indicative mood.

G5632

Got Healing?

A moment in time action; with the subject as performing the action, as being a possibility or a potentiality, describing what may or may not occur, depending upon circumstances.

G5780 - **Tense-Second Aorist** - The "second aorist" tense is identical in meaning and translation to the normal or "first" aorist tense. The only difference is in the form of spelling the words in Greek, and there is no effect upon English translation.

G5784 - **Voice-Active** - The active voice represents the subject as the doer or performer of the action.

G5792- **Mood-Subjunctive** - The subjunctive mood is the mood of possibility and potentiality. The action described may or may not occur, depending upon circumstances.

G5633

A moment in time action; with the subject as performing the action, as being a possibility or a potentiality, an action really occurs or has occurred or will occur.

G5780 - **Tense-Second Aorist** - The "second aorist" tense is identical in meaning and translation to the normal or "first" aorist tense. The only difference is in the form of spelling the words in Greek, and there is no effect upon English translation.

G5788 - **Voice-Middle Deponent** - The middle deponent forms in almost all cases are translated as being in the active voice. The active voice represents the subject as the doer or performer of the action.

G5791 - **Mood-Indicative** - The indicative mood is a simple statement of fact. If an action really occurs $^{\{Present\}}$ or has occurred $^{\{Past\}}$ or will occur $^{\{Future\}}$, it will be rendered in the indicative mood.

G5634

Tense-Second Aorist	See [G5780]
Voice-Middle Deponent	See [G5788]
Mood -Imperative	See [G5794]

G5635

A moment-in-time action, with the subject as performing the action; adding prefixes (such as "to" in "to believe") reflecting purpose or result.

G5780 - **Tense-Second Aorist** - The "second aorist" tense is identical in meaning and translation to the normal or "first" aorist tense. The only difference is in the form of spelling the words in Greek, and there is no effect upon English translation.

G5788 - **Voice-Middle Deponent** - The middle deponent forms in almost all cases are translated as being in the active voice. The active voice represents the subject as the doer or performer of the action.

G5795- **Mood-Infinitive** - The Greek infinitive mood in most cases corresponds to the English infinitive, which is basically the verb with "to" prefixed, as "to believe." Like the English infinitive, the Greek infinitive can be like a noun phrase ("It is better to live than to die"), as well as to reflect purpose or result ("This was done to fulfil what the prophet said").

G5637

A moment-in-time action, with the subject as performing the action; reflecting "- ing" or "- ed" being suffixed to the basic verb for, and can be either like a verb or a noun.

<u>G5780</u> - *Tense-Second Aorist* - The "second aorist" tense is identical in meaning and translation to the normal or "first" aorist tense. The only difference is in the form of spelling the words in Greek, and there is no effect upon English translation.

<u>G5788</u> - *Voice-Middle Deponent* - The middle deponent forms in almost all cases are translated as being in the active voice. The active voice represents the subject as the doer or performer of the action.

<u>G5796</u>- *Mood-Participle* - Corresponds for the most part to the English participle, reflecting "- ing" or "- ed" being suffixed to the basic verb form. The participle can be either like a verb or a noun.

G5639

A moment-in-time action, with the subject performing the action upon themselves or for their own benefit; a s then action really occurs {Present} or has occurred {Past} or will occur {Future}.

<u>G5780</u> - *Tense-Second Aorist* - The "second aorist" tense is identical in meaning and translation to the normal or "first" aorist tense. The only difference is in the form of spelling the words in Greek, and there is no effect upon English translation.

<u>G5785</u> - *Voice-Middle* - The middle voice indicates the subject performing an action upon himself (reflexive action) or for his own benefit. E.g., "The boy groomed himself." Many verbs which occur only in middle voice forms are translated in English as having an active sense; these are called "deponent" verbs, and do not comply with the normal requirements for the middle voice.

<u>G5791</u> - *Mood-Indicative* - The indicative mood is a simple statement of fact. If an action really occurs [Present] or has occurred [Past] or will occur [Future], it will be rendered in the indicative mood.

G5642

A moment-in-time action, with the subject performing the action upon themselves or for their own benefit; reflecting "- ing" or "- ed" being suffixed to the basic verb form.

<u>G5780</u> - *Tense-Second Aorist* - The "second aorist" tense is identical in meaning and translation to the normal or "first" aorist tense. The only difference is in the form of spelling the words in Greek, and there is no effect upon English translation.

<u>G5785</u> - *Voice-Middle* - The middle voice indicates the subject performing an action upon himself (reflexive action) or for his own benefit. E.g., "The boy groomed himself." Many verbs which occur only in middle voice forms are translated in English as having an active sense; these are called "deponent" verbs, and do not comply with the normal requirements for the middle voice.

Got Healing?

G5796- *Mood-Participle* - Corresponds for the most part to the English participle, reflecting "- ing" or "- ed" being suffixed to the basic verb form. The participle can be either like a verb or a noun.

G5643

T=A moment-in-time action; V=with the subject performing the action upon themselves or for their own benefit; as the mood of possibility and potentiality. M=The action described may or may not occur, depending upon circumstances.

G5780 - *Tense-Second Aorist* - The "second aorist" tense is identical in meaning and translation to the normal or "first" aorist tense. The only difference is in the form of spelling the words in Greek, and there is no effect upon English translation.

G5785 - *Voice-Middle* - The middle voice indicates the subject performing an action upon himself (reflexive action) or for his own benefit. E.g., "The boy groomed himself." Many verbs which occur only in middle voice forms are translated in English as having an active sense; these are called "deponent" verbs, and do not comply with the normal requirements for the middle voice.

G5792- *Mood-Subjunctive* - The subjunctive mood is the mood of possibility and potentiality. The action described may or may not occur, depending upon circumstances.

G5648

A moment-in-time action, with the subject receiving the action, in the past, present, or future, .

G5780 - *Tense-Second Aorist* - The "second aorist" tense is identical in meaning and translation to the normal or "first" aorist tense. The only difference is in the form of spelling the words in Greek, and there is no effect upon English translation.

G5786 - *Voice-Passive* - The passive voice represents the subject as being the recipient of the action. Passive is being willing to wait for the manifestation.

G5791 - *Mood-Indicative* - The indicative mood is a simple statement of fact. If an action really occurs $^{\{Present\}}$ or has occurred $^{\{Past\}}$ or will occur $^{\{Future\}}$, it will be rendered in the indicative mood.

G5651

A moment-in-time action, with the subject receiving the action, , reflecting "- ing" or "- ed" being suffixed to the basic verb form. The participle can be either like a verb or a noun.

G5780 - *Tense-Second Aorist* - The "second aorist" tense is identical in meaning and translation to the normal or "first" aorist tense. The only difference is in the form of spelling the words in Greek, and there is no effect upon English translation.

G5786 - *Voice-Passive* - The passive voice represents the subject as being the recipient of the action. Passive is being willing to wait for the manifestation.

Got Healing?

<u>G5796</u>- *Mood-Participle* - Corresponds for the most part to the English participle, reflecting "- ing" or "- ed" being suffixed to the basic verb form. The participle can be either like a verb or a noun.

G5656

A simple fact or reality occurring in real time, with the subject performing the action, in the past, present, or future.

<u>G5777</u> – *Tense-Aorist* - The aorist tense characterizes by its emphasis on punctiliar action; that is, the concept of the verb is without regard for past, present, or future time. There is no direct or clear English equivalent for this tense, though it generally renders as a simple past tense in most translations.

<u>G5784</u> - *Voice-Active* - The active voice represents the subject as the doer or performer of the action.

<u>G5791</u> - *Mood-Indicative* - The indicative mood is a simple statement of fact. If an action really occurs {Present} or has occurred {Past} or will occur {Future}, it will be rendered in the indicative mood.

G5657

A simple fact or reality occurring in real time, with the subject performing the action; and expresses a command to the hearer to perform a certain action by the order and authority of the one commanding.

<u>G5777</u> – *Tense-Aorist* - The aorist tense characterizes by its emphasis on punctiliar action; that is, the concept of the verb is without regard for past, present, or future time. There is no direct or clear English equivalent for this tense, though it generally renders as a simple past tense in most translations.

<u>G5784</u> - *Voice-Active* - The active voice represents the subject as the doer or performer of the action.

<u>G5794</u> - *Mood-Imperative* - The imperative mood corresponds to the English imperative, and expresses a command to the hearer to perform a certain action by the order and authority of the one commanding.

G5658

A simple fact or reality occurring in real time, with the subject performing the action, being used like noun phrase, as well as to reflect purpose of result.

<u>G5777</u> – *Tense-Aorist* - The aorist tense characterizes by its emphasis on punctiliar action; that is, the concept of the verb is without regard for past, present, or future time. There is no direct or clear English equivalent for this tense, though it generally renders as a simple past tense in most translations.

<u>G5788</u> - *Voice-Middle Deponent* - The middle deponent forms in almost all cases are translated as being in the active voice. The active voice represents the subject as the doer or performer of the action.

<u>G5795</u>- *Mood-Infinitive* - The Greek infinitive mood in most cases corresponds to the English infinitive, which is basically the verb with "to" prefixed, as "to believe." Like the English

infinitive, the Greek infinitive can be like a noun phrase ("It is better to live than to die"), as well as to reflect purpose or result ("This was done to fulfil what the prophet said").

G5660

A simple fact or reality occurring in real time, with the subject performing the action; which is basically the verb with "to" prefixed, as "to believe." Like the English infinitive, the Greek infinitive can be like a noun phrase ("It is better to live than to die"), as well as to reflect purpose or result.

G5777 – **Tense-Aorist** - The aorist tense characterizes by its emphasis on punctiliar action; that is, the concept of the verb is without regard for past, present, or future time. There is no direct or clear English equivalent for this tense, though it generally renders as a simple past tense in most translations.

G5784 - **Voice-Active** - The active voice represents the subject as the doer or performer of the action.

G5795- **Mood-Infinitive** - The Greek infinitive mood in most cases corresponds to the English infinitive, which is basically the verb with "to" prefixed, as "to believe." Like the English infinitive, the Greek infinitive can be like a noun phrase ("It is better to live than to die"), as well as to reflect purpose or result ("This was done to fulfil what the prophet said").

G5661

A simple fact or reality occurring in real time, with the subject being passive of the action; as being a possibility or a potentiality, describing what may or may not occur, depending upon circumstances.

G5777 – **Tense-Aorist** - The aorist tense characterizes by its emphasis on punctiliar action; that is, the concept of the verb is without regard for past, present, or future time. There is no direct or clear English equivalent for this tense, though it generally renders as a simple past tense in most translations.

G5789 - **Voice-Passive Deponent** - The passive deponent forms in almost all cases are translated as being in the passive voice.

G5792- **Mood-Subjunctive** - The subjunctive mood is the mood of possibility and potentiality. The action described may or may not occur, depending upon circumstances.

G5662

A simple fact or reality occurring in real time, with the subject as the doer/performer of the action; occurring in the Present, Past, or Future.

G5777 – **Tense-Aorist** - The aorist tense characterizes by its emphasis on punctiliar action; that is, the concept of the verb is without regard for past, present, or future time. There is no direct or clear English equivalent for this tense, though it generally renders as a simple past tense in most translations.

G5788 - **Voice-Middle Deponent** - The middle deponent forms in almost all cases are translated as being in the active voice. The active voice represents the subject as the doer or performer of the action.

Got Healing?

<u>G5791</u> - *Mood-Indicative* - The indicative mood is a simple statement of fact. If an action really occurs $^{\{Present\}}$ or has occurred $^{\{Past\}}$ or will occur $^{\{Future\}}$, it will be rendered in the indicative mood.

G5666

A simple fact or reality occurring in real time, with the subject as the doer/performer of the action; corresponding for the most part to the English participle, reflecting " - ing" or " - ed" being suffixed to the basic verb form. The participle can be either like a verb or a noun,

<u>G5777</u> – *Tense-Aorist* - The aorist tense characterizes by its emphasis on punctiliar action; that is, the concept of the verb is without regard for past, present, or future time. There is no direct or clear English equivalent for this tense, though it generally renders as a simple past tense in most translations.

<u>G5788</u> - *Voice-Middle Deponent* - The middle deponent forms in almost all cases are translated as being in the active voice. The active voice represents the subject as the doer or performer of the action.

<u>G5796</u>- *Mood-Participle* - Corresponds for the most part to the English participle, reflecting "- ing" or "- ed" being suffixed to the basic verb form. The participle can be either like a verb or a noun.

G5667

A simple fact or reality occurring in real time, with the subject as the doer/performer of the action; as the mood of possibility and potentiality. The action described may or may not occur, depending upon circumstances,

<u>G5777</u> – *Tense-Aorist* - The aorist tense characterizes by its emphasis on punctiliar action; that is, the concept of the verb is without regard for past, present, or future time. There is no direct or clear English equivalent for this tense, though it generally renders as a simple past tense in most translations.

<u>G5788</u> - *Voice-Middle Deponent* - The middle deponent forms in almost all cases are translated as being in the active voice. The active voice represents the subject as the doer or performer of the action.

<u>G5792</u>- *Mood-Subjunctive* - The subjunctive mood is the mood of possibility and potentiality. The action described may or may not occur, depending upon circumstances.

G5668

A simple fact or reality occurring in real time, with the subject as the doer/performer of the action, upon himself (reflexive action) or for his own benefit; being an action that really occurs or has occurred or will occur,

<u>G5777</u> – *Tense-Aorist* - The aorist tense characterizes by its emphasis on punctiliar action; that is, the concept of the verb is without regard for past, present, or future time. There is no direct or clear English equivalent for this tense, though it generally renders as a simple past tense in most translations.

Got Healing?

<u>G5785</u> - *Voice-Middle* - The middle voice indicates the subject performing an action upon himself (reflexive action) or for his own benefit. E.g., "The boy groomed himself." Many verbs which occur only in middle voice forms are translated in English as having an active sense; these are called "deponent" verbs, and do not comply with the normal requirements for the middle voice.

<u>G5791</u> - *Mood-Indicative* - The indicative mood is a simple statement of fact. If an action really occurs ^{Present} or has occurred ^{Past} or will occur ^{Future}, it will be rendered in the indicative mood.

G5672

A simple fact or reality occurring in real time, with the subject as the doer/performer of the action, upon himself (reflexive action) or for his own benefit; being an action described that may or may not occur, depending upon circumstances.

<u>G5777</u> – *Tense-Aorist* - The aorist tense characterizes by its emphasis on punctiliar action; that is, the concept of the verb is without regard for past, present, or future time. There is no direct or clear English equivalent for this tense, though it generally renders as a simple past tense in most translations.

<u>G5785</u> - *Voice-Middle* - The middle voice indicates the subject performing an action upon himself (reflexive action) or for his own benefit. E.g., "The boy groomed himself." Many verbs which occur only in middle voice forms are translated in English as having an active sense; these are called "deponent" verbs, and do not comply with the normal requirements for the middle voice.

<u>G5792</u>- *Mood-Subjunctive* - The subjunctive mood is the mood of possibility and potentiality. The action described may or may not occur, depending upon circumstances.

G5675

A simple fact or reality occurring in real time, with the subject performing the action, in the past, present, or future.

<u>G5777</u> – *Tense-Aorist* - The aorist tense characterizes by its emphasis on punctiliar action; that is, the concept of the verb is without regard for past, present, or future time. There is no direct or clear English equivalent for this tense, though it generally renders as a simple past tense in most translations.

<u>G5789</u> - *Voice-Passive Deponent* - The passive deponent forms in almost all cases are translated as being in the passive voice. Passive is being willing to wait for the manifestation.

<u>G5791</u> - *Mood-Indicative* - The indicative mood is a simple statement of fact. If an action really occurs ^{Present} or has occurred ^{Past} or will occur ^{Future}, it will be rendered in the indicative mood.

G5679

A simple fact or reality occurring in real time, with the subject performing the action. Corresponds for the most part to the English participle, reflecting "-

ing" or "- ed" being suffixed to the basic verb form. The participle can be either like a verb or a noun.

G5777 – *Tense-Aorist* - The aorist tense characterizes by its emphasis on punctiliar action; that is, the concept of the verb is without regard for past, present, or future time. There is no direct or clear English equivalent for this tense, though it generally renders as a simple past tense in most translations.

G5789 - *Voice-Passive Deponent* - The passive deponent forms in almost all cases are translated as being in the passive voice. Passive is being willing to wait for the manifestation.

G5796- *Mood-Participle* - Corresponds for the most part to the English participle, reflecting "- ing" or "- ed" being suffixed to the basic verb form. The participle can be either like a verb or a noun.

G5680

A simple fact or reality occurring in past tense, with the subject receiving the action, in the mood of possibility and potentiality; with action described as may or may not occur, depending upon circumstances.

G5777 – *Tense-Aorist* - The aorist tense characterizes by its emphasis on punctiliar action; that is, the concept of the verb is without regard for past, present, or future time. There is no direct or clear English equivalent for this tense, though it generally renders as a simple past tense in most translations.

G5789 - *Voice-Passive Deponent* - The passive deponent forms in almost all cases are translated as being in the passive voice. Passive is being willing to wait for the manifestation.

G5792- *Mood-Subjunctive* - The subjunctive mood is the mood of possibility and potentiality. The action described may or may not occur, depending upon circumstances.

G5681

A simple fact or reality occurring in past tense, with the subject receiving the action, in the past, present, or future.

G5777 – *Tense-Aorist* - The aorist tense characterizes by its emphasis on punctiliar action; that is, the concept of the verb is without regard for past, present, or future time. There is no direct or clear English equivalent for this tense, though it generally renders as a simple past tense in most translations.

G5786 - *Voice-Passive* - The passive voice represents the subject as being the recipient of the action. Passive is being willing to wait for the manifestation.

G5791 - *Mood-Indicative* - The indicative mood is a simple statement of fact. If an action really occurs [Present] or has occurred [Past] or will occur [Future], it will be rendered in the indicative mood.

G5682

A simple fact or reality occurring in past tense, with the subject receiving the action; expresses a command to the hearer to perform a certain action by the order and authority of the one commanding.

<u>G5777</u> – *Tense-Aorist* - The aorist tense characterizes by its emphasis on punctiliar action; that is, the concept of the verb is without regard for past, present, or future time. There is no direct or clear English equivalent for this tense, though it generally renders as a simple past tense in most translations.

<u>G5786</u> - *Voice-Passive* - The passive voice represents the subject as being the recipient of the action. Passive is being willing to wait for the manifestation.

<u>G5794</u> - *Mood-Imperative* - The imperative mood corresponds to the English imperative, and expresses a command to the hearer to perform a certain action by the order and authority of the one commanding.

<u>G5683</u>

A simple fact or reality occurring in past tense, with the subject receiving the action; adding prefixes (such as "to" in to believe") reflecting purpose or result.

<u>G5777</u> – *Tense-Aorist* - The aorist tense characterizes by its emphasis on punctiliar action; that is, the concept of the verb is without regard for past, present, or future time. There is no direct or clear English equivalent for this tense, though it generally renders as a simple past tense in most translations.

<u>G5786</u> - *Voice-Passive* - The passive voice represents the subject as being the recipient of the action. Passive is being willing to wait for the manifestation.

<u>G5795</u>- *Mood-Infinitive* - The Greek infinitive mood in most cases corresponds to the English infinitive, which is basically the verb with "to" prefixed, as "to believe." Like the English infinitive, the Greek infinitive can be like a noun phrase ("It is better to live than to die"), as well as to reflect purpose or result ("This was done to fulfil what the prophet said").

<u>G5685</u>

A simple fact or reality occurring in real time, with the subject receiving the action; reflecting " - ing" or " - ed" being suffixed to the basic verb form.

<u>G5777</u> – *Tense-Aorist* - The aorist tense characterizes by its emphasis on punctiliar action; that is, the concept of the verb is without regard for past, present, or future time. There is no direct or clear English equivalent for this tense, though it generally renders as a simple past tense in most translations.

<u>G5786</u> - *Voice-Passive* - The passive voice represents the subject as being the recipient of the action. Passive is being willing to wait for the manifestation.

<u>G5796</u>- *Mood-Participle* - Corresponds for the most part to the English participle, reflecting "- ing" or "- ed" being suffixed to the basic verb form. The participle can be either like a verb or a noun.

<u>G5686</u>

T=A simple fact or reality occurring in real time; V=with the subject receiving the action; M=in the past, present, or future.

<u>G5777</u> – *Tense-Aorist* - The aorist tense characterizes by its emphasis on punctiliar action; that is, the concept of the verb is without regard for past, present, or future time. There is no direct

or clear English equivalent for this tense, though it generally renders as a simple past tense in most translations.

G5789 - Voice-**Passive Deponent** - The passive deponent forms in almost all cases are translated as being in the passive voice. Passive is being willing to wait for the manifestation.

G5791 - Mood-**Indicative** - The indicative mood is a simple statement of fact. If an action really occurs ${}^{\{Present\}}$ or has occurred ${}^{\{Past\}}$ or will occur ${}^{\{Future\}}$, it will be rendered in the indicative mood.

G5691

A simple fact or reality occurring in real time, represents the subject as being the recipient of the action. Passive is being willing to wait for the manifestation.

G5781 – Tense-**Second Future** - The second future tense corresponds to the English future, and indicates the contemplated or certain occurrence of an event which has not yet occurred.

G5786 - Voice-**Passive** - The passive voice represents the subject as being the recipient of the action. Passive is being willing to wait for the manifestation.

G5791 - Mood-**Indicative** - The indicative mood is a simple statement of fact. If an action really occurs ${}^{\{Present\}}$ or has occurred ${}^{\{Past\}}$ or will occur ${}^{\{Future\}}$, it will be rendered in the indicative mood.

G5692

A simple fact or reality occurring in real time, with the subject performing the action, in the past, present, or future.

G5776 – Tense-**Future** - The future tense corresponds to the English future, and indicates the contemplated or certain occurrence of an event which has not yet occurred.

G5784 - Voice-**Active** - The active voice represents the subject as the doer or performer of the action.

G5791 - Mood-**Indicative** - The indicative mood is a simple statement of fact. If an action really occurs ${}^{\{Present\}}$ or has occurred ${}^{\{Past\}}$ or will occur ${}^{\{Future\}}$, it will be rendered in the indicative mood.

G5694

Indicating the contemplated or certain occurrence of an event, which has not yet occurred; with the subject performing the action, Corresponds for the most part to the English participle, reflecting " - ing" or " - ed" being suffixed to the basic verb form. The participle can be either like a verb or a noun.

G5776 – Tense-**Future** - The future tense corresponds to the English future, and indicates the contemplated or certain occurrence of an event, which has not yet occurred.

G5784 - Voice-**Active** - The active voice represents the subject as the doer or performer of the action.

G5796- Mood-**Participle** - Corresponds for the most part to the English participle, reflecting "- ing" or "- ed" being suffixed to the basic verb form. The participle can be either like a verb or a noun.

Got Healing?

G5695

Indicating the contemplated or certain occurrence of an event, which has not yet occurred; with the subject performing the action, a simple statement of fact; as an action really occurs or has occurred or will occur.

G5776 – *Tense-Future* - The future tense corresponds to the English future, and indicates the contemplated or certain occurrence of an event, which has not yet occurred.

G5788 - *Voice-Middle Deponent* - The middle deponent forms in almost all cases are translated as being in the active voice. The active voice represents the subject as the doer or performer of the action.

G5791 - *Mood-Indicative* - The indicative mood is a simple statement of fact. If an action really occurs $^{\{Present\}}$ or has occurred $^{\{Past\}}$ or will occur $^{\{Future\}}$, it will be rendered in the indicative mood.

G5697

A simple fact or reality occurring in real time, with the subject performing the action, in the past, present, or future.

G5776 – *Tense-Future* - The future tense corresponds to the English future, and indicates the contemplated or certain occurrence of an event which has not yet occurred.

G5784 - *Voice-Active* - The active voice represents the subject as the doer or performer of the action.

G5791 - *Mood-Indicative* - The indicative mood is a simple statement of fact. If an action really occurs $^{\{Present\}}$ or has occurred $^{\{Past\}}$ or will occur $^{\{Future\}}$, it will be rendered in the indicative mood.

G5701

A fact or reality indicates the contemplated or certain occurrence of an event which has not yet occurred; representing the subject as the doer/receiver of the action; as an action really occurs or has occurred or will occur.

G5776 – *Tense-Future* - The future tense corresponds to the English future, and indicates the contemplated or certain occurrence of an event which has not yet occurred.

G5786 - *Voice-Passive* - The passive voice represents the subject as being the recipient of the action. Passive is being willing to wait for the manifestation.

G5791 - *Mood-Indicative* - The indicative mood is a simple statement of fact. If an action really occurs $^{\{Present\}}$ or has occurred $^{\{Past\}}$ or will occur $^{\{Future\}}$, it will be rendered in the indicative mood.

G5703

A fact or reality indicates the contemplated or certain occurrence of an event which has not yet occurred; representing the subject as the doer/receiver of the action; as an of possibility and potentiality. The action described may or may not occur, depending upon circumstances.

G5776 – *Tense-Future* - The future tense corresponds to the English future, and indicates the contemplated or certain occurrence of an event which has not yet occurred.

Got Healing?

G5786 - *Voice-Passive* - The passive voice represents the subject as being the recipient of the action. Passive is being willing to wait for the manifestation.

G5792- *Mood-Subjunctive* - The subjunctive mood is the mood of possibility and potentiality. The action described may or may not occur, depending upon circumstances.

G5704

A fact or reality indicates the contemplated or certain occurrence of an event which has not yet occurred; representing the subject as the doer/performer of the action; as an action really occurs or has occurred or will occur.

G5776 – *Tense-Future* - The future tense corresponds to the English future, and indicates the contemplated or certain occurrence of an event which has not yet occurred.

G5799 - *No Tense or Voice Stated* - In almost all of these cases, one can assume that the tense is Present and the voice is Active, especially when the sense is that of a command (Imperative).

G5791 - *Mood-Indicative* - The indicative mood is a simple statement of fact. If an action really occurs $^{\{Present\}}$ or has occurred $^{\{Past\}}$ or will occur $^{\{Future\}}$, it will be rendered in the indicative mood.

G5707

T=A fact or reality representing continual or repeated action; V=with the subject performing the action; M=in the past, present, or future.

G5775 – *Tense-Imperfect* - represents continual or repeated action. Where the present tense might indicate "they are asking, " the imperfect would indicate "they kept on asking." In the case of the verb "to be, " however, the imperfect tense is used as a general past tense and does not carry the connotation of continual or repeated action.

G5784 - *Voice-Active* - The active voice represents the subject as the doer or performer of the action.

G5791 - *Mood-Indicative* - The indicative mood is a simple statement of fact. If an action really occurs $^{\{Present\}}$ or has occurred $^{\{Past\}}$ or will occur $^{\{Future\}}$, it will be rendered in the indicative mood.

G5711

A fact or reality representing continual or repeated action; with the subject performing the action, in the past, present, or future.

G5775 – *Tense-Imperfect* - represents continual or repeated action. Where the present tense might indicate "they are asking, " the imperfect would indicate "they kept on asking." In the case of the verb "to be, " however, the imperfect tense is used as a general past tense and does not carry the connotation of continual or repeated action.

G5790 - *Voice-Middle or Passive Deponent* - The middle or passive deponent forms in almost all cases are translated as being in the active voice. Passive is being willing to wait for the manifestation.

G5791 - *Mood-Indicative* - The indicative mood is a simple statement of fact. If an action really occurs {Present} or has occurred {Past} or will occur {Future}, it will be rendered in the indicative mood.

G5713

A fact or reality representing continual or repeated action; with the subject performing the action, as it really occurs or has occurred or will occur.

G5775 – *Tense-Imperfect* - represents continual or repeated action. Where the present tense might indicate "they are asking," the imperfect would indicate "they kept on asking." In the case of the verb "to be," however, the imperfect tense is used as a general past tense and does not carry the connotation of continual or repeated action.

G5799 - *No Tense or Voice Stated* - In almost all of these cases, one can assume that the tense is Present and the voice is Active, especially when the sense is that of a command (Imperative).

G5791 - *Mood-Indicative* - The indicative mood is a simple statement of fact. If an action really occurs {Present} or has occurred {Past} or will occur {Future}, it will be rendered in the indicative mood.

G5719

T=A simple fact or reality occurring in real time; V=with the subject performing the action; M=in the past, present, or future.

G5774 – *Tense-Present* - The present tense represents a simple statement of fact or reality viewed as occurring in actual time

G5784 - *Voice-Active* - The active voice represents the subject as the doer or performer of the action.

G5794 - *Mood-Imperative* - The imperative mood corresponds to the English imperative, and expresses a command to the hearer to perform a certain action by the order and authority of the one commanding.

G5720

A simple fact or reality occurring in actual time, showing the subject as the doer, expressing a command to the hearer to realize a certain action through the authority of the One commanding.

G5774 – *Tense-Present* - The present tense represents a simple statement of fact or reality viewed as occurring in actual time

G5784 - *Voice-Active* - The active voice represents the subject as the doer or performer of the action.

G5791 - *Mood-Imperative* - The imperative mood expresses a command to the hearer to realize a certain action by the order and authority of the one commanding.

G5721

A simple fact or reality occurring in real time, with the subject performing an action, adding prefixes (such as "to" in "to believe") reflecting purpose or result.

G5774 – *Tense-Present* - The present tense represents a simple statement of fact or reality viewed as occurring in actual time

G5784 - *Voice-Active* - The active voice represents the subject as the doer or performer of the action.

G5795- *Mood-Infinitive* - The Greek infinitive mood in most cases corresponds to the English infinitive, which is basically the verb with "to" prefixed, as "to believe." Like the English infinitive, the Greek infinitive can be like a noun phrase ("It is better to live than to die"), as well as to reflect purpose or result ("This was done to fulfil what the prophet said").

G5723

T=A simple fact or reality occurring in real time; V=with the subject performing an action; M=reflecting "- ing" or "- ed" being suffixed to the basic verb form. The participle can be like a verb or a noun.

G5774 – *Tense-Present* - The present tense represents a simple statement of fact or reality viewed as occurring in actual time

G5784 - *Voice-Active* - The active voice represents the subject as the doer or performer of the action.

G5796- *Mood-Participle* - Corresponds for the most part to the English participle, reflecting "- ing" or "- ed" being suffixed to the basic verb form. The participle can be either like a verb or a noun.

G5725

A simple fact or reality occurring in actual time, with the subject performing an action; being in mood as a possibility or potentiality; the action described may or may not occur, depending upon circumstances.

G5774 – *Tense-Present* - The present tense represents a simple statement of fact or reality viewed as occurring in actual time

G5784 - *Voice-Active* - The active voice represents the subject as the doer or performer of the action.

G5792- *Mood-Subjunctive* - The subjunctive mood is the mood of possibility and potentiality. The action described may or may not occur, depending upon circumstances.

G5729

A simple fact or reality occurring in actual time, with the subject performing the action; reflecting purpose or result, either actively or passively.

G5774 – *Tense-Present* - The present tense represents a simple statement of fact or reality viewed as occurring in actual time

G5787 - *Voice-Either Middle or Passive* - Many of the so-called "deponent" verbs can have either a middle or passive form. These are normally translated as having an active voice, since they have no active form in their outward spelling. At times, however, they retain their middle or passive significance.

G5795- *Mood-Infinitive* - The Greek infinitive mood in most cases corresponds to the English infinitive, which is basically the verb with "to" prefixed, as "to believe." Like the English infinitive, the Greek infinitive can be like a noun phrase ("It is better to live than to die"), as well as to reflect purpose or result ("This was done to fulfil what the prophet said").

G5730

A simple fact or reality occurring in actual time, with the subject performing the action; reflecting "- ing" or "- ed" being suffixed to the basic verb form. The participle can be either like a verb or a noun, as in English, and thus is often termed a "verbal noun."

G5774 – *Tense-***Present** - The present tense represents a simple statement of fact or reality viewed as occurring in actual time

G5787 - *Voice-***Either** *Middle* **or** *Passive* - Many of the so-called "deponent" verbs can have either a middle or passive form. These are normally translated as having an active voice, since they have no active form in their outward spelling. At times, however, they retain their middle or passive significance.

G5796 - *Mood-***Participle** - The Greek participle corresponds for the most part to the English participle, reflecting "- ing" or "- ed" being suffixed to the basic verb form. The participle can be either like a verb or a noun, as in English, and thus is often termed a "verbal noun."

G5731

A simple fact or reality occurring in real time, with the subject performing an action upon one's own self (reflexive action) or for their own benefit; expresses a simple statement of fact; as it will be an action that really occurs or has occurred or will occur.

G5774 – *Tense-***Present** - The present tense represents a simple statement of fact or reality viewed as occurring in actual time.

G5785 - *Voice-**Middle*** - The middle voice indicates the subject performing an action upon himself (reflexive action) or for his own benefit. E.g., "The boy groomed himself." Many verbs which occur only in middle voice forms are translated in English as having an active sense; these are called "deponent" verbs, and do not comply with the normal requirements for the middle voice.

G5791 - *Mood-**Indicative*** - The indicative mood is a simple statement of fact; as an action really occurs or has occurred or will occur.

G5732

A simple fact or reality occurring in real time, with the subject performing an action upon one's own self (reflexive action) or for their own benefit; expresses a command to the hearer to perform a certain action by the order and authority of the one commanding.

G5774 – *Tense-***Present** - The present tense represents a simple statement of fact or reality viewed as occurring in actual time.

G5785 - *Voice-**Middle*** - The middle voice indicates the subject performing an action upon himself (reflexive action) or for his own benefit. E.g., "The boy groomed himself." Many verbs which occur only in middle voice forms are translated in English as having an active sense; these are called "deponent" verbs, and do not comply with the normal requirements for the middle voice.

G5794 - *Mood-Imperative* - The imperative mood corresponds to the English imperative, and expresses a command to the hearer to perform a certain action by the order and authority of the one commanding.

G5733

A simple fact or reality occurring in real time, with the subject performing an action upon one's own self (reflexive action) or for their own benefit, adding prefixes (such as "to" in "to believe") reflecting purpose or result.

G5774 – *Tense-Present* - The present tense represents a simple statement of fact or reality viewed as occurring in actual time.

G5785 - *Voice-Middle* - The middle voice indicates the subject performing an action upon himself (reflexive action) or for his own benefit. E.g., "The boy groomed himself." Many verbs which occur only in middle voice forms are translated in English as having an active sense; these are called "deponent" verbs, and do not comply with the normal requirements for the middle voice.

G5795- *Mood-Infinitive* - The Greek infinitive mood in most cases corresponds to the English infinitive, which is basically the verb with "to" prefixed, as "to believe." Like the English infinitive, the Greek infinitive can be like a noun phrase ("It is better to live than to die"), as well as to reflect purpose or result ("This was done to fulfil what the prophet said").

G5734

A simple fact or reality occurring in actual time, indicating the subject performing an action upon themselves (reflexive action), or for their own benefit, reflecting either an "-ing" or "-ed" being suffixed to the basic verb form, becoming a "verbal noun,

G5774 – *Tense-Present* - The present tense represents a simple statement of fact or reality viewed as occurring in actual time.

G5785 - *Voice-Middle* - The middle voice indicates the subject performing an action upon himself (reflexive action) or for his own benefit. E.g., "The boy groomed himself." Many verbs which occur only in middle voice forms are translated in English as having an active sense; these are called "deponent" verbs, and do not comply with the normal requirements for the middle voice.

G5796 - *Mood-Participle* - The Greek participle corresponds for the most part to the English participle, reflecting "- ing" or "- ed" being suffixed to the basic verb form. The participle can be either like a verb or a noun, as in English, and thus is often termed a "verbal noun."

G5735

A simple fact or reality occurring in actual time, indicating the subject performing an action upon themselves (reflexive action), or for their own

Got Healing?

benefit, the mood of possibility and potentiality. The action described may or may not occur, depending upon circumstances.

G5774 – Tense-Present - The present tense represents a simple statement of fact or reality viewed as occurring in actual time.

G5785 - Voice-Middle - The middle voice indicates the subject performing an action upon himself (reflexive action) or for his own benefit. E.g., "The boy groomed himself." Many verbs which occur only in middle voice forms are translated in English as having an active sense; these are called "deponent" verbs, and do not comply with the normal requirements for the middle voice.

G5792- Mood-Subjunctive - The subjunctive mood is the mood of possibility and potentiality. The action described may or may not occur, depending upon circumstances.

G5736

A simple fact or reality, with the subject as performing the action, as it will be an action that really occurs or has occurred or will occur.

G5774 – Tense-Present - The present tense represents a simple statement of fact or reality viewed as occurring in actual time.

G5790 - Voice-Middle or Passive Deponent - The middle or passive deponent forms in almost all cases are translated as being in the active voice. Passive is being willing to wait for the manifestation.

G5791 - Mood-Indicative - The indicative mood is a simple statement of fact. If an action really occurs $^{\{Present\}}$ or has occurred $^{\{Past\}}$ or will occur $^{\{Future\}}$, it will be rendered in the indicative mood.

G5737

A simple fact or reality occurring in actual time; with the subject as performing the action, and being willing to wait; accepting that this verb expresses a command to the hearer to perform a certain action by the order and authority of the one commanding.

G5774 – Tense-Present - The present tense represents a simple statement of fact or reality viewed as occurring in actual time.

G5790 - Voice-Middle or Passive Deponent - The middle or passive deponent forms in almost all cases are translated as being in the active voice. Passive is being willing to wait for the manifestation.

G5794 - Mood-Imperative - The imperative mood corresponds to the English imperative, and expresses a command to the hearer to perform a certain action by the order and authority of the one commanding.

G5738

A simple fact or reality, with the subject as performing the action; which is basically the verb with "to" prefixed, as "to believe." Like the English infinitive, the Greek infinitive can be like a noun phrase ("It is better to live than to die"), as well as to reflect purpose or result.

Got Healing?

<u>G5774</u> – *Tense-* **Present** - The present tense represents a simple statement of fact or reality viewed as occurring in actual time.

<u>G5790</u> - *Voice-* **Middle** *or* **Passive Deponent** - The middle or passive deponent forms in almost all cases are translated as being in the active voice. See "Active" [*G5784*] Passive is being willing to wait for the manifestation.

<u>G5795</u>- *Mood-* **Infinitive** - The Greek infinitive mood in most cases corresponds to the English infinitive, which is basically the verb with "to" prefixed, as "to believe." Like the English infinitive, the Greek infinitive can be like a noun phrase ("It is better to live than to die"), as well as to reflect purpose or result ("This was done to fulfil what the prophet said").

G5740

A simple fact or reality, with the subject as performing the action; reflecting "-ing" or "-ed" being suffixed to the basic verb form, used as either a verb or noun.

<u>G5774</u> – *Tense-* **Present** - The present tense represents a simple statement of fact or reality viewed as occurring in actual time.

<u>G5790</u> - *Voice-* **Middle** *or* **Passive Deponent** - The middle or passive deponent forms in almost all cases are translated as being in the active voice. See "Active" [*G5784*] Passive is being willing to wait for the manifestation.

<u>G5796</u> - *Mood-* **Participle** - The Greek participle corresponds for the most part to the English participle, reflecting "- ing" or "- ed" being suffixed to the basic verb form. The participle can be either like a verb or a noun, as in English, and thus is often termed a "verbal noun."

G5741

A simple fact or reality, with the subject as performing the action; with the mood of possibility and potentiality. The action described may or may not occur, depending upon circumstances.

<u>G5774</u> – *Tense-* **Present** - The present tense represents a simple statement of fact or reality viewed as occurring in actual time.

<u>G5790</u> - *Voice-* **Middle** *or* **Passive Deponent** - The middle or passive deponent forms in almost all cases are translated as being in the active voice. See "Active" [*G5784*] Passive is being willing to wait for the manifestation.

<u>G5792</u>- *Mood-* **Subjunctive** - The subjunctive mood is the mood of possibility and potentiality. The action described may or may not occur, depending upon circumstances.

G5743

A simple statement of fact/reality occurring in actual time; commanding the hearer and expresses a command to the hearer to perform; If as an action really occurs {Present} or has occurred {Past} or will occur {Future}.

<u>G5774</u> - *Tense-* - The present tense represents a simple statement of fact or reality viewed as occurring in actual time.

<u>G5786</u> - Voice-**Passive** - The passive voice represents the subject as being the recipient of the action. Passive is being willing to wait for the manifestation.

<u>G5791</u> - Mood-**Indicative** - The indicative mood is a simple statement of fact. If an action really occurs ^{Present} or has occurred ^{Past} or will occur ^{Future}, it will be rendered in the indicative mood.

G5744

A simple statement of fact/reality occurring in actual time, commanding the hearer and expresses a command to the hearer to perform a certain action by the order and authority of the one commanding.

<u>G5774</u> - Tense- - The present tense represents a simple statement of fact or reality viewed as occurring in actual time.

<u>G5786</u> - Voice-**Passive** - The passive voice represents the subject as being the recipient of the action. Passive is being willing to wait for the manifestation.

<u>G5794</u> - Mood-**Imperative** - The imperative mood corresponds to the English imperative, and expresses a command to the hearer to perform a certain action by the order and authority of the one commanding.

G5745

A simple statement of fact/reality occurring in actual time, commanding the hearer and expresses a command to the hearer to perform the verb with "to" prefixed, as in "to believe." It can be like a noun phrase ("It is better to live than to die"), as well as to reflect purpose or result.

<u>G5774</u> - Tense- - The present tense represents a simple statement of fact or reality viewed as occurring in actual time.

<u>G5786</u> - Voice-**Passive** - The passive voice represents the subject as being the recipient of the action. Passive is being willing to wait for the manifestation.

<u>G5795</u>- Mood-**Infinitive** - The Greek infinitive mood in most cases corresponds to the English infinitive, which is basically the verb with "to" prefixed, as "to believe." Like the English infinitive, the Greek infinitive can be like a noun phrase ("It is better to live than to die"), as well as to reflect purpose or result ("This was done to fulfil what the prophet said").

G5746

A simple statement of fact/reality occurring in actual time, commanding the hearer to receive certain action(s) reflecting "-ing" or "-ed" being suffixed to the basic verb form, used as either a verb or noun.

<u>G5774</u> - Tense- - The present tense represents a simple statement of fact or reality viewed as occurring in actual time.

<u>G5786</u> - Voice-**Passive** - The passive voice represents the subject as being the recipient of the action. Passive is being willing to wait for the manifestation.

<u>G5796</u> - Mood-**Participle** - The Greek participle corresponds for the most part to the

Got Healing?

English participle, reflecting "- ing" or "- ed" being suffixed to the basic verb form. The participle can be either like a verb or a noun, as in English, and thus is often termed a "verbal noun."

G5748

A simple statement of fact/reality occurring in actual time; commanding the hearer to perform certain action(s) in the past, present, or future.

G5774 - *Tense* - The present tense represents a simple statement of fact or reality viewed as occurring in actual time.

G5799 - *No Tense or Voice Stated* - In almost all of these cases, one can assume that the tense is Present and the voice is Active, especially when the sense is that of a command (Imperative).

G5791 - *Mood-Indicative* - The indicative mood is a simple statement of fact. If an action really occurs $^{\{Present\}}$ or has occurred $^{\{Past\}}$ or will occur $^{\{Future\}}$, it will be rendered in the indicative mood.

G5749

A simple statement of fact/reality occurring in actual time, commanding the hearer to perform certain action(s) by order of the one commanding.

G5774 - *Tense-Perfect* - The present tense represents a simple statement of fact or reality viewed as occurring in actual time.

G5799 - *No Tense or Voice Stated* - In almost all of these cases, one can assume that the tense is Present and the voice is Active, especially when the sense is that of a command (Imperative).

G5794 - *Mood-Imperative* - The imperative mood corresponds to the English imperative, and expresses a command to the hearer to perform a certain action by the order and authority of the one commanding.

G5750

A simple statement of fact/reality occurring in actual time, commanding the hearer to perform certain action(s) corresponding to the English infinitive, which is basically the verb with "to" prefixed, as "to believe." Like the English infinitive, the Greek infinitive can be like a noun phrase ("It is better to live than to die"), as well as to reflect purpose or result.

G5774 - *Tense-Perfect* - The present tense represents a simple statement of fact or reality viewed as occurring in actual time.

G5799 - *No Tense or Voice Stated* - In almost all of these cases, one can assume that the tense is Present and the voice is Active, especially when the sense is that of a command (Imperative).

G5795- *Mood-Infinitive* - The Greek infinitive mood in most cases corresponds to the English infinitive, which is basically the verb with "to" prefixed, as "to believe." Like the English infinitive, the Greek infinitive can be like a noun phrase ("It is better to live than to die"), as well as to reflect purpose or result ("This was done to fulfil what the prophet said").

G5752

Got Healing?

A simple statement of fact/reality occurring in actual time, reflecting "- ing"
or "- ed" being suffixed to the basic verb form; and can be either like a verb
or a noun.

<u>G5774</u> - *Tense-**Perfect*** - The present tense represents a simple statement of fact or reality viewed as occurring in actual time.

<u>G5799</u> - *No Tense or Voice Stated* - In almost all of these cases, one can assume that the tense is Present and the voice is Active, especially when the sense is that of a command (Imperative).

<u>G5796</u> - *Mood-**Participle*** - The Greek participle corresponds for the most part to the English participle, reflecting "- ing" or "- ed" being suffixed to the basic verb form. The participle can be either like a verb or a noun, as in English, and thus is often termed a "verbal noun."

<u>G5753</u>

A simple statement of fact/reality occurring in actual time, with the subject
performing the action; which action may or may not occur, depending upon the
circumstances.

<u>G5774</u> - *Tense-**Perfect*** - The present tense represents a simple statement of fact or reality viewed as occurring in actual time.

<u>G5799</u> - *No Tense or Voice Stated* - In almost all of these cases, one can assume that the tense is Present and the voice is Active, especially when the sense is that of a command (Imperative).

<u>G5792</u>- *Mood-**Subjunctive*** - The subjunctive mood is the mood of possibility and potentiality. The action described may or may not occur, depending upon circumstances.

<u>G5754</u>

Represents continual or repeated action; with the subject as the
doer/performer of the action; occurring in as Present, Past, or Future tense.

<u>G5775</u> – *Tense-**Imperfect*** - represents continual or repeated action. Where the present tense might indicate "they are asking, " the imperfect would indicate "they kept on asking." In the case of the verb "to be, " however, the imperfect tense is used as a general past tense and does not carry the connotation of continual or repeated action.

<u>G5799</u> - *No Tense or Voice Stated* - In almost all of these cases, one can assume that the tense is Present and the voice is Active, especially when the sense is that of a command (Imperative).

<u>G5791</u> - *Mood-**Indicative*** - The indicative mood is a simple statement of fact. If an action really occurs [Present] or has occurred [Past] or will occur [Future], it will be rendered in the indicative mood.

<u>G5755</u>

describes an action viewed as completed in the past, once and for all, not
needing to be repeated; with the subject as the doer/performer of the action;
basically the verb with "to" prefixed, as "to believe." Like the English

---

infinitive, the Greek infinitive can be like a noun phrase ("It is better to live than to die"), as well as to reflect purpose or result.

G5778 – Tense-**Second Perfect** - describes an action viewed as completed in the past, once and for all, not needing to be repeated.

G5784 - Voice-**Active** - The active voice represents the subject as the doer or performer of the action.

G5795- Mood-**Infinitive** - The Greek infinitive mood in most cases corresponds to the English infinitive, which is basically the verb with "to" prefixed, as "to believe." Like the English infinitive, the Greek infinitive can be like a noun phrase ("It is better to live than to die"), as well as to reflect purpose or result ("This was done to fulfil what the prophet said").

G5756

Represents continual or repeated action; with the subject as the doer/performer of the action; corresponding for the most part to the English participle, reflecting "- ing" or "- ed" being suffixed to the basic verb form. The participle can be either like a verb or a noun.

G5775 – Tense-**Second Perfect** - The second perfect is identical in meaning to that of the normal or "first" perfect tense, and has no additional effect on English translation. The classification merely represents a spelling variation in Greek.

G5784 - Voice-**Active** - The active voice represents the subject as the doer or performer of the action.

G5796- Mood-**Participle** - Corresponds for the most part to the English participle, reflecting "- ing" or "- ed" being suffixed to the basic verb form. The participle can be either like a verb or a noun.

G5758

An action of the past, once and for all, not needing to be repeated with the subject performing the action; as really occurring or has occurred or will occur.

G5778 - Tense-**Perfect** - The perfect tense in Greek corresponds to the perfect tense in English, and describes an action which is viewed as having been completed in the past, once and for all, not needing to be repeated.

G5784 - Voice-**Active** - The active voice represents the subject as the doer or performer of the action.

G5791 - Mood-**Indicative** - The indicative mood is a simple statement of fact. If an action really occurs $^{\{Present\}}$ or has occurred $^{\{Past\}}$ or will occur $^{\{Future\}}$, it will be rendered in the indicative mood.

G5760

An action of the past, once and for all, not needing to be repeated with the subject performing the action; as really occurring {Present} or has occurred {Past} or will occur {Future}

G5778 - _Tense-Perfect_ - The perfect tense in Greek corresponds to the perfect tense in English, and describes an action which is viewed as having been completed in the past, once and for all, not needing to be repeated.

G5784 - _Voice-Active_ - The active voice represents the subject as the doer or performer of the action.

G5791 - _Mood-Indicative_ - The indicative mood is a simple statement of fact. If an action really occurs $^{\{Present\}}$ or has occurred $^{\{Past\}}$ or will occur $^{\{Future\}}$, it will be rendered in the indicative mood.

G5761

An action of the past not repeated, with the subject performing the action, as an action really occurs or has occurred or will occur.

G5778 - _Tense-Perfect_ - The perfect tense in Greek corresponds to the perfect tense in English, and describes an action which is viewed as having been completed in the past, once and for all, not needing to be repeated.

G5784 - _Voice-Active_ - The active voice represents the subject as the doer or performer of the action.

G5791 - _Mood-Indicative_ - The indicative mood is a simple statement of fact. If an action really occurs $^{\{Present\}}$ or has occurred $^{\{Past\}}$ or will occur $^{\{Future\}}$, it will be rendered in the indicative mood.

G5762

An action of the past not repeated, with the subject performing the action, as the mood of possibility and potentiality. The action described may or may not occur, depending upon circumstances.

G5778 - _Tense-Perfect_ - The perfect tense in Greek corresponds to the perfect tense in English, and describes an action which is viewed as having been completed in the past, once and for all, not needing to be repeated.

G5784 - _Voice-Active_ - The active voice represents the subject as the doer or performer of the action.

G5792- _Mood-Subjunctive_ - The subjunctive mood is the mood of possibility and potentiality. The action described may or may not occur, depending upon circumstances.

G5769

An action of the past not repeated, with the subject receiving the action, reflecting "-ing" or "-ed" being suffixed to the basic verb form, used as either a verb or noun.

G5778 - _Tense-Perfect_ - The perfect tense in Greek corresponds to the perfect tense in English, and describes an action which is viewed as having been completed in the past, once and for all, not needing to be repeated.

G5786 - _Voice-Passive_ - The passive voice represents the subject as being the recipient of the action. Passive is being willing to wait for the manifestation.

Got Healing?

<u>G5791</u> - *Mood-**Indicative*** - The indicative mood is a simple statement of fact. If an action really occurs ^{Present} or has occurred ^{Past} or will occur ^{Future}, it will be rendered in the indicative mood.

G5771

*An action of the past not repeated, with the subject performing an action
upon themselves, or for their own benefit; reflecting "-ing" or "-ed" being
suffixed to the basic verb form, used as either a verb or noun.*

<u>G5777</u> – *Tense-**Aorist*** - The aorist tense is characterized by its emphasis on punctiliar action; that is, the concept of the verb is considered without regard for past, present, or future time. There is no direct or clear English equivalent for this tense, though it is generally rendered as a simple past tense in most translations.

<u>G5785</u> - *Voice-**Middle*** - The middle voice indicates the subject performing an action upon themselves (reflexive action) or for their own benefit. E.g., "The boy groomed himself." Many verbs which occur only in middle voice forms are translated in English as having an active sense; these are called "deponent" verbs, and do not comply with the normal requirements for the middle voice.

<u>G5796</u>- *Mood-**Participle*** - Corresponds for the most part to the English participle, reflecting "- ing" or "- ed" being suffixed to the basic verb form. The participle can be either like a verb or a noun.

G5772

*Describes an action which is viewed as having been completed in the past,
once and for all, not needing to be repeated; represents the subject as being
the recipient of the action; as action really occurs or has occurred or will
occur.*

<u>G5778</u> - *Tense-**Perfect*** - The perfect tense in Greek corresponds to the perfect tense in English, and describes an action which is viewed as having been completed in the past, once and for all, not needing to be repeated.

<u>G5786</u> - *Voice-**Passive*** - The passive voice represents the subject as being the recipient of the action. Passive is being willing to wait for the manifestation.

<u>G5791</u> - *Mood-**Indicative*** - The indicative mood is a simple statement of fact. If an action really occurs ^{Present} or has occurred ^{Past} or will occur ^{Future}, it will be rendered in the indicative mood.

<u>G5777</u> - *Tense-**Aorist*** - The aorist tense is characterized by its emphasis relating to a moment in time action; that is, <u>the concept of the verb is considered without regard for past, present, or future time</u>. There is no direct or clear English equivalent for this tense, though it is generally rendered as a simple past tense in most translations.

The events described by the aorist tense are classified into a number of categories by grammarians. The most common of these include a view of the action as having begun from a certain point ("inceptive aorist"), or having ended at a certain point ("cumulative aorist"), or merely existing at a certain point ("punctiliar aorist"). The categorization of other cases can be found in Greek reference grammars.

The English reader need not concern himself with most of these finer points concerning the aorist tense, since in most cases they cannot be rendered accurately in English translation, being fine points of Greek exegesis only. The common practice of rendering an aorist by a simple English past tense should suffice in most cases.

Appendix 4:
Hebrew = Old Testament

H8675

S=Simple, causative, sometimes reflexive action; M=as an order, or a command.

H8818 *Stem -Hiphil* = expresses causative action, sometimes reflective.

H8810 *Mood -Imperative* = expresses an order or a command.

H8685

S=Simple, causative, sometimes reflexive action; M=as an order, or a command.

H8818 *Stem -Hiphil* = expresses causative action, sometimes reflective.

H8810 *Mood -Imperative* = expresses an order or a command.

H8686

S=Simple, causative, sometime reflexive action;
M=as an action, process, or condition incomplete.

H8818 *Stem -Hiphil* = expresses causative action, sometimes reflective.

H8811 *Mood -Imperfect* = expresses an action, process, or condition which is incomplete.

H8687

S=Simple, causative, sometime reflexive action; M=as an action, process, or condition incomplete.

H8818 *Stem -Hiphil* = expresses causative action, sometimes reflective.

H8812 *Mood -Infinitive* = expresses combination of a word plus a verb, and therefore it expresses action or a state of being.

H8688

S=Simple expressing of causative action, process/condition, in its unbroken continuity, M=and may be used of present, past, or future time.

H8818 *Stem -Hiphil* = expresses causative action, sometimes reflective.

H8813 *Mood -Participle* = represents an action or condition in its unbroken continuity, and may be used of present, past or future time.

H8689

S=Simple, causative, sometime reflexive action, M=completed at a time or the present.

H8818 *Stem -Hiphil* = expresses causative action, sometimes reflective.

H8816 *Mood -Perfect* = expresses a completed action; referring to a time, or the present.

H8690

Got Healing?

A reflexive, reciprocal, or simple action, expressing a completed action;
referring to a time, or the present.

H8819 Stem -Hithpael = expresses a reflexive, reciprocal, or simple action.

H8816 Mood -Perfect = expresses a completed action; referring to a time, or the present.

H8691

S=A reflexive, reciprocal, or simple action, M=as being an action,
process, or condition which is incomplete.

H8819 Stem -Hithpael = expresses a reflexive, reciprocal, or simple action.

H8811 Mood -Imperfect = expresses an action, process, or condition which is incomplete.

H8714

Simple expressing of passive action, process/condition, incomplete, while
having a wide range of meaning.

H8825 Stem -Hophal = expresses passive causative action, sometimes passive reflective. Passive is being willing to wait for the manifestation.

H8811 Mood -Imperfect = expresses an action, process or condition which is incomplete, and it has a wide range of meaning.

H8734

S=Expresses simple action, sometimes reflective; M=expressing an order
or a command/directive/mandate.

H8833 Stem -Niphal = expresses simple action, sometimes reflective.

H8810 Mood -Imperative = expresses an order or a command/directive/man-date.

H8735

S=Simple, sometimes reflexive action, either a verbal noun with verb;
M=expressing a verbal idea; or expressing a finite form of the verb.

H8833 Stem -Niphal = expresses simple action, sometimes reflective.

H8811 Mood -Imperfect = expresses an action, process, or condition which is incomplete.

H8736

S=Simple, sometimes reflexive M=uncompleted action, process, or
condition.

H8833 Stem -Niphal = expresses simple action, sometimes reflective.

H8812 - Mood -Infinitive = expresses either a verbal noun with verb; expressing a verbal idea; or expressing a finite form of the verb.

EXTENDED DEFINITION: *It is very difficult to define infinitive, and there is not a single definition. We generalize and say that infinitives are non-finite/unlimited verbs, namely, they are not conjugated(inflected) by pronoun(person), number(singular or plural), tense, etc. An infinitive includes a combination of a word plus a verb, and therefore it expresses action or a state of being.*

Got Healing?

H8737

S=Simple, sometime reflexive uncompleted action, process, or condition ;in its unbroken continuity; M=and may be used of present, past, or future time.

H8833 Stem -Niphal = expresses simple action, sometimes reflective.

H8813 Mood -Participle = represents an action or condition in its unbroken continuity, and may be used of present, past or future time.

H8738

S=Simple, sometime reflexive completed action M=referring either to a time, or the present.

H8833 Stem -Niphal = expresses simple action, sometimes reflective.

H8816 Mood -Perfect = expresses a completed action; referring to a time, or the present.

H8761

An intensive or intentional, a repeated or extended action as an order/command/directive/mandate..

H8840 Stem -Piel = expresses intensive or intentional, a repeated or extended action.

H8810 Mood -Imperative: = expresses an order or a command/directive/mandate.

H8762

S=An intensive or intentional, a repeated or extended action, process, or condition M=which is incomplete.

H8840 Stem -Piel = expresses intensive or intentional, a repeated or extended action.

H8811 Mood -Imperfect = expresses an action, process, or condition which is incomplete.

H8763

S=An intensive or intentional action, representing an action or condition in its unbroken continuity, M=expresses either a verbal noun with verb; expressing a verbal idea; or expressing a finite form of the verb.

H8840 Stem -Piel = expresses intensive or intentional, a repeated or extended action.

H8812 - Mood -Infinitive = expresses either a verbal noun with verb; expressing a verbal idea; or expressing a finite form of the verb.

H8764

S=An intensive or intentional action, representing an action or condition in its unbroken continuity, M=and may be used of present, past or future time.

H8840 Stem -Piel = expresses intensive or intentional, a repeated or extended action.

H8813 Mood -Participle = represents an action or condition in its unbroken continuity, and may be used of present, past or future time.

Got Healing?

S=Simple expressing intensive/intentional, repeated/extended action;
M=completed referring to a time, or the present.

H8840 Stem -Piel = expresses intensive or intentional, a repeated or extended action.

H8816 Mood -Perfect = expresses a completed action; referring to a time, or the present.

H8768

S=Simple expressing intensive/intentional, repeated/extended action;
M=completed referring to a time, or the present.

H8841 Stem -Piel = This form is equivalent to the Piel intensive form, and occurs due to reduplication of the final root letter

H8816 Mood -Plerfect = expresses a completed action; referring to a time, or the present.

H8775

S=Represents an action or condition in its unbroken continuity, and corresponds to the English verb, "to be" with the present participle. M=It may be used of present, past or future time.

H8843 Stem -Poal = This form is the passive of the Poel, and functions much like the normal Pual.

H8813 Mood -Participle = represents an action or condition in its unbroken continuity, and may be used of present, past or future time.

H8792

S=Passively expressing a causative action being intensive or intentional,
as repeated or extended; action; M=expresses an action, process, or
condition which is incomplete.

H8849 Stem -Pual = expresses the passive of being intensive or intentional, a repeated or extended action. Passive is being willing to wait for the manifestation.

H8811 Mood -Imperfect = expresses an action, process, or condition which is incomplete.

H8794

S=Passively expressing a causative action being intensive or intentional,
as repeated or extended; action or condition in its unbroken continuity,
M=and may be used of present, past or future time.

H8849 Stem -Pual = expresses the passive of being intensive or intentional, a repeated or extended action. Passive is being willing to wait for the manifestation.

H8813 Mood -Participle = represents an action or condition in its unbroken continuity, and may be used of present, past or future time.

H8795

Got Healing?

Passively expressing a causative action being intensive or intentional, as repeated or extended; action or a completed action; referring to a time, or the present.

H8849 Stem -Pual = expresses the passive of being intensive or intentional, a repeated or extended action. Passive is being willing to wait for the manifestation.

H8816 Mood -Plerfect = expresses a completed action; referring to a time, or the present.

H8798
S=Expressing a causative action; M=by a command/directive/mandate.

H8851 Stem -Qal = expresses the "simple" or "causal" action of the root in the active voice.

H8810 Mood -Imperative: = expresses an order or a command/directive/man-date.

H8799
S=A simple/causal action, or process, or condition of the root, M=which is incomplete.

H8851 Stem -Qal = expresses the "simple" or "causal" action of the root in the active voice.

H8811 Mood -Imperfect = expresses an action, process or condition which is incomplete, and it has a wide range of meaning.

H8800
S=A combination of a word plus a verb, M=expressing an action or a state of being.

H8851 - Stem -Qal = expresses the "simple" or "causal" action of the root in the active voice.

H8812 - Mood -Infinitive = expresses either a verbal noun with verb; expressing a verbal idea; or expressing a finite form of the verb.

<u>EXTENDED DEFINITION:</u> *It is very difficult to define infinitive, and there is not a single definition. We generalize and say that infinitives are non-finite/unlimited verbs, namely, they are not conjugated(inflected) by pronoun(person), number(singular or plural), tense, etc. An infinitive includes a combination of a word plus a verb, and therefore it expresses action or a state of being.*

H8801
S=Expressing a causative action being intensive or intentional, as repeated or extended; M=action or condition in its unbroken continuity, and may be used of present, past or future time.

H8851 - Stem -Qal = expresses the "simple" or "causal" action of the root in the active voice.

H8813 Mood -Participle = represents an action or condition in its unbroken continuity, and may be used of present, past or future time.

H8802

Got Healing?

S=Expresses the "simple" or "causal" action of the root in the active voice;
M=through an action or condition in its unbroken continuity.

H8851 - Stem -Qal = expresses the "simple" or "causal" action of the root in the active voice.

H8814 - Mood -Participle Active = expresses an action or condition in its unbroken continuity.

H8803

S=Expresses the "simple" or "causal" action of the root in the active
voice; M=represents an action or condition in its passive unbroken
continuity; in its passive/inert/inactive/reflexive activity.

H8851 - Stem -Qal = expresses the "simple" or "causal" action of the root in the active voice.

H8813 Mood -Participle = represents an action or condition in its passive unbroken continuity, in its passive/inert/inactive/reflexive activity.

H8804

S=A simple/causal action M=referring to a time, or the present.

H8851 Stem -Qal = expresses the "simple" or "causal" action of the root in the active voice.

H8816 Mood -Perfect = expresses a completed action; referring to a time, or the present.

H8809

S=A simple/causal action M=referring to a time, or the present.

H8853 Stem -Qal = reflects a causative like the Hebrew Hiphil, but with a Tau prefixed rather than the usual He. It otherwise functions like the Hebrew Hiphil.

H8816 Mood -Perfect = expresses a completed action; referring to a time, or the present.

Appendix 5:

Hebrew-Aramaic Alphabets
Symbols Explained

ALEPH=OX'S **HEAD**=connect/**BOND**/effect/power/**INFLUENCE**/leader/**AUTHORITY**

BEYT=TENT-FLOOR-**PLAN**=**THOUGHTS**/family/house/**PATTERN**/mark/**DWELLING**

GIMAL= **FOOT**=gather/**COMPREHEND**/carry/**EXPERIENCE**/walk/**PROGRESS**

DALET=TENT-**DOOR**=move/**OPPORTUNITY**/hang/**ARRANGE**/entrance/**ENTER**

HEY=MAN-W/RAISED-**ARMS**=**BREATH**/look/**REVEAL**/sight/**INSIGHT**

VAV=**TENT-PEG**=add/secure/**ANCHOR**/hook/**ASSURE**/assign/**MEASURE**

ZAYIN=**PLOUGH**/MATTOCK=**ENCOURAGE**/cut/**ALTER**/weapon/**INSTRUMENT**

HHETS=TENT **WALL**=**OUTSIDE**/external/**SEPARATE**/divide/trail/**BEYOND**/exclude

THET=BASKET=**SURROUND**/**CONTAIN**/basket/mud/**MIXTURE**

YUD=HAND&ARM-**MOVING**=work/**EFFORT**/worship/**BEHAVIOR**/**PURPOSE**

KAPH=PALM-OF-THE-HAND=bend/**SURRENDER**/**OPEN**/expose/**ALLOW**/tame

LAMED=SHEPHERD'S-STAFF=teach/**IMPART**/yoke/**CHANNEL**/bind

MEM=WATER=chaos/**QUESTION**/conflict/**CHALLENGE**/ mighty/blood/**PROVOKE**

NUN=SPROUTING-SEED=**CONTINUE**/heir/son/**DEVELOP**/mature/**IMPROVE**

SAMECH=THORN=**ADVANTAGE**/seed/**SOURCE**/take-hold/**APPREHEND**

AYIN=EYE(of)=watch/**DISTINGUISH**/know/**PERCEIVE**/shade/**INSIGHT**

PEY=OPEN-**MOUTH**=blow/**TRANSCEND**/scatter/**BROADCAST**/strength/**SPEAK**

TsAD=TRAIL=path/**JOURNEY**/hunt/chase/**PURSUIT**/wait/**ANTICIPATE**

QUPH=SUNRISE/SUNSET=condense/circle/**ESSENCE**/time/**COMPARE**/**CONTRAST**

RESH= HEAD-OF-MAN=first/top/**BEGINNING**/**POSSESS**/**INCREASE**

SHIN=TWO-FRONT-TEETH=sharp/press/eat/**CONSUME**/two/**COMPEL**/**PRESSURE**

TAW=TWO-CROSSED-STICKS=mark/**DEMONSTRATE**/sign/**EVIDENCE**/**PROVE**

Appendix 6:
Chronological Order Of
The Books Of The New Testament.

While no arrangement of these books can be made with absolute confidence, the following dates are sufficiently reliable to serve the purpose of the Bible student.

James - 50 A.D.

First Thessalonians - 52-53.

Second Thessalonians - 52-53.

Galatians - 55.

First Corinthians - 57.

Second Corinthians - 57.

Romans - 57-58.

Philippians - 62-63.

Colossians - 62-63.

Philemon - 62-63.

Ephesians - 62-63.

Luke - 63.

Acts - 64.

First Timothy - 65.

Titus - 65.

Second Timothy - 66.

Mark - 66.

Matthew - 67.

Hebrews - 67.

First Peter - 67-68.

Second Peter - 68.

Jude - 68.

Apocalypse - 68.

John - c. 85.

Epistles of John - 90-95.

Appendix 7:
Bibliography

Barth, Karl; *Christ and Adam: Man and Humanity in Romans 5.* Wipf & Stock, an Imprint of Wipf and Stock Publishers.

Bosworth, F.F. *Christ, the Healer* Fleming Revell/Baker Book House, Grand Rapids, MI.

Braden, Gregg. *The God Code*. Hay House.

Braden, Gregg. *The Spontaneous Healing of Belief: Shattering the Paradigm of False Limits*. Hay House.

Capps, Charles. *God's Creative Power for Healing* Capps Publishing.

Clark, Randy. *Authority to Heal: Restoring the Lost Inheritance of God's Healing Power.* Destiny Image, Inc.

Dyer, Wayne W. *Everyday Wisdom For Success*. Hay House.

Eldredge, John. *Walking with God: Talk to Him. Hear from Him. Really*. Thomas Nelson.

Frangipane, Francis. *Discerning of Spirits*.

Goddard, Neville. *Feeling Is The Secret*; Hillary Hawkins Production.

Goddard, Neville. *I Know My Father*.

Hunter, Charles & Frances Hunter. *How to Heal the Sick*. Whitaker House

Hunter, Joan. Healing The Whole Man Handbook. Whitaker House.

Jacobsen, Wayne. *He Loves Me!: Learning to Live in the Father's Affection*. Windblown Media.

Kenyon, E. W. *The Blood Covenant*. Book Baby.

Kruger, C. Baxter. *Across All Worlds: Jesus Inside Our Darkness* Perichoresis, Inc.

Kruger, C. Baxter (2011-08-09). *God Is For Us*.

Lockyer, Herbert. *The Gospel in the Pentateuch*. Chariot Ebooks.

Murdock, Mike. *Dream Seeds* Wisdom International, Inc.

Murray, Andrew. *Abide in Christ*. Scriptura Press.

Ridout, Samuel. *The Collected Works of Samuel Ridout - Nine books in one*. Jawbone Digital.

Got Healing?

Stone, Dan; Gregory, David; *The Rest of the Gospel*. Harvest House Publishers.

Sagan, Carl (2011-07-06). *Cosmos.* Random House Publishing Group.

Toit, Francois Du (2014-01-08). *Mirror Bible: A selection of key New Testament texts paraphrased from the Greek*. Mirror Word Publishing.

Tozer, A. W.. *The Pursuit of God*: Updated Edition (Annotated) Aneko Press.

Young, Wm. Paul. *Lies We Believe About God*. Atria Books.

Other Books Available by Dwaine Thomas Martin:

Anchoring In Safe Harbor:

The Functional Gifts(an 8-volume series)

...*explore the gifting given by God to you at birth, empowered at salvation, and released by prayer; this information will set the soul free to soar above the challenges of life and attain destiny...*

Ebb N' Flow

...*discover the three-folded cord within every person, uncovering the fullness of who you are, what you are about, and whose you are; as God is a three-folded BE-ing, so is each person as Spirit and Soul and Body...*

Got Love?

...*This is the aspect, the character of His LOVE that bewilders, and at times, overwhelms the psyche of men. HE FIRST LOVED US. Though we betray this LOVE multiple times throughout our living, He CONTINUES to LOVE us. Learn more about this happening called, LOVE...*

By The Mercies Of God

...*Discover a dimension in Christ, a side of the Father, a kingdom in Spirit that supersedes, or goes beyond anything that you have witnessed, or experienced. In the fullness of the Godhead, the Spirit promises wealth untold, wisdom yet to be found, and MERCIES unmerited, yet always abounding in the compassions of our God....*

Proverbs: God's Wisdom Today

...*verse-by-verse, these volumes offer insight by experience; living life can only be taught by perspective, insight, and tenacity.*

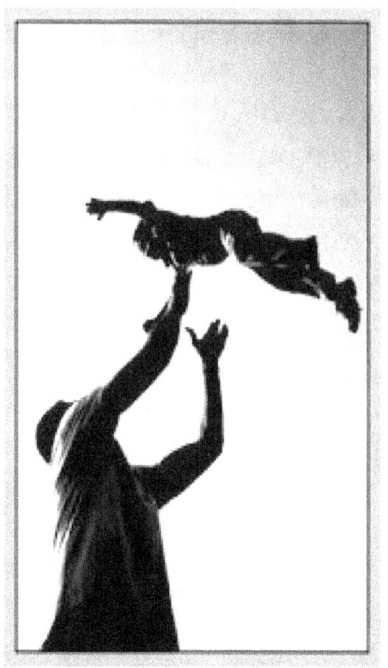

COMING SOON:

Beginnings: Genesis - Precept Starts With Covenant

... At the outset, Genesis is a beginning outline preceding even the most current of events. Yet, because of MIS-taken Identities, the Body of Christ has forged mentalities that robs us of the power necessary to overcome our surroundings and renature the world around us. We have not been the nation changing the world, because we do not believe in an earth manifestation and spiritual assignment significant enough to blow the breath away from the world system.......

PUBLISHED BY:

SPIRIT-WIND HOUSE
14338 Hwy. 49 – SPC. #70
Grass Valley, CA 95949
dwaine07@hotmail.com

Got Healing?

*O*s HEALING a valid promise or just an illusion created by some magician, or minister wanting a *"fast buck"*? Charlatans abound; and magicians like *"Simon [Acts 8:9]"* constantly mesmerize the unwitting soul into believing what their ministry has, is what everyone needs.

*R*ESTORATION of Health is about a GREAT EXCHANGE in one's LIVING! By many creeds and dogmas, the pilgrim in pursuit of God begins an arduous excursion, leading them toward many pitfalls of unsound and unscriptural beliefs. Most dogmas are about one man's control over others. These things are <u>NOT OF GOD</u>! WHY? Because they do not produce a lifestyle that exemplifies THE RESURRECTED LIFE OF CHRIST JESUS through the believer.

Healing is one of those topics that demands answers, as well as a response to such answers. Regardless of whether or not we believe what we have been told, the WILL OF GOD IS TO HEAL!. This is the fact of the Scriptures read and studied. Without such assurance, there is no security available enough to override one's personal concerns, or fears. Wherever Jesus went, He ministered with compassion and healed the sick.

Christ's example showed an interconnection with salvation as many believed following their healing. Healing is for the physical ills of the human body, and the psyche of the human mind. If the life-force/spirit in man GENESIS 2:7; 1CORINTHIANS 6:17, is joined as ONE with the Holy Spirit as God; then, there is no lack, no error, no need in this joining to/of SPIRIT for training of any kind. Healing is about LEARNING to adapt, LEARNING to accept, and LEARNING to agree with what God SPOKE, since before time, or humanity began.

Higher Dimension Community Fellowship

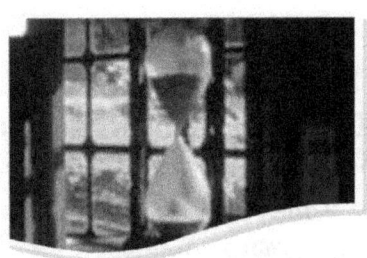

Meeting: 671 Maltman Drive—Unit #6
Grass Valley, CA 95949

Mailing: 14338 HWY 49 SPC #70
Grass Valley, CA 95949-9215

Church Phone: (530) 575-4204
Cell Phone: (530) 798-9538

E-mail: dwaine@higherdimension.us

www.ingramcontent.com/pod-product-compliance
Lightning Source LLC
Chambersburg PA
CBHW081106170526
45165CB00008B/2345